My Mysterious Son

My Mysterious Son

Son

A Life-Changing Passage
Between Schizophrenia and Shamanism

DICK RUSSELL

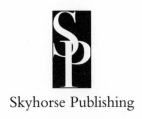

Skyhorse Publishing

Skyhorse Publishing books may be purchased in bulk at special discounts for sales promotion, corporate gifts, fund-raising, or educational purposes. Special editions can also be created to specifications. For details, contact the Special Sales Department, Skyhorse Publishing, 307 West 36th Street, 11th Floor, New York, NY 10018 or info@skyhorsepublishing.com.

Skyhorse® and Skyhorse Publishing® are registered trademarks of Skyhorse Publishing, Inc.®, a Delaware corporation.

Visit our website at www.skyhorsepublishing.com.

10 9 8 7 6 5 4 3 2 1

Library of Congress Cataloging-in-Publication Data is available on file.

Cover design by Jane Shepard
Cover photo credit Thinkstock

ISBN: 978-1-62914-487-0
Ebook ISBN: 978-1-62914-957-8

Printed in the United States of America

To the Ancestors

Contents

I'm a gust on the sea,
I'm a footfall of a wave,
I'm a roar of the sea....
I'm a hawk on a cliff,
I'm a tear of sunlight,
I'm a cry of love,
I'm a boar in rage....
I'm the god who kindles fire in your head
Who makes smooth the mountain's stones?
Who can count the ages of the moon?
Who finds the place where the sun goes down?

—Excerpt from *The Mystery* by Amergin Glangel,
chief poet of the Giodelic Celts

Prologue: The Tell-Tale Heart

If we are not going to expect that all should be alike and are to agree instead that the psyche has its own strange ways of accomplishing its ends, then perhaps what were called symptoms and syndromes may call for a different interpretation and evaluation.

—Dr. John Weir Perry, *The Far Side of Madness*[1]

THIS IS A BOOK ABOUT a "different interpretation" of schizophrenia, based upon almost twenty years of one father's experiences with his son's struggle against mental illness. Experiences fraught with desperation, confusion, incomprehension, and pain. Experiences also filled with surprise, humor, adventure, and hope. Experiences that ultimately go beyond (but do not discard) the Western "medical model" for treating mental illness.

This book is also an account of a father-and-son journey. Externally down hospital corridors and through therapy sessions and halfway houses; eventually embarking on travels together in Africa, Jamaica, and New Mexico. Internally to the depths of the psyche, as well as to the recognition of clairvoyance and another dimensionality to what is called schizophrenia. And ultimately into a shamanic quest—divination, ritual, ancestral invocation—that has opened unforeseen new possibilities toward recovery and reconciliation.

• • •

When I was young, I remember being so captivated by Edgar Allen Poe's short story, "The Tell-Tale Heart," that I would read it aloud to myself. It began:

> True!—nervous—very, very dreadfully nervous I had been and am! but why will you say that I am mad? The disease had sharpened my

senses—not destroyed—not dulled them. Above all was the sense of hearing acute. I heard all things in the heaven and in the earth. I heard many things in hell. How, then, am I mad? Harken! and observe how healthily—how calmly—I can tell you the whole story.

Coming upon that passage again all these years later, I realize that the lines are so familiar I seem to have memorized them. I wonder if, when I read this short story, I was around the same age as my son would be when, at seventeen, he experienced his first "psychotic episode," as the medical professionals called it.

The terms *insanity* and *psychosis* are largely interchangeable, although psychosis is today the common medical term. Symptomatic are delusions, hallucinations, or disorganized thoughts (sometimes all three). The occurrence may be short-lived. . . . Or it may become chronic, often characterized by poor social skills, diminished motivation, and difficulty in expressing emotions.

Of course, parents never think that such a terrible circumstance can happen to them, no matter what traits a child may have displayed in earlier years that can later be seen as precursors. As Andrew Solomon writes in his book, *Far from the Tree*:

> The shock of schizophrenia is that it manifests in late adolescence or early adulthood, and parents must accept that the child they have known and loved for more than a decade may be irrevocably lost, even if that child looks much the same as ever. Initially, parents almost universally believe that schizophrenia is invasive, an added layer masking their beloved child, who must somehow be liberated from the temporary conquest.[2]

I was no exception, though I would later see much of my son's condition mirrored in the accounts of others labeled schizophrenic, as Dr. E. Fuller Torrey quoted them in his book, *Surviving Schizophrenia*:

- "An outsider may see only someone 'out of touch with reality.' In fact we are experiencing so many realities that it is often confusing and sometimes totally overwhelming."[3]
- "Sometimes when people speak to me my head is overloaded. It's too much to hold at once. It goes out as quick as it goes in. It makes you forget what you just heard because you can't get

hearing it long enough. It's just words in the air unless you can figure it out from their faces."[4]

- "I was extremely unhappy. I felt myself getting younger; the system wanted to reduce me to nothing. Even as I diminished in body and in age, I discovered that I was nine centuries old. For to be nine centuries old actually meant being not yet born. That is why the nine centuries did not make me feel at all old; quite the contrary."[5]

Depression as a common early symptom . . . a preoccupation with messianic ideas . . . difficulty in distinguishing what is real from unreal . . . neologisms, or made-up words . . . inappropriate or flattened emotions . . . breaking out in laughter for no apparent reason . . . withdrawal from others and sometimes complete isolation . . . the notion that you can control someone else's mind, or vice versa . . . a frequent inability to sort, interpret, or respond. "I used to get the sudden thing that I couldn't understand what people said, like it was a foreign language."[6]

I was no stranger to any of that. "*Strangeness* has typically been the key feature in the fractured dialogues that go on, or the silences that intrude, between the 'mad' and the 'sane.' Madness is a foreign country,"[7] wrote Roy Porter in *A Social History of Madness*. That was certainly not foreign territory to me.

But where does it come from? This is the question that plagues thousands of parents. Is a predisposition for schizophrenia genetically passed on? Is it related to a traumatic event in childhood? Or, more generally, to the way a child was raised? In other words, is it somehow "our fault?"

Psychologist Julian Jaynes of Princeton University set forth this summary of how the various disciplines view the subject:

The socio-environmental researcher sees the schizophrenic as the product of a stressful environment. The biochemist insists that the stressful environment has its effect only because of an abnormal biochemistry in the patient. Those who speak in terms of information processing say that a deficit in this area leads directly to stress and counterstress defenses. The defense-mechanism psychologist views the impaired information processing as a self-motivated withdrawal from contact with reality. The geneticist makes hereditary interpretations from family history data, while others might develop interpretations about the role of schizophrenogenic parental influence from the same data.[8]

As Dr. Pablo Gejman, director of the Center for Psychiatric Genetics at Northwestern University, has said: "The complexity of schizophrenia is very great. We're probably talking about hundreds of individual factors—many genetic, some the result of environmental exposures. We actually have a profound ignorance on the specific molecular mechanisms of schizophrenia."[9] In short, nobody knows just how the brain circuits happen to misfire. It's a scientific enigma.

Recent research reveals that some adults taking antipsychotic medication for schizophrenia have been misdiagnosed and should more accurately be assessed for an autism spectrum disorder. As well, a fine line exists between the "thought disorder" that characterizes schizophrenia, the "mood disorder" associated with bipolar illness, and "schizoaffective disorder" that displays qualities of both. My son had been diagnosed with each at different times by different doctors.

Genetic studies reveal that more than 80 percent of an individual's vulnerability to schizophrenia is heritable. For several decades, researchers have pursued a "schizophrenia gene," in hopes this would lead toward a potential cure. However, a major study released in 2008, examining fourteen "candidate genes" considered prime suspects behind schizophrenia, found not a single one of these to have a significant association to the disease.[10]

A study appearing in the medical journal *Lancet* in February 2013 detected the same underlying genetic changes in the five most common mental illnesses or disorders: schizophrenia, bipolar, major depression, autism, and ADHD. But these same genes show simply a predisposition, with hundreds or even thousands of different genes contributing to someone developing one of these problems.[11]

• • •

The upshot is that schizophrenia remains as mysterious today as it's been throughout human history. Some evidence points to the disorder existing even prior to *Homo sapiens'* exodus from Africa around 50,000 years ago. In recorded history, the fifth-century BC king of Sparta was apparently schizophrenic, and similar individuals are cited in 2,000-year-old Chinese and Indian texts. Socrates apparently experienced auditory hallucinations, and his pupil Plato believed that "divine madness" lay behind poetic inspiration. Pythagoras's unusual beliefs included having "inhabited the bodies of important people from past generations" and giving "mystical properties to various numbers."[12] Aristotle said: "No great genius has ever existed without some touch of madness."

"In Western Europe, from 500 to 1500 AD, people who heard voices or saw visions considered themselves, and were considered by their contemporaries, to have had actual perceptual experiences of either divine or satanic inspiration. They were not considered mad and were not dealt with as such."[13] (John Milton and later William Blake fell into this category).

This viewpoint changed during the late Middle Ages, when the yet-unnamed disease was linked to witchcraft or possession by the devil, and often resulted in serious punishments being meted out to those afflicted. The most humane included exorcising the demons in religious ceremony, but the evil spirits could also be "released" by drilling holes in a patient's skull—not unlike the frontal lobotomies practiced on some labeled as schizophrenic in the mid-twentieth century.

King Henry VI, who governed both England and France during the first half of the fifteenth century, seems to have had his first schizophrenic breakdown in his early thirties—apparently an inheritance from earlier generations on his mother's side, including his maternal grandfather, King Charles VI of France, whose initial bout occurred at twenty-four. Henry VI became the subject of Shakespeare's first play, to be followed later by such "mad" characters as Ophelia in *Hamlet* and Poor Mad Tom in *King Lear*.

The advent of the nineteenth-century Industrial Age saw a marked increase in observed schizophrenic symptoms. (It has been noted that enthusiastically working fixed long hours is especially difficult for people so diagnosed). In modern psychology, it was first called *dementia praecox*—meaning, in effect, "precocious madness," to differentiate it from the absence of emotion that also can occur with the aging process. The term "schizophrenia" was introduced in 1911 by Swiss psychiatrist Eugen Bleuler, derived from two Greek roots—*schizo* (split) and *phrene* (mind).

Freudian analysts sought to show that schizophrenia was caused by early childhood experiences, such as abuse or dysfunctional families.

C. G. Jung, Freud's protégé who ultimately broke from him, saw it differently. Jung wrote in 1939:

> These forces . . . are most emphatically not the result of poisoned brain cells, but are normal constituents of our unconscious psyche. They appeared in numberless dreams, in the same or a similar form, at a time of life when seemingly nothing was wrong. And they appear in dreams of normal people who never get anywhere near a psychosis. . . . Through my work with patients I realized that paranoid ideas and hallucinations contain a gem of meaning.[14]

Harry Stack Sullivan, an important post-Freudian thinker in the 1930s and 1940s, developed a theory of psychiatry based on interpersonal relationships. He possessed an uncanny ability to communicate with schizophrenic patients, whom Sullivan believed suffered from some form of early childhood behavioral disturbance. He postulated that their mental functions were impaired, but not permanently damaged, and could be recovered through talk therapy.

The writings of a Sullivan contemporary, Frieda Fromm-Reichmann, "made clear that schizophrenia is a human experience with meaning, meaning that is hard to uncover, but it only takes patience, kindness, a tolerance for not understanding as well as for the patient's desperate defenses, and a willingness to understand the human condition at its most painful and to take psychoanalytic ideas seriously when patients talk about them. Understanding persons with schizophrenia means facing facts about ourselves, our families, and our society that we do not want to know, or to know again (in the case of repressed feelings and experiences)."[15]

These benign approaches, however, coincided with the most brutal of interventions for schizophrenia—tens of thousands of lobotomies performed in the 1940s and early 1950s. Only after two French psychiatrists discovered that a compound intended for pre-anesthesia (chlorpromazine) could be remarkably effective for schizophrenics did the combination of medications and talking therapy come to the foreground.

By the mid-1960s, biological psychiatry recognized schizophrenia as a medical condition that didn't result from traumatic life experiences. It was not the fault of someone's upbringing, but a brain-based illness similar to other mental and neurological diseases; a developmental disorder inscribed in the brain even before the child was born. Paralleling this was a more holistic view of schizophrenia among certain psychiatrists. Thomas Szasz, a severe critic of his own profession in *The Myth of Mental Illness*, famously said: "If you talk to God, you are praying; if God talks to you, you have schizophrenia."[16] To Szasz, labeling someone as mentally ill places them in a dependent and therefore inferior role in our society, stigmatizing them.

An even more radical psychiatrist, R. D. Laing, believed that "no age in the history of humanity has perhaps so lost touch with this natural healing process that implicates some of the people we label schizophrenic."[17] And Jungian analyst John Weir Perry started an experimental residence facility called Diabasis in San Francisco, where following acute schizophrenic episodes, young adults could reside and explore their situations together without using medications.

Today, about 2.2 million Americans are considered to have schizophrenia in any given year (about eight out of every thousand people).[18] "In Western societies, occupational impairment is usually severe, as evidenced by unemployment rates approaching 90 percent."[19] The tragic reality of our time is that at least as many are homeless, living in shelters, or serving time in jails and prisons as there are in all hospitals and related facilities.[20]

And the medical treatment model, in alliance with the big pharmaceutical companies, continues to dominate current thinking. Schizophrenics have often been found with a damaged or poorly functioning prefrontal cortex in the brain, believed to contribute to the disorganized thoughts and lack of a "social filtration system" for their ideas. Someone's DNA is also tied to how the body processes and utilizes a neurotransmitter called dopamine, which determines the way we perceive relevancy in our environment. Many diagnoses of schizophrenia coincide with too-high levels of dopamine, and the advent of psychotropic medications that reduce dopamine levels made the illness more treatable, if not curable. (As a brain chemical associated with energy and motivation, low dopamine levels are often found in people suffering from depression.) There is growing evidence implicating abnormalities of another neurotransmitter, glutamate, in schizophrenia.

Since his breakdown at seventeen, my son has been prescribed antipsychotics, mood stabilizers, and antidepressants with varying rates of success. But over the years, while engaging in periodic battles with the mental health system and its pharmacological methodology, I've moved away from accepting at face value what therapists and drug companies push—their implication being to spend a lifetime on strong medication or to face becoming permanently institutionalized. I've come to realize that there are powerful alternatives that can lead to a greater understanding and better life for the person afflicted. I've also come to realize that my son's sometimes "delusional thinking" is not what might be dismissed as meaningless babble, but contains poetic gems and a different kind of truth—one that is simply beyond the "normal" ways that our everyday reality is understood.

Such changes in one father's perception are ultimately what this book is about. In a way, it takes off from a statement by John Nash, subject of the book and film *A Beautiful Mind*, recipient of the 1994 Nobel Prize in economics, and a long-ago-diagnosed schizophrenic. Nash was once asked how he, as a mathematician, "a man devoted to reason and logical proof . . . could believe that extraterrestrials are sending you messages? How could you believe that you are being recruited by aliens from outer space to save the world?" To which Nash replied matter-of-factly: "Because the ideas I had about supernatural beings came to me the same way that my mathematical ideas did. So I took them seriously."[21]

Joseph Campbell, America's greatest scholar of comparative mythology, came to conclude "that the imagery of schizophrenic fantasy perfectly matches that of the mythological hero journey" which he had elucidated in his classic 1949 book, *The Hero with a Thousand Faces*. Campbell's hero first separates from the established social order, embarking upon a long inward and backward journey, where in the depths of his psyche he must confront chaotic and terrifying forces. If fortunate, the hero finds courage at a harmonious center and, as Campbell wrote, "comes back from this mysterious adventure with the power to bestow boons on his fellow men." The schizophrenic, wrote Campbell, "is actually experiencing inadvertently that same beatific ocean deep which the yogi and saint are ever striving to enjoy: except that, whereas they are swimming in it, he is drowning."[22]

In 2012, Dr. Joseph Polimeni, a Canadian professor and internationally recognized evolutionary psychiatrist, published a book titled *Shamans Among Us*. He writes in the first chapter:

In its simplest form, the shamanistic theory of schizophrenia says that people with schizophrenia are the modern manifestation of prehistoric tribal shamans. In other words, the inborn cognitive factors or personality style that would have predisposed certain people to become shamans is the same psychological mindset that underlies schizophrenia.[23]

Polimeni's thesis focuses around similarities such as genetic predisposition, onset during young adulthood, intensified symptoms during periods of stress, and preponderance among males. The resemblance, Dr. Polimeni writes, "surpasses coincidence." While schizophrenia "does not fit neatly under the rubric of classic neuropsychiatric diseases," it clearly mimics shamanism. "The personal histories of shamans so often contain episodes of serious mental disturbance, including numerous accounts of spiritual hallucinations. Shamans become engrossed with magico-religious beliefs and suspicions of otherworldly threats. They have the reputation of being solitary, unsociable, and odd."[24]

And, of course, shamans are diviners and healers still held in great esteem by indigenous societies. I believe my son has elements of that same capacity. Colin Campbell, an African healer, puts it like this: "People hearing voices for instance or feeling certain things are in touch with other realities, especially the whole mythic realm, that Western society does not have a time or place for. Who is going to give voice to those parts of us?"[25]

Ultimately, this book is my attempt to do that. And, in so doing, give families in similar situations the message that there can indeed be light at the end of those many dark tunnels. Mental illness is one of these, autism and Alzheimer's are others. In each of these situations, we live with the human conditions of expectation and hope, never being able to quite let go of those, if we even should. In each, too, we are dealing with connection and how to maintain it amid situations that often prove unfathomable.

Beyond such conditions, we are all raising children in a world where our advances in technology are forging minds very different than the ones we had half a century ago; where there is today a "natural" attunement to other realms of existence. You need only to think of video games and virtual reality. In a sense, the mythic realm is upon all of us, try as we might to disclaim it.

The first part of this book, which I've called "The Desperate Years," is my recollection of the fifteen-year-long period following Franklin's first breakdown and hospitalization. I could best describe what I went through as an ongoing mixture of hopelessness and acceptance, desperation and denial, bafflement and expectation, failure to perceive and flashes of insight. None of which broke the pattern in his life of rejecting and then acquiescing to a series of antipsychotic and other medications, of long stints in hospitals and assorted group homes, of mood swings ranging from anger to compassion.

It took a long time before I stopped cringing at his seeming delusions, especially when expressed in public, alongside my obsessive desire to "crack the code" of their often repetitive patterns. All the while, I jotted notes in my effort to understand . . . and because it is my nature as a journalist. My son wrote, too, prodigiously on occasion. And it took a long time for me to see that, in Franklin's poetically evocative fashion, he was quite a remarkable writer . . . through the pain of it all. Perhaps it's no coincidence that one of his most consistent fantasies is owning a company that will publish our books. With his permission, a number of passages from his journal will appear in these pages.

Part two is the story of what transpired when I took Franklin, at the age of thirty-two, on a trip to witness the wildlife migration across the Serengeti Plain in East Africa—a trip that changed both of us in ways and through means that I could never have anticipated. These chapters focus not only on our relationship to nature, but the nature of relationships as we embark with my son's boyhood pediatrician and a Maasai guide (the same age as Franklin).

The third section of this book describes the subsequent exploration with my son of the shamanic realm. As the years passed, I had observed that Franklin could be remarkably psychic—able to read my thoughts and feelings in astonishing ways, as if he had a direct pipeline to a parallel reality. Our spending time with a renowned West African shaman not only brought recognition of the other-worldly nature of Franklin's experiences, but simultaneously helped to ground him more in the earthly dimension that he currently must inhabit.

I have always loved mysteries. As a youngster, I devoured the thirty-some volumes of *The Hardy Boys* and much of Sherlock Holmes. Later I became intrigued by metaphysical mysteries, and probing the likelihood of conspiracy in the assassination of President Kennedy. And still later, the mystery of why gray whales choose to approach humans in the wild at a particular lagoon in Mexico.

Now, as I turn sixty-five, I explore perhaps the greatest mystery of all—my own son. Franklin may be torn, confused, afflicted, or any number of other adjectives. But above all, he is not merely a victim but a person, his own person, with appeal, wit, grit, personality . . . and, perhaps, a vehicle for something profound. I don't believe saying that is over-romanticizing. But even if it is, I have learned—my son has taught me—to appreciate who he is, and what he has to offer. That, I hope, is a story worth telling.

Notes

1. "If we are not going to expect….": John Weir Perry, *The Far Side of Madness*, Prentice-Hall, 1974, p. 109.
2. Andrew Solomon, *Far from the Tree: Parents, Children, and the Search for Identity*, Scribner, 2012, p. 295.
3. "An outsider may see only someone….": E. Fuller Torrey, *Surviving Schizophrenia*, Quill, 2001, p. 36.
4. "Sometimes when people speak to me….": Torrey, p. 37.
5 "I was extremely unhappy….": Torrey, p. 49.
6. "I used to get the sudden thing….": Torrey, p. 43.
7. "Strangeness has typically been….": Porter quoted in Torrey, p. 31.
8. "The biochemist insists….": Julian Jaynes, *The Origin of Consciousness in the Breakdown of the Bicameral Mind*, Mariner Books, 2000, p. 431.
9. "The complexity of schizophrenia….": Pablo Gejman, see "The Role of Genetics in the Etiology of Schizophrenia," *Psychiatric Clinics of North America,* Mar 2010; 33(1): 35–66.
10. "No genes for schizophrenia? What gives?" article by Randolph Nesse, *The Evolution & Medicine Review*, May 28, 2008, citing a study published in the *American Journal of Psychiatry*, Saunders et al.
11. Study in *Lancet*: "5 Disorders Share Genetic Risk Factors, Study Finds," *New York Times*, February 28, 2013; "5 Mental Disorders Share Genetic Links," Associated Press, February 28, 2013.
12. Pythagoras: Van Doren, 1991, cited in Joseph Polimeni, *Shamans Among Us: Schizophrenia, Shamanism, and the Evolutionary Origins of Religion*, 2012, p. 92.
13. View of schizophrenia in Western Europe, 500 to 1500: Kroll and Bachrach, 1982, cited in *Shamans Among Us*, p. 38.

14. *Collected Works of C. G. Jung, Volume 3:* "Psychogenesis of Mental Disease," p. 239.

15. Frieda Fromm-Reichmann: Bertram P. Karon, "The Tragedy of Schizophrenia without Psychotherapy," *Journal of the American Academy of Psychoanalysis and Dynamic Psychiatry,* 31 (1), 89–118, 2003.

16. "If you talk to God....": Thomas Szasz, *The Second Sin,* Anchor/Doubleday, 1973, p. 113.

17. "no age in the history of humanity....": "Dr. R. D. Laing: The Experience of Schizophrenia," cited in spiritualrecoveries.blogspot.com, January 13, 2007.

18. Statistics on schizophrenia: Torrey, p. 5.

19. Psychosis and schizophrenia: Polimeni, *Shamans Among Us,* p. 2.

20. Homeless vs. hospitals: Torrey, p. 1.

21. John Nash, quoted in Torrey, *Surviving Schizophrenia,* p. 54.

22. Joseph Campbell, "Schizophrenia: The Inward Journey," published in *Myths to Live By,* 1970, http://www.mindspring.com/~berks-healing/campbell-schiz.pdf

23. "In its simplest form, the shamanistic theory....": *Shamans Among Us,* p. 1.

24. Shamans and schizophrenics: *Shamans Among Us,* p. 216.

25. Interview with Colin Campbell—African Sangoma, by Niyati Evers, www.theicarusproject.net, August 17, 2008.

PART 1

• • •

The Desperate Years

CHAPTER 1

• • •

Two Faces

Fatherhood, in the sense of conscious begetting, is unknown to man. It is a mystical estate, an apostolic succession, from only begetter to only begotten.
—James Joyce, *Ulysses*

IT'S THE END OF THE day at a safari lodge in northern Tanzania. My son and I are atop a high bluff that marks the northern boundary of Tarangire National Park, seated in wrought-iron chairs along a panoramic veranda. Southeast of the park lie the plains of the Maasai Steppe, to the north and west are the lakes of East Africa's Great Rift Valley. Approaching dusk, the overlook view from the Tarangire Safari Lodge is at its most breathtaking. For miles below, a coral sunset bathes the acacia thickets and savannah plains that brush the Tarangire River as it meanders through gently rolling terrain. Numerous families of elephants can be seen approaching the river to drink. Solitary giraffes browse the leaves of the flat-topped acacia trees. The flutter of Southern ground hornbills and white buffalo-weavers caresses the gathering twilight.

We have come here, in mid-January of 2012, to witness the annual wildlife migration across the Serengeti Plain . . . the same month that my son will turn thirty-three . . . almost sixteen years since he was given a hospital diagnosis of probable schizophrenia. Uncertainty has been the one constant since Franklin suffered his first breakdown as an adolescent. You never know what to expect from day to day, only that you must try to give up all expectation. And I know that bringing my son on this trip is a risky thing to do.

3

In Boston, Franklin lived about a half-hour from me, in a group home alongside others with similar mental illnesses. There were many days when he rarely left his room. Some time ago I came to terms with the fact that, even staying on his medication, he might never be free of his delusional thinking, be able to hold a steady job, or have much semblance of a "normal" life. Where he lived, he didn't seem to mind residing amid the taciturn, sometimes almost spectral, presences of two older men on the same floor. But did he look at them and see his own dismal future? Could there be anything in his life that would make it different? Was I too late in coming to certain realizations about my son's deeper nature?

Yet I never quite gave up hope. Perhaps a father cannot. So I have taken the chance of uprooting my son from all he knows, toward the possibility that here together, in Africa, something might change.

There is a reason for choosing Africa, beyond the wonder of seeing multitudes of animals. Franklin is African American on his mother's side, Caucasian on mine. He's never before been in a predominantly black culture. This gives rise to still more questions: Will he be fascinated? Perhaps apprehensive? And how will we fare, the two of us, living for almost three weeks in as intimate a circumstance as we've known together since he was a baby?

After years of conflict and struggle, could it be that Africa might mark some kind of turning point—in the relationship between father and son, and in our individual lives?

• • •

We're in a Land Rover driving past a flamingo-filled lake, some 2,000 feet down inside the Ngorongoro Crater. This is one of the wonders of the world, a wildlife sanctuary as big as Paris. The crater formed some 2.5 million years ago, when Ngorongoro was still a large active volcano that rivaled Mount Kilimanjaro in size. Following a major eruption of molten lava, its cone had collapsed inward, leaving behind the vast, unbroken caldera whose 100-plus square miles we're traversing.

I was here long ago, just over forty years, a young man of the sixties generation, hitchhiking my way around. I'd told Franklin some of the stories of that exciting period of my life. Now it's he who aims a camera as our guide slows down and asks him, "Frank, you are going to spot a rhino today, right?"

"Yeah, maybe," my son replies.

"Maybe a cheetah," our guide says.

"Absolutely!" Frank exclaims. "And take a picture!"

It's hard to believe that, only the day before, my son was so far removed from taking a picture that I wasn't sure if he'd end up having to be hospitalized in East Africa. He wouldn't eat. As darkness descended, he merely stared at the canopy atop his bed. He only spoke when I demanded to know what was going on. And then it was with a venom directed at life in general—and me in particular.

I didn't know if we'd make it through the night.

• • •

How to describe Franklin? He expresses his thoughts and feelings through some form of art—be it writing, cooking, music, woodworking, or painting, all of which he has definite gifts for. He possesses an intuitive and sharp sense of humor. His physical presence is quite commanding, whether he is in a positive or negative attitude. Big, but capable of moving with the grace of a dancer, surprisingly agile, sometimes reminiscent of a boxer. The body has a power not quickly seen, because while Frank loves clothes, he tends to wear things that are big and that cover him up, although he doesn't always put on a belt and folks will sometimes get an unintentional (or maybe intentional?) "mooning" from him. As his mother once pointed out, Franklin is blessed with incredibly beautiful hands and feet. Sometimes she said she just liked to watch him move those long fingers with the differently shaped nails.

Yet Franklin can also be sullen and extremely willful. When he gets agitated, which can be triggered by a look from someone or a sudden movement, his speech may speed up to the point of being unintelligible. Or his gait may take on a strange shuffling-and-skipping quality. Occasionally he moves his lips as if talking to an invisible someone or waves his hand impulsively at a passing stranger. His mood can shift rapidly and unpredictably, and his thought patterns sometimes make no logical sense. And there have been times when, due to the medication he was on, he has been terribly overweight.

Like many people of mixed race, Frank could easily be taken for Latino or Middle Eastern—the skin color and hair texture being that of many peoples of the earth. My son has always been "multicultural," in the sense of imagining himself as someone at home in many geographical locations. Some years ago, he wrote: "In today's society, can we obtain happiness amongst one another. Or, are we permanently separated by race, ethnicity, and religion? Why can't we obliterate the notion of race? How could we travel over the whole world and feel comfortable?"

Such was Franklin's dream . . . not all that long ago . . . though sometimes it has seemed like lifetimes.

• • •

Early in 1979, Etta and I had been together for almost two years when our beautiful baby boy was born. We were each part of a large extended family, initially a group of close friends who had come together out of the sixties' folk music world in Boston. After fixing up a series of run-down houses in Roxbury's Fort Hill neighborhood and beginning to raise children together, the group had expanded to have homes in Los Angeles and New York, as well as a farm in Kansas. A family-run construction business provided our main means of support. Franklin, in a short autobiographical piece written in his teens, would describe growing up "in an extended family that is like a Chinese commune but more like a tribe in that it is more personal. We don't just work together. We live together, eat together, and try to share each other's lives."

Etta was one of two African American women in our predominantly white family. We'd gotten to know each other when I moved from the East Coast out to LA, to be a staff writer in *TV Guide* magazine's Hollywood bureau. She happened to be working as a secretary on the same block, and we'd have lunch together among the fossil excavations at the La Brea Tar Pits right across Wilshire Boulevard. Before too long, we were sharing more than just lunch.

Our backgrounds were vastly different. I'd been raised in upper-middle-class Midwestern suburbs, where watching and writing about sports was my passion. Etta came from inner-city Philadelphia, with a rich and diverse cultural education although her family often struggled to make ends meet. Music was a common bond. She was a marvelous cellist who'd once played with both the Louisville and Oakland symphony orchestras; each of my parents were classically trained musicians, and I enjoyed singing and playing guitar. Etta and I, too, were comfortable in a wide range of social situations, and enjoyed attending Hollywood events as part of my working for *TV Guide.*

We were in our early thirties and very much wanted to have a child. But it was an extremely difficult birth, hours of labor followed by a caesarean. Perhaps it was the soul's premonition of hard times ahead. Our new baby and the American President Franklin D. Roosevelt, one of our heroes, were born one day apart. So our family suggested naming him Franklin Delano Russell. "Little FDR." He was such a striking and awake child, and I couldn't have been more proud. A close friend, upon seeing a photograph taken of him in the hospital the day after his birth, told Etta a curious thing: "I think Franklin is really your teacher."

From a Neuropsychological Evaluation, late 1997: "Frank reports he weighed 9 lbs 2 oz when born and was an early talker. Not aware of complications at time of mother's pregnancy. Foot problem as infant that necessitated his wearing a cast for a period."

As a little boy, Franklin possessed an uncanny ability to find fossils; either while walking on a beach or in the Flint Hills of Kansas. One of these, a prehistoric shark's tooth, still graces one of our family mantelpieces. He was also an avid collector of quartz crystals, revered by many Native Americans as the "brain cells" of Grandmother Earth. In certain of their traditions, anyone able to attune to the power of the quartz crystal obtains the capability to communicate directly with spiritual worlds.

Years later, Franklin would reminisce about the Landmark books he read as a boy—specifically on Washington, Jefferson, and Lincoln. From a letter, dictated at age three:

Dear Daddy,

I started a book.
I learn to do letters.
Then I do books.
Me and my daddy type on the type writer.
Now I beginning to write like my daddy.

From the Neuropsychological Evaluation, late 1997: "Age 7 enrolled in speech class to work on pronunciation of S's and R's. Suspended in 3rd 4th and 6th grades for fighting/disruptive behavior and indicated he was 'always moving around' (hyperactive) and that it was hard for him to stay focused. Asked what precipitated fighting: 'I had the illusion I could fight so I wanted to.'"

Etta would never forget the day she realized that Franklin was no longer reading with comprehension. This is something, she came to consider long afterward, that often happens to children on the autism spectrum. They may come into the world very bright and learning to read early, and then abruptly lose that ability. In retrospect, Franklin wasn't being stubborn about doing his school work; he really couldn't do it. But no one could understand, because he was so incredibly smart; even the word recognition and verbal reading were fine. But the comprehension was scattered.

When Franklin was nine months old, Etta and I split up. I ended up quitting the magazine and returning to our family's place in Boston. We both continued to live as part of the community, but often in different locations. So, during much of his early life, I didn't see Franklin on a consistent basis. I told myself that others in the family were more experienced at raising children than I was, which was true—but also an excuse for my leading a purposeful life as a journalist and environmental activist. Etta was with our son far more regularly but, having come from a family in which there was seldom physical demonstration of affection, she often felt like other and more demonstrative women whom she knew must be better mothers. "There were times I had so little faith in myself that I followed what other people suggested, and not my own feelings and instincts," she would recall. She also reflected years later on how strong the bond is between parent and child, despite all the difficulties and mistakes that are made along the way.

How deeply my son felt abandoned by me, I don't really know. Neither retrospection nor guilt can resolve all questions. I do know that, since his early years, he'd felt "different." Being the youngest boy growing up in an unconventional type of family was one thing. Another had to do with race. We'd never talked about the realities that a mixed-race child would face in the larger American society. Even though Etta and I were no longer together, we remained friends sharing a bigger life, which we believed was paramount.

But when Frank was about five, I remember walking with him along a riverbank in Kansas, and his persistently asking about what happens when you mix two parts together. He was talking about genes, black and white, his mother's and mine. Was this somehow against the way of nature? he wondered. I don't recall exactly what I said, although I reassured him that this was not something to worry about—and then secretly hoped that the subject would not come up again. (When it comes to racial issues, this is perhaps the case with many well-intentioned white Americans.)

Later, when my son entered third grade in the Boston public school system, he had to fill out one of those forms where you must list your ethnicity. He was confused and didn't know what to do. "But I'm both," he told the teacher, almost in tears. They made him choose anyway. He checked off "Black." I had encountered a similar situation when I enrolled him. I, too, was in a quandary. Finally I had checked off "White."

Only as Franklin approached adolescence did I become aware that, in the eyes of the world, he was definitely not "white." We were living together in LA that school year. I used to pick him up every afternoon at the sixth-grade playground. He hated it when I sometimes got out of the car and called his name, and he insisted I not do that. Eventually he revealed that his schoolmates were taunting him because his father was white. "No, that can't be your dad," they would say. "You must be adopted."

I didn't know how to handle this. Just as I hadn't known what to do about the "ethnic choice" forced upon him earlier. I tried to put it out of my mind. I tried not to call Franklin's name again. But sometimes I had to get out of the car and find him in the schoolyard, and he would glare at me as I approached—mutual silence—then walk either ahead of or behind me, but always apart.

For the first time, though, as Franklin neared his teens, I was very much a steady part of his life. I took him to the redwood forest and to an early electric car operation I was writing an article about. One night, after he'd been suspended from school for fighting, I asked Frank if he had a problem with me. "Oh no, I think you're a much better dad than you used to be," he said. "I used to think you were kind of lazy. I know you were real busy, but . . ." Did he mean lazy in terms of my spending more time with him? Yes, he did.

But his periodic rages, sometimes accompanied by violent head-aches that he'd had from the time he was little, seemed to increase as he grew older. Etta and I started some family counseling with a psychiatrist at Cedars Sinai Hospital. Franklin brought up the issue of race right away, asking the doctor—who was originally from India—whether she saw him as black or white. He explained that he saw himself as black, yet his skin was much lighter and so this caused some confusion.

Franklin's sixth-grade IQ test score had come back between 155 and 160, at the "genius" level. He talked to the doctor about think-ing too much, and Etta recalled his having three different answers to the same question simultaneously when he was very small. His precociousness—and his wanting always to have the last word—sur-faced in amusing ways with the doctor. When she made astute obser-vations about some drawings he'd brought to the appointment, Frank responded: "Oh, now I see what you do. At first I thought you weren't very professional." The doctor laughed and said, "That's a left-handed compliment." At one point she told a personal story about her father making her wear long dresses as a child instead of short skirts like the other kids, and her letting dad know how she felt, and while he didn't give in, it was better than keeping all her anger inside. "I guess that's how you became a psychologist," Frank said. And the doctor cracked up laughing.

During another session, Franklin was adamant that what he does *has* to be perfect, otherwise he'll abandon it. He was fascinated with the way things are put together, especially machines and electronics in general. But while he could always start something, he had a terrible time bringing anything to completion. I viewed him as a dreamer. I tried disciplining him into finishing school projects, and Frank did manage to complete a go-kart in the garage. The school psychologist told me that such perfectionist tendencies are often seen in mixed-parent children, and that it has to do with low self-esteem in the sense that the child believes the only way to win approval is to do some-thing perfectly.

A close friend, whose older brother had been diagnosed with a mental illness as a teenager, noted how Franklin's thoughts seemed so disconnected. Nor could Frank often tell the difference between what he thinks and his emotions; he used the word *embarrassed* a lot to express what he feels. In an earlier letter to me, the same friend had written that Frank was "a bit of a manic-depressive." He was eleven at the time.

Still, there were periods of considerable achievement, particularly in the arts. I enrolled Franklin in a weekly musical children's chorus, which was visited periodically by Hollywood studios needing kids for productions. Frank ended up appearing on the Academy Awards with members of his group, running onto the stage and singing a nominated song from the movie *Home Alone*.

When Frank was twelve, he and I spent part of the summer together on our family's Kansas farm, I took him along on a story assignment to the Lakota Sioux reservation in the Black Hills of South Dakota. It proved a powerful experience for Frank, one that he would often make reference to in the years to come. Not only did he make friends among the Native American children, our visit coincided with a Sun Dance, which we were invited to attend. When storm clouds gathered overhead, the announcement came that rain must not inter-rupt the ceremony. We spectators all needed to come together, share a pipe, and pray. As we did so, and the drumming and dancing intensified, and the wind howled, the thunderhead divided and moved off across the surrounding hills. A few miles away, we learned, four inches of rain and hail had fallen. But nothing landed on the Sun Dance. Franklin was quietly but profoundly moved by the mystery, and he never forgot it.

· · ·

The next fall, he received a nearly full scholarship to Park School, a private school in Boston, for seventh grade. And that winter, with his mother, he took part in a gospel-style annual Christmas pageant called "Black Nativity." Etta was always there for him, sitting through rehearsals, visiting with his teachers, whatever came up.

We'd had Franklin tested for a learning disability the previous summer. When his end-of-semester reports at Park School came up short, Etta and I wrote a letter to his teachers.

> Ever since Franklin was very young he had a seemingly contradic-
> tory learning pattern. He was always very outgoing and interested in
> things, especially to do with math or science, constantly thinking up
> new "inventions" . . . but asking for help on the smallest reading assign-

ments. He would get into trouble both in school and at home for not finishing work. He would sit for maybe three hours in front of any given assignment and not do it . . . maybe just get a sentence written. He'd get extremely grumpy and develop terrible migraine headaches. There was always some reason he could not do it . . . "It's so boring," "I can't think of anything." Up until the last few years we had looked upon this as a behavior problem; not being able to understand how and why a child who is so bright and interested in so many things, knows vocabulary and reads fairly well, scores well on standard achievement tests etc. . . . would not be able to look up ten words for vocabulary and write a few sentences in anything less than two hours . . . knowing full well that he was missing doing some other activity he really wanted to do. Now we know there is a definite brain dysfunction at work. It is called Concept Imagery Dysfunction.

That had been the conclusion of the test results, with the woman administering it saying, "This child has been doing a lot of cover up"—compensating in many ways for a lack of quickness and focus. In a demanding middle-school academic environment, there was no way to hide it. The teachers were understanding. Instead of going on Ritalin, which they'd formerly suggested, my son began twice-weekly tutoring and seeing a school psychologist who he liked. This, too, was problematic. The psychologist was a nice enough fellow, but not deep; Franklin basically ran the sessions.

Generally speaking, though, Frank's eighth and ninth grade years at Park School were the most we could have hoped for. His grades picked up; he started on the varsity basketball team and his track coach felt he had the potential to be a college high-jumper; he took drum lessons and wrote poetry; he spent two expense-paid weeks in Spain with his class and two summers in Baja, Mexico, at a beautiful place our extended family was starting to build above the Sea of Cortés.

Some years later, Frank wrote a reminiscence about that period in his life:

On his way to Barcelona, he makes a stop in Leon Spain. The city is beautiful at night. The Cathedrals hold a dark gaunt and ancient air. Gambling casinos line the streets. Beautiful fountains gush sparkling water into the air and over succulent plants. As he is walking in the city he sees an old round open building. Peering inside one of the columns, he is opened up to a whole world of shouting, hissing, fans, and lunging kicking soccer players. They are dressed in the colors of the Spanish flag. How patriotic, he ponders. There is a certain beauty in the martiality of the game. . . . In this sport the men have legs like horses with the acceleration of a cheetah after its prey.

At Frank's graduation from Park School in June of 1994, a number of his teachers came up to Etta and me raving about the change they'd seen in our son. The ones with whom he'd gone through the most hell over the three middle-school years ended up being the ones who loved him the most. His social studies instructor took me aside and said, "Yes, Frank's still got to work on his study skills, but he's got the soul, and that's a quality you can't teach." The headmaster said to him, "Well, after all, Frank, we really got to *know* each other. Some of these kids, I never knew much more about than their names." To me, the headmaster said he was more proud of Frank than anyone else in the class. His poetry was featured in the school's "Day of Appreciation," and Franklin inscribed personal poems as bookmark gifts to all of his teachers.

One of his poems was published by the school, and was untitled:

Fire scorches the ground.
Hot air screams out of the earth,
condensing to make water that streams
over the cliff dripping into my thought processes.
    An idea takes root in the mind.
    Expression is the key, maybe not one of a kind
       but original for me.
It can't be contained—
comes down like the rain—might not make sense
but I'm trying in vain.

I don't recall exactly when I came across another piece of my son's, but my handwritten notation at the top of the page says: "This was written '93–'94 sometime." It was typed, and on first reading seemed occult and obscure. It was headed:

SYMBOLS:
Core: White triangle with golden wings—thoughts from my inner self reaching people universally. Green circle inside the white triangle and rays in four directions. I want to give my mind to the world and the

earth, to save them both. Circle is the earth. The rays are pathways for these thoughts.

Limits: Person enclosed in the North—My ideas are trapped in my head. Sometimes I can't express them. I spend a lot of time trying to get them out. Lightning bolts are the ideas that are trying to get out of my head. Closed eye in the West—sometimes I only see the outside of a person and can't see myself clearly. Open eye in the East—it is easier for me to see far-away things, and things on the outside. Person enclosed in the South—sometimes I don't feel connected to people. They could be having fun while I'm on my own.

Attributes: Star in the East—the need to understand people—Tree in the South—I have more growing to do. Two faces—one black and one white represent the two parts of me learning to live with each other.

The angst of a teenager? Yes, it was that. Yet the way Franklin described it—the colors, the shapes, the differences in what he saw by turning to each of the four directions, the desire to "save the world"— all this in a symbol language that he identified as such: years later, I realized, it bore the mark of some strange initiatory journey.

• • •

Shortly before his sixteenth birthday, Franklin handed me a type-written sheet of paper with some trepidation. I read it while he sat across from me in his room. Then I glanced up at him, and read it again.

This is something that I saw last night (December 30, 1994) while I was lying in bed. My eyes were closed, but I wasn't asleep, when I saw a square. I went through the square, and a circle appeared with a spiral like a camera lens in the center. From it protruded rays, not like the sun but like lines. Outside of it there was another circle, that cut the lines. It was at least three times as large as the first circle. Then the center circle turned into a sun, which was yellow and orange. As I came closer, all the time I was moving; it became a tunnel. This tunnel was as if it was in space and nothing else existed, like a long cable in space. I moved slowly along it and through it. All around, it was glowing, a green yellowish color. I kept going. Each time I opened my eyes, this picture would disappear. Then when I closed them again, it would reappear.

Then there was an opening into something that I've never seen be-fore, and that is so beautiful I couldn't even imagine. First I saw one column. In front of it there was a pyramid. As I steadily moved forward, I saw the other columns on both sides of it. I moved through them. At this point I was about ten feet above the ground. There was an open eye on the ground, like the one on the dollar bill. I was going higher and higher. To my right there was water glistening with the light of the sun. The two little jewels that I picked up on Martha's Vineyard were together in the dream. The one that I have now is separate from the other one, because I have given one to an old friend from school. I went on further and I saw another tunnel. This tunnel was like a cave, with dips in the earth, although it wasn't musty. It was shiny and full of colors like the ones you could see on a computer screen. Nothing seemed real. I opened my eyes, then fell asleep, and the last thing I remember is going through that tunnel slowly.

At the time my son's vision occurred—if that's what it was—I didn't know what to make of it. A parent could never be sure, but I didn't think Franklin had been using any psychedelic drugs. Coming of age during the sixties, I'd tried mescaline and LSD and had what I considered profound experiences, but nothing like he was describing. Adolescents are generally a mystery to the older generation, but this seemed something else entirely. What he saw was also similar to what a number of people have reported about "near death experiences." My rational mind wondered if this could be related to a minor operation Franklin had over that Christmas break. He had never gone under anesthesia before.

For his tenth-grade year, with our consent, our larger group decided to home-school Frank and two other boys close to his age, on our property in LA. They hadn't all been together for some time, and public high school choices seemed limited. Frank loved writing poetry and even started his own school paper, *Dominions*. But overall, he wasn't happy, and I wasn't there much. One night in the spring he ran away from home, spending the night with some homeless people, and when he came back said he wanted to drop out and get a job. Maybe even start a business with the men he'd met on the street. I flew out from Boston and, in accord with his teachers, Etta and I decided to let him quit school. Frank stayed in LA with his mom while I headed back to Boston.

It was a pivotal time in my life, entering a new relationship within the family. Alice and I had long been good friends when we found ourselves falling in love, and were now living together in Boston. Her friendship with Etta went way back, having met in a macrobiotic food store in Illinois shortly before they independently came to Boston to live as part of the community twenty-five years before.

That summer in 1995, Etta and Frank both returned to the East Coast, where he landed work bagging groceries at a Stop & Shop. We all started seeing Dr. G., a psychiatrist in Cambridge—initially Etta and me together and Franklin separately. The doctor made it clear from the outset that this was late to be initiating family therapy, because at sixteen a young person is moving away from their parents toward defining themselves, with different sets of issues. Also, as he put it, "you don't have an intimate relationship but come together because of him, which can be very confusing to him." Still, we delved into some important matters. Was I compensating for my lack of time with Frank as a little boy by always trying to be "understanding?" Did I then blame his mother for his difficulties? I admitted that a part of me wanted to place Franklin in my private world; when he wasn't talking to Etta, I didn't care so long as he was communicating with me. Unconsciously, I cut her out.

I'd gone into our first session with an agenda, things I wanted to bring up; afterward, I could remember everything in sequence and came away quite pleased with myself. But I'd left Etta feeling utterly alone. The next time, we'd talked openly about her dysfunctional family background in contrast to my upper-middle-class upbringing. She felt I was "so white," and I said I was afraid of "the darkness" in her. (In retrospect, we were both wrong.) I wanted our son to be "successful"; his mother was terribly afraid that he would fail. I always wanted things to be "all right"; she lived with the constant worry that they never are. He was caught in the gulf between the two of us, between what we reinforce in him, while we live from crisis to crisis.

Afterward, I found myself completely undone. My mind went blank, which terrified me.

What I wrote in my journal had nothing to do with the session *per se*. I described what I termed Franklin's mood swings, saying that "what was true between us yesterday, when I felt close to him, is suddenly not there." But at the time, I turned the problem into self-reflection. "Why is it so hard for me to react to him in a moment? I want everything to be rational, reasonable, harmonious. I think I am seeking to give him understanding, but is it only understanding on my terms? There is so much I overlook. The way he comes into a room, sits disinterested at the dinner table, answers the telephone coldly . . ." I was also afraid of my son, I had to admit, because I never knew what to expect.

I had a dream about being beside a body of water, holding a child in my arms. Curiously, Franklin told Dr. G. about a very similar dream, also holding a child, but while riding on a bus. They were crossing a bridge, and the child wanted to jump out the window into the water below. At the front of the bus was a white girl, and at the back was a black girl. He'd known them both at Park School and, as he spoke of their different personalities, the doctor suggested that they represented parts of himself. Not just the fact of the two races, but the one in front as moving forward and seeking to find out who he was, while the one in back represented the part that tries to mold himself into what he thinks other people want to hear or want him to be.

All of the analysis appeared to help. A woman Franklin met at the grocery store liked him immensely, and suggested he apply to a Boston private high school called Commonwealth. He made it happen, doing especially well on math and Spanish placement tests. That August, the school said it would not only accept Frank, but give him a substantial scholarship. It felt like a miracle. He would need to repeat the tenth grade that he'd dropped out of, and while Franklin wasn't happy about that, he did accept it. He worked hard at his new school and the teachers were pleased. This, I wrote in a letter, "is just the kind of challenge he needed."

At the same time, that winter, my son began immersing himself in the study of astrology. Our family didn't make a religion out of it, but found that keeping up with the planetary alignments to one's birth chart could be very useful in figuring out what was going on at particular junctures in life. Franklin seemed to possess an amazing knack for astrology, being able to memorize almost instantly the signs and houses where the seven planets in our solar system had been positioned at the time of someone's birth.

One night Franklin asked me, "Dad, do you think I'm a walking mind?" This, it turned out, was what an astrological guide called *Heaven Knows What* says about those, like himself, who are born under the Zodiac sign of Aquarius. Then he began running through the various elements: "Water, that means emotion or feeling; air, that's mind; earth, your structure I guess; fire, would that be spirit?" There he paused and exclaimed, "Well, I'm an Aquarius with an Aries moon, I guess that's why I've got so many *hot ideas!*" He cracked himself up, adding that of course this was why those other qualities were definitely necessary. I loved that he was developing a sense of humor about himself.

Early in 1996, in the course of writing the book *Black Genius,* which I would dedicate to my son, I took Frank along to New York on a research trip. We went to a play about the life of Paul Robeson and to interviews I conducted with Stanley Crouch and Norman Mailer, with whom I was already acquainted. It turned out that Franklin, Mailer, and his wife Norris shared the same birthday, January 31. Afterward I wrote in a letter: "Mailer got totally into this, figuring out the odds of all three people being in one room at the same time, which is something like forty million to one. Norman served us up a fine lunch himself and told fascinating stories about his experiences with Ralph Ellison, James Baldwin, and Muhammad Ali." Yet for Franklin, it came down to his wondering aloud to an older friend: "Why is my dad introducing me to all these famous people?" Hearing about this, I confided to my journal: "Perhaps what he needs from me is not the 'together' father who takes him into the world of my ambition and career, but the human side." How prescient that was, but how long it would take to manifest . . .

Frank wrote his history term paper on Gandhi, and fulfilled a school "community service" requirement by helping put together a new exhibit at Roxbury's Museum for Afro-American Artists, not far from our home. He would study long into the night, and the Commonwealth School noted he'd made "substantial progress," and awarded him an even bigger scholarship for the next term.

Privately, my son made this entry in his journal:

5/6/96: The spirit. What am I to do with this spirit of mine. This dissatisfied ball of clay without shape.

Franklin again spent most of that summer at the beautiful, remote spot our family was continuing to develop along Mexico's southern Baja peninsula. He wrote me several letters, including a sketch of the columned *ramada* he was helping erect. He was doing some summer reading for school, including *Huckleberry Finn* and Ellison's *Invisible*

Man. I sent him Dostoevsky's *Notes from Underground* and *The Autobiography of Malcolm X.* On a lighter note, he said in his letter:

> Sometimes we go surfing, and sometimes fishing.
> I've been fishing three or four times since I've been here.
> I try to do some art once in awhile.
> I miss you and Boston and folks.

He appeared to have had a marvelous summer. Shortly before Frank returned for his junior year at Commonwealth School, a friend wrote me:

> He's wrestling with a lot of questions that start to get very real at seventeen and he's certainly a lot more open about them than I was at his age. He has his sullen and reclusive times but not too bad and they don't last too long. I just think you need to make sure you keep him talking.

The school had written his mother and me that "all of his teachers have nothing but praise for Franklin's incredible work ethic. . . . We all have confidence that he will complete Commonwealth successfully." However, his teachers also pointed to "a certain difficulty that shows up both in class and in his reading. In class, Franklin sometimes seems to be out of touch with the discussion and unable to focus his mind."

> *Things are rough, I've had enough, I want independence, but I can't muster up a declaration. I don't have the words or the balls, I want to cry and scream through the halls. Am I at the beginning or at the end, are you my foe or my friend. Heaven help me.*
>
> —Franklin's Journal

CHAPTER 2

• • •

Breakdown

I felt a Cleaving in my Mind—
As if my Brain had split—
I tried to match it—Seam by Seam—
But could not make it fit. . . .

—Emily Dickinson, *The Lost Thought*

W HEN AN ADOLESCENT "BREAKDOWN" HAPPENS—AND, with diagnoses of schizophrenia, generally this occurs in the late teens—there is no way for a parent to be prepared for what seems to erupt from nowhere. Franklin was midway through his seventeenth year when, less than a month into the fall term at school, one day coming home in the car he told me: "I don't know what's happening. I can't find my old self again."

Another time, to my surprise and dismay, he said he was even having suicidal thoughts. "What?! You'd never do that, would you Frank?"

"No, I wouldn't," he'd said.

"Well, if you keep having those kinds of thoughts, you'll tell me, won't you?"

"Yes," he'd said. I told myself this would surely pass, it must be something many teenagers went through, and I decided not to tell his mother.

Early that October, I found Franklin watching TV and refusing to do his homework. We argued, and it ended with my yelling at him to go to his room. The next day, he told me that he'd taken a razor blade and tried to cut himself. Also, that he'd written something on the wall next to his bed. There, in an un-erasable black magic marker, I read: "I am going to die and the world will be a better place."

I was appalled and scared, and we talked for a long time. But I ended up feeling that Frank was not in any immediate danger, and so again let things ride. I was, assuredly, in denial. I don't even remember the episode that a hospital document had later described, which was: "A few days later Franklin reportedly went out to buy some marijuana from the brother of a friend. In the process, someone pulled a knife. Franklin became extremely upset and ran home. Following this, he was afraid to leave the home, stating repeatedly that the world was not safe, and that he was scared to take the 'T' to school."

I do recall that, a week after the talk we'd had, Franklin stayed home from school and said he was going to the library to study. Instead, he packed a bag and, without anyone knowing, ran away. In Charlestown's Sullivan Square, he said something that angered another young man, who told Franklin he had a gun and was going to shoot him. My son called me from a nearby subway and asked that I come get him. As we drove home, he was sure that people on the street were staring at him.

He seemed to calm down when we got to the house. We talked some more. I suggested, only partly in jest, that maybe he just needed to lose his virginity. That night, at my suggestion, he agreed to go visit a college-age friend with whom he'd grown up and discuss how to go about this. But soon after I dropped him off at the apartment, Franklin had a beer and became increasingly paranoid. Fearing that his friends were going to kill him, he ran home, about two miles through a sometimes dangerous neighborhood. When Franklin burst through the front door, he was clearly "out of his mind."

Several months earlier, he had written in his journal:

So he runs.
Through the streets.
Through the rain.
Through his pain. . .
He runs home, and goes straight to his bed.
His last words are "Good night Lord, and where is my salvation."

He spent that night crouched in a corner of his mother's room, afraid to venture outside it. I believe he was clutching a stuffed animal to his chest, as if regressing to his childhood. I called Dr. G., who said we should contact a colleague right away who specialized in adolescents. We did, and at the appointment early the next afternoon, Franklin asked to be hospitalized. The doctor was able to find a bed for him at nearby Cambridge Hospital. His mother and I drove him there, the longest half-mile of silence I can remember.

• • •

Reason for referral: a three week period of . . . increase in psychotic symptoms, including paranoid thoughts, command hallucinations telling him to hurt himself. . . . In addition, Franklin has been experiencing some depressive symptomatology, including difficulty concentrating, decreased appetite, decreased energy, increased sadness, and suicidal ideation.
—Cambridge Hospital Evaluation, October 1996.

His academic adviser at Commonwealth School tells the hospital: "Franklin had few friends, alienating peers (both male and female) with his bizarre sense of humor and his inability to read social cues and situations." I wish they'd told his parents.

I keep copious notes on a daily basis, trying to make sense of what's happened.

It's an adolescent ward. He's given a cot in the hallway, so that staff can check on him every five minutes, as he's considered a suicide risk. "Why don't you just get it over with?" he says to me. Then, to both his mother and me, "why don't you put me to sleep like a dog." There's a quiet fury in his words.

I am sitting with Frank on the cot, leaning against a wall. "Nobody wants to feel pain," my son says and adds: "You will. Everybody in this room will." He gestures around at a few other young people either sleeping or pacing about. I tell him I don't know what to do to help him, but I wish I did.

It's almost surreal. We could all have been a dream, a terrible nightmare—everything we knew or thought we knew seemingly turned upside down.

He looks at Etta and says, "Should we go back to Africa? To Europe?"

All the places he came from. Franklin is still very aware of what he's saying and the reactions of people around him—and he doesn't have to care.

Etta begins singing from "Black Nativity," the annual Christmas pageant in which she and Franklin had both participated. He sings along.

He turns to me and says, "We've had some of the best times. You've taught me a lot, about love."

My gratitude in that moment knows no bounds.

"You won't hurt me now because you need me," he continues. "A lot of people need my help. I can help them."

Then he says, "When you had me, I was more than both of you."

He asks, did Jimi Hendrix and his other heroes really live? We assure him they did.

"I'm being crucified," he says. "It's inevitable."

He looks at his palm, says he sees a circle that's emerged at his life-line, which he adds indicates a crisis point.

"None of your reassurances help me," he says.

"You're not in control. I'm in control," he says.

I listen in amazement to the articulate but frightening new voice that is coming from my son, and I tell him I am getting to know him. I can't believe how lame, how hollow, I sound.

Before we leave, he is talking again about dying and killing himself. I lean forward, right into his face, and tell him in a whisper: "Swear to me you'll never do that."

"I swear it," he says, taking a deep breath.

Then, as I back away from him, he says: "I thought that moment would never happen."

Was my son truly suicidal at that time? Or was this more dramatic, desperately seeking attention and confirmation that someone cared? He was certainly smart enough to know the big trigger words to make parents snap to attention.

That night, I come across a crumpled piece of paper on the floor of Franklin's room at home. It was typed up and said:

> Shame on society for . . . the idolatry, the bigotry, the duality, fast food, the clichés, the music, the internet and mass culture, better known as mass torture for the man who does not know and is innocent or the one that is morally respectful. Shame on the false inspiration without hesitation, the quick success. . . . Shame on the man [who] knows how to do right but does wrong. Shame on the sorrowful selfishness that still persists when the man resists.

Cruel cycle within a cycle. It takes knowledge to be enlightened. It takes enlightenment to find your way out of the dark. Maybe the light is the natural things, that means everything under the sun. Maybe the darkness began in the cave the first man dwelt in. Natural beauty, smooth and shiny, natural destruction and decay, the leaves in the swamps, the crocodile in the mud of the Nile, bless him for eyes that see, but do not know. . . .

Are you just a pawn in a chess game controlled by your maker, or are you your maker? Shame on words for they do not entirely convey a human message or a human moment. Shame on this poem for attempting to advocate any creed—the world is filled with evil deeds. A man must do what he needs take heed, beware of greed. . . .

By a young man looking for meaning while life is demeaning….I'm about to have a fit for I am wondering if it is just my big ego that makes the whole tree that is me grow, and know. Shame on me for being aware.

The last line seems the crux. He's so aware, yet with no foundation.

• • •

I speak to a hospital psychiatrist the next morning. She tells me that she's very worried because Franklin has been hearing voices of people telling him to hurt himself. He thinks someone may be poisoning him. He believes he's being sent special messages through the newspaper or the radio. The first step, the doctor says, is to quiet the paranoia. She suggests one of several medications, with Risperdal being the top choice. There is less chance, she says, of muscular problems than with Haldon or Trilafon. Reluctantly, we go along with her assessment.

I go to see Frank that afternoon. He says he was convinced the other night, when he saw me talking on the phone, that we were conspiring against him. He talks, as well, about a government conspiracy, and that he's getting messages from the TV. We watch a movie, *The Karate Kid*, in the ward with several other young people about a teenager who learns karate to overcome school bullying. I wonder what else Franklin might be picking up from the movie? There is one girl he keeps glancing at. He tells me when we're alone that, even though there's never been a girl who loved him, he's not giving up. I tell him it will happen eventually. He says he hopes so. I tell him I love him very much. "Of course you do," he says, consolingly. I am weeping in front of him, perhaps for the first time.

The hospital psychiatrist tells me the next morning that Franklin's thoughts are more organized, but he remains in what they call a "flight from reality," where someone withdraws into inactivity, fantasy, or detachment. They are considering putting him on a second drug, Depakote, to help control his mood swings. The preoccupation with hurting himself has not gone away either.

I find myself disoriented. My sense of direction is gone when I drive, I am missing turns at streets. At dinner, talking with friends about what's been happening, I burst into tears.

Five days into his hospitalization, a doctor asks Franklin to rank his level of paranoia on a scale of one-to-ten. It was eight when he was admitted, now it's at four. He's not sleeping out in the hallway anymore, but in a shared room. When Etta and I go to see him in the early evening, we tell him about us visiting Commonwealth School and how they said he shouldn't worry about catching up at this point. He asks his mother whether she felt spiritually connected to him during that day. She says yes, and he agrees.

"The things I said last night weren't true," he says, turning to me, "about you learning from me."

"But in a way, it *is* true, Franklin," I say.

Later, alone with me, he asks if I believe in psychic fields, saying that he's getting a lot of "intrusion" happening with other kids here in the hospital. "We know what each other is thinking," he says, then asks: "Can you read my thoughts?" He seems to believe me when I say I can't. "Does either of us have more of a right to survive than the other?" he asks. I say no.

He goes on: "We're both men, right? Our struggle is the same." He says he's still very afraid, knows he needs to balance out, feels paranoid right now, thinking about conspiracy again. Then, looking long and direct into my eyes, he says: "My spirit is still strong."

"You will get even stronger through this," I tell him.

The three of us have dinner together downstairs in the hospital cafeteria. Afterward we listen to classical music in his room for awhile. Etta reads aloud to him from a book on the history of painting. Toward the end, she says she feels like he needs a hug. He thinks so, too. But after the hug, he freezes, lying on the bed with his arms extended into the air. He asks why she is looking at him like that?

"Why are you keeping your hands like that?" she responds.

"I'm afraid of you—that you're gonna kill me. I need you to love me. What's all this time been here? Just words. Just talking."

"Sometimes I don't know how to show you that I love you, Franklin," Etta says.

"Yeah, you do," he says. "You're working at it."

All through this visit, he often looked back and forth between the two of us—as if at the parts that created him. I am beginning to tell when a mood swing begins because his sentences become clipped, his responses quick.

The next day, the doctor says Franklin's symptoms are getting better, but this could take a couple of months. The relapse rate, he warns, is quite high.

A week in, Frank is given a pass and the three of us go to dinner together at Legal Seafoods. "This is breaking down barriers in me, too," I tell him. What I don't say is that somehow I'm realizing—through what's happening now between Franklin, Etta, and me—how competitive I am; how I'd chosen to exclude his mother from the painful conversations he and I had leading up to this hospitalization. Later in the room when I am talking too abstractly, he says: "Let's not talk about that. I'm bored." He continues, "I'm ashamed of how I've been feeling." Then he asks about the TV. "People can't really change it, right?" meaning the messages it might be secretly imparting. Of course, there is some validity to this; TV, among other technologies, is constantly sending out messages.

The following day, based on how Frank seems to be improving, the hospital gives him another pass for a Saturday afternoon. Five of us go to the movies, including one of his peers and one of ours. Frank wanted to see *Get on the Bus*, the new Spike Lee movie. It's a story about fifteen disparate African American men on a cross-country trip to take part in the Million Man March—including a young man who's been allowed to break probation and go, providing he remains hand-cuffed to his father the whole time.

In the middle of the film, Franklin gets up and says he needs to go to the bathroom. He walks off down the aisle. I ask Etta, "Do you think he's all right?" She doesn't know.

Uncertain of what to do, but suddenly paranoid myself about "messages" he might be picking up from the film that could cause him to bolt, I follow him out. I stand outside the men's room for a moment, then decide to go in. The minute he sees me, Franklin is instantly paranoid and demands to know what I'm doing there. I had to pee, too, I lie.

"Are people out there laughing at me?" he says, and sits down beside the urinal against the wall. He only moves when another man enters, and Frank lets me take his arm, and we walk out to the hallway.

"Why did you come in there?" he demands again.

This time I tell him the truth: that I was worried he might wander off.

"Why were you watching me during the movie? Why do you only laugh when other people laugh?"

Maybe sometimes I do, I say.

"I'm talking about now." Then he asks: "Why are you standing like that?"

I realize how awkward I must look, hands tucked unnecessarily into my pockets.

Finally I say, "I don't have enough faith in you." Franklin agrees. That's the truth he's been waiting to hear. We return to our seats next to one another in the darkened theater. In the meantime, Etta has panicked and gone out to look for us, but eventually returns. As she would later point out about the things he'd said to me, it wasn't necessarily psychotic. The mental instability simply opened the door for him to say what many teenagers might be thinking, but couldn't say before.

The movie, as it continues to unfold, blows me away. It seems to be directed straight at me. A scene between the father and son, who's chained to him and then runs away into the woods, is devastating. I am shaking, crying, barely able to keep it together. The film ends at the Lincoln Memorial; in the shadow of the great man, with the father removing his son's handcuffs.

So much, I am thinking as we leave the theater, emanates from the feeling that passes between father and son. How could I not have known?

I talk to the doctor on-call that Sunday at Cambridge Hospital about what happened at the movie theater. I write down what he says. "The situation is inherently fraught with contradiction or paradox. You would've been a nervous wreck staying in your seat, so the answer was not necessarily to sit and sweat it out when your son went to the bathroom. On the other hand, he's a big boy, and how will he feel about being accompanied? The problem is in the ambiguous way you're responding; so he wonders, *why am I being followed?* Not going immediately expressed your own ambivalence. Instead of his hearing from you, 'I'll trust you, okay?' Or your straightforwardly saying, 'Because of the extraordinary nature of these circumstances, you'll have to understand why I'm coming along with you'—but instead, you ended up in the middle ground. The unstated message is, 'I don't know if I trust you.'"

With Etta and one of his younger friends from our family, we soon take another outing, this time to a Taco Bell and then the Museum of Fine Arts. I'm hoping to do better than I did at the movies: be quicker, more honest. On the drive back to the hospital, Franklin expresses frustration that none of the hospital doctors are really helping him work through his problems. I mention the psychiatrist he saw just before his hospitalization as someone who specializes in "kids." Franklin bridles. "I'm not a kid," he says angrily. I've blown it again.

"What makes the difference between an adolescent and adults?" he asks.

"Because you're still growing," his mother tells him.

He doesn't buy that one bit. "How do you know? What do you know about people my age?" He's furious. Etta suggests we pull over, but he doesn't want to. The only thing that goes anywhere is my finally talking to him about how the psychiatrist he saw really thought he could help him.

We sit in the car in the hospital parking lot. He brings up whether he looks more like me or his mother. He says everybody who knows him says he looks like his dad, but people who don't know him—like this girl Tara in the hospital—say he looks like his mom. He wants to know what characteristic we each see that looks like us. "The color of your skin," I tell him, "is more like your mom." He accepts that, though it's the most surface thing I could have said and only partly true.

"Sometimes I'm afraid I'll just go into oblivion and stay there," Franklin says. "But I can get out of that place when I remember people I care about. If I could just see in someone's face what I feel for them, it would be different." He adds that it's pretty late, now that he's seventeen, to establish something between us.

He's refusing to go back inside, and Etta gets out of the car to walk around, and my son and I are alone together. Desperately, I bare my guts to him about how I'm a human being and make mistakes and don't know what to do, but how much I have seen in him this past week—his "soul qualities"—and the moments we've had that *are* there to build upon. Afterward I can't remember all the things I said, except that they were painful, beautiful, and terrifying to me.

"Okay, let's go," he says. The sound of the car doors opening and closing feels almost deafening. I realize how much Franklin identifies with someone's weaknesses and vulnerabilities when you are willing to expose them. At the same time, he is rarely able to express his own deepest feelings and fears.

When I return home, I come across something else Franklin had written earlier in the year.

> Teenage years, seeing the same things pass my eyes, nothing *new* because I detach myself from the world. I classify the infinite possibilities of life under truth, pain, suffering, devoutness. Pettiness, falsity, normality, and death.
>
> Dissatisfaction with my life brings me into my own mind. There, I lose track of my heart that wants me to be boundless, searching, living, doing, succeeding, feeling. I decline the opportunities I am offered envisioning them as hardships, difficulties, despair. I become depressed, guilty, gloomy, resentful, nebulous.
>
> Then, as if a guardian angel has a hand in my fate, I break free, in sacrifice, humility, devotion, or hatred, impudence, accident, or rage. Then I reawaken or resurrect; the light inside of me shines brightly in new birth.
>
> Hopefully, as time is my bookkeeper, and I the businessman, I will accomplish my business.
>
> After speculation, errors, and bankruptcy, hopefully, I will expand into an empire.
>
> *Now* is not the time to worry about the end of the road. For as night is the absence of light, it casts a shadow on the road of destiny.
>
> My life is before me.

· · ·

"I'm not like other kids," he tells his mother and me at the outset of our next visit in the hospital. We play cards as we often do—crazy eights, sometimes 21 or Go Fish. He doesn't like it when Etta teases him, and responds: "You know, I don't have a lot of confidence."

The doctors see signs of progress, including an ability to have an "observing ego"—meaning Frank could *see* that some of his thoughts are delusions. However, on the negative side, the delusional system could be quite paranoid and widespread—hypervigilance, seeing conspiracies, believing he can influence the TV. He's talked recently about fear of death—and that all of history might not be true. I wonder if the doctors might ever have considered that themselves about history.

Twelve days since he was hospitalized, I pick up my son and take him down the street for an MRI. He wants me to stay with him as, wearing a helmet, he's wheeled inside a big machine. We're told the magnetization in the room is so strong that, if not shielded, it would pull all the cars going by to this side of the building. It's so loud that both Frank and I need earplugs. Afterward, on our way back to the car, he talks about being able to "mind read," like knowing when the man running the MRI machine would stop it. At lunch his mood changes. "Is my whole life a setup?" he asks. He questions my honesty. "If I do what I want to, I'll be happy," he says, adding, "a son you can be proud of."

The preliminary MRI results come back essentially normal in terms of any neurological condition. However, a number of symptoms often related to the onset of schizophrenia were indicated by the hospital assessment: considerable difficulty regarding association with the brain's frontal lobe or "executive system"; also with multi-step planning on a maze test and shifting from one way of problem solving to another. When telling a story, my son did a good job but, toward the end, his thoughts "loosened" and moved into "the supernatural or nature." At one point, the doctors said, Frank reported seeing an endless tunnel. Just like in the visionary experience he wrote down almost two years before.

Two days after the MRI, he says he read the mind of a nurse who knocked on the bathroom door, and who was wondering if he was in the shower with a girl. He talks of society deteriorating and a sense of impending anarchy. "Then you would have a choice," I say. "Between black and white?" he asks. "No, between the side of anarchy or helping restore order," I say. He says he could envision playing a role "if I live." His mother had said to him the evening before, "I won't see you again," meaning that night, but he wants to know what she meant by that. Etta explains. Today when we depart, trying facetiously to validate this, I say, "Be seeing you for a long time." The next day, he will ask why I said that.

I'm alone with Frank for most of a Saturday, just over two weeks into his hospitalization. Did I ever dream of being king of the world? he asks, but doesn't wait for my reply. He says he does, but emphasizes that he'd be a *benevolent* dictator. He tells me of dreaming about a rug inside a large ice cream maker, the machine creating a new energy source from the generated static. He's allowed another outing, and we go to a gym and sit in a whirlpool. He comes home and plays the drums. We feel close, crossing the bridge back to Cambridge. But in the hospital elevator, I express what a difference today is from the previous night when I felt so frustrated. What do I mean by that? Frank asks back in his room. Our arguments, the inability to talk, I say. This sets him off again; he's all over me about abandonment, lack of love, wanting to hurt him. Anything I might say to Franklin at this time could cause him to blow up. "There's nowhere to take this," I tell him, "I'll see you tomorrow." I confide to my diary: "I had 'played' psychiatrist all day, pursuing things he would bring up with questions, was left nowhere."

The next day, out of the blue, Frank says: "When God gave man fire, that was when man received values." I'm struck by this, but have no time to ponder its meaning, as he goes on about fire as capable of being both controlled and tamed; the paradox of humanity was that someone could never escape from the negative forces. He warns me that if I look primarily for the positive, things will be harder in my next lifetime. His insights and eloquence astonish me. "You're really an amazing person, Franklin," I say. "Thanks, Dad," he says.

A couple of days later, Frank tells Etta and me that he's having trouble. He'd gone walking outside with a group, and all these thoughts came about how holy he was. He strutted around feeling this way, but doesn't think anyone noticed. Still, he is down on himself for feeling messianic. Finishing dinner at a nearby restaurant, Frank goes into a deep silence and says, "Let's go." Back in his room, he speaks about a feeling suddenly coming over him when everyone grew quiet in the restaurant—that it was all about him, especially troublesome when Etta and I looked around at other people.

A handwritten note left on a bedside table in the hospital:

Feeling nebulous, like nothing in the world can help me. Just want to go back to the way things were. I keep reading things into what people are saying and I get so paranoid. Sometimes I feel like nothing is grounding me. I have extreme paranoias. I just want to get better.

It's so very terrible, that when a person is blown wide open the way Franklin was, there is no sanctuary except drugs. Besides the Risperdal for psychosis, he's on Depakote for mood swings and now Zoloft to combat depression. My son enjoys being onstage with an audience of psychiatrists, and is full of blame. He also says at a "family night" among a few other parents that he lets his own control him because he doesn't want to disappoint us. We sit apart from him in the cafeteria while he's with some of the other kids. We leave depressed, feeling that if he comes home, he'll just run away.

On Halloween, Frank puts on the costume of an African chief. In the ward, a teacher assigns him to do some study about Africa.

Home again soon after that for a visit, Frank starts work on a bench in our shop and says he wants to have a business selling such. In his room he pauses in front of a full-length mirror and wants me to stand beside him to see how much we look alike. I tell him I look old. No you don't, he says. In the car back to the hospital, he points at a passerby out the window and asks: "What is God? Is God those businessmen in their suits?" I answer with the first thought that comes: "God is the highest aspirations of mankind" and then add, "Universal love." We ride along in silence. He wants to hang out in the car in the hospital parking lot. He's a megalomaniac, he says, how can that be cured? Upstairs he tells a nurse that he did not enjoy his visit.

A Sunday, just over three weeks since being hospitalized: Frank asks me to please tell him when he's rude, and says he feels badly that he's put me through so much. The next night, he switches again, wants to get an apartment with one or both of his mother and me, but again talks of killing himself. Later, he tells me candidly, "I'm looking for something to blame."

The way he tunes in to things inside me is too fast, I can't handle it: "Really proud, aren't you? You don't care about people the same way I don't. . . . You have a paranoid complex yourself." There's a frightening meeting with him and two staff members, where it appears

Franklin is resigned to staying in the hospital. At a Pizza Hut, he talks about having an "analytical disorder"—his mind analyzing everything into the ground—and of his inability to put something back together after taking it apart and how this feeds into his obsessions. Later, in the hospital parking lot again, he speaks of how he feels like a mirror, reflecting what's inside people; how hard it is to sort out what's him and what's them.

If he'd lived in another time, he probably would have been one of those mad artists like Van Gogh, he says.

> *Meditation as opposed to medication. Is it the answer or a combination of meditation and counseling [sic]? Where does bipolar illness come from and why do so many people have it? Is it from abuse, is it intense desire, is it a chemical difference from the norm?*
>
> —Franklin's Journal, Autumn 1996

He knew then that there was another way. We did, too. But it would take us a long time to figure it out.

CHAPTER 3

. . .

Beam Me Up, Scottie

The relation of fathers and sons is mysterious and terrifying. It has never been rational, nor will it ever be.

—Weston La Barre, American anthropologist[1]

A MONTH AFTER BEING ADMITTED to Cambridge Hospital, Frank felt he was "becoming part of the walls" on the unit, and anxious to get the hell out of there. That would happen, I would think in retrospect, to any "normal person" who perhaps had a nervous break-down and was given antipsychotics and locked up for a month. His discharge summary, however, reflects concerns from neurophysiologi-cal testing that could indicate "an acute deterioration in his cogni-tive functioning, consistent with symptoms associated with the onset of schizophrenia."

Frank returns to our family's home in Roxbury on Fort Hill, from where he is to attend an adolescent day program. But the medications he's on are clearly taking a toll. It's hard for him to wake up even after fourteen hours of sleep. This can be terribly frustrating, both for him and for Etta and me. One night he storms away from the dinner table up to his room on the third floor and I follow him. I tell him I can't tolerate this kind of behavior, but nothing I say can penetrate my son's sullen distance. Then I notice that, on the radio beside his bed, a talk show is discussing parent-and-child psychiatry. And I decide to "join" the discussion. I'm talking fast, responding to the questions posed by the host, doing a voice-over on the guest. This goes on for perhaps a minute before Franklin, wide-eyed and breathless, interrupts to ask: "Dad, what's happening?!"

"I'm talking to the radio! I'm getting messages from the radio!" I exclaim.

I continue my rapid-fire monologue while gesturing wildly with my arms and imagining my eyes must be glazed over. I have no idea how Franklin will react. But after a timeless passing of what must be several more minutes, he gets up from his bed, comes to stand beside me, and puts an arm around my shoulder.

"Everything's going to be all right," Frank assures me. The next morning, I overhear him telling Etta: "Mom, Dad went crazy on me last night."

Years later, I would come across *The Fifty-Minute Hour*, a 1955 book by psychotherapist Dr. Robert Lindner, describing how he had decided "in a sudden flash of inspiration" to try and pry a patient loose from his psychosis by entering the fantasy with him. The evidence he offered "of total acceptance—even of conspiracy—had, for the first time, made him question it," Lindner wrote. The doctor's participation served another purpose as well: ". . . when the therapist engages in the same behavior as the patient—and expresses the same ideas in the same language—the patient's own image and activities are projected before him as on a screen. He is thus, in one bold maneuver, thrust to the side of reality, forced to take up a critical position vis-à-vis what he observes, i.e., his own behavior, and compelled to adopt an attitude."[2]

• • •

A woman in charge of the day program says of Franklin: "He presents a very grounded piece mixed up with all the distortion, paranoia, tangential intrusive thinking. There is a continuous struggle between those two factions inside his head." Re-reading these notes as I write, I wonder if that "continuous struggle between those two factions"— never settling on either side—was what, with guidance, my son was *supposed* to be listening to.

Etta and I meet with the headmistress at Commonwealth School. She doesn't see any way he could possibly return. The school is simply too stressful academically and he would be too far behind to catch up. It's a painful meeting, but realistically I know she is right. We're told there are high schools in the area that specialize in teenagers with difficulties like Frank's.

One of these is Beacon High in nearby Brookline, a small "alternative" private school with about 45 students and a good arts program. They have no openings, but Frank goes through the preliminary testing anyway and does well. And sure enough, when a girl drops out, he gets accepted in mid-February 1997, shortly after turning eighteen.

> *I want to make it for my sake. I want to be strong and awake. I want to teach love not hate, learn not to frustrate.*
>
> —Franklin's Journal

I, too, am keeping a regular journal, in hopes of making more sense of what's happening to Frank. He's started weekly therapy sessions with Dr. L., the adolescent specialist who'd been so helpful getting him admitted to the hospital. The doctor tells me: "Frank said he had been doing some self-testing, thinking one thing and saying something else to the kids at school. This is a way of finding his boundaries"—seeing how others would react to him.

Alice has been a huge help, too. We've now been living together for almost two years, and eventually will get married. When in her early twenties, she had been hospitalized for "manic depression" (today called bipolar disorder). Alice still takes medication, and she well understands what Franklin is going through.

After the school year ends, Frank spends the summer on our family's farm in Kansas, where the outdoor environment seems to help. A friend writes me that, while he's "still struggling with paranoid thoughts and is very vulnerable," he's also beginning to accept his condition as an illness with no quick cure.

Back in Boston that fall, when Franklin stays occupied, his bouts with paranoid thoughts become fewer and farther between. He's starting to fit well into school and singing in the choir of a local church's youth group. But he's put on considerable weight, about forty pounds, over the past six months. It will be a few years before I realize this is likely due to a newly prescribed antipsychotic medication called olanzapine, sold under the brand name of Zyprexa. Soon after entering the twelfth grade in December, Frank starts experiencing rapid mood swings and must spend a week at McLean's Hospital, where he "explained that he feels different from others his age, feels he can't think of things to say fast enough, and has no real 'crowd' or close friends to spend time with." Returning home, disjointed thoughts continue to plague him. "He seizes on little things and magnifies them," I write in my diary.

Sometimes I accompany him to his therapy with Dr. L. On the way to one appointment, Frank asks: "Am I my brother's keeper?" I'm carrying a book by John Edgar Wideman titled *Brothers and Keepers*, and presume that's why he raised the question. Now, during the session with Dr. L., Frank brings up the same question: "Am I my brother's keeper?" He says that he'd not seen the title of the book until after he first mentioned this, and so the sequence made him paranoid. I suggest that maybe he tunes into things in mysterious ways. Dr. L. counters that my son probably glimpsed the book earlier but wasn't conscious of it. I wonder to myself which of these realities is true. I'd be wondering for a long time.

> *As soon as he realized he was bound to earth, he realized that he was an alien from another planet. He was thrown into earth to teach lessons of a godly nature.*
>
> —Franklin's Journal

So many conundrums to wrestle with. . . . One day dropping him off at school, he says he wants to go back to the hospital. I end up giving him a slap on the arm and telling him to wake up. And that seems to shift Franklin's negativity. When this comes up during an intense mutual therapy hour, Dr. L. terms it a "complicated moment" and asks what had changed how Frank felt. "When he hit me," Frank says, because this had shown him I was concerned. The doctor asks Frank to demonstrate on a chair how hard the "hit" had been. He taps the armrest. Dr. L. glares at me and says I should never do that again. Frank looks at me and shrugs, as if to say, "Well, I tried, Dad." Such a response might bring short-term gain, the doctor says, but in the long run could cause greater difficulties, with Franklin projecting his anger toward me onto others and increasing the paranoia factor. Instead, I should examine my own fears and express *that* to him. All this is making him very depressed, my son responds. Dr. L. fires back that he's sure it is, but this is something important to discuss.

Earlier in the session, Frank had mentioned: "I just thought of, 'White is right.'" The next day, his mother's birthday, he's in an "angry mood" and wants to talk. "I hate you," he tells me, "because you're white." Later, he hates me because my name is Dick. This makes me laugh. "Give me something real to hate me about," I say. I end up telling him that our conversation is boring, and now he can hate me legitimately.

Is my son saying things simply to get my goat? Or am I ignoring what may be the painful truth in what he expresses? Is any of this getting us anywhere? I have no idea. And part of me is glad to escape. My work often requires research trips—sometimes lengthy ones—and I have not only close family but beautiful places to write in both LA and Baja. Over the years, in addition to living with his mother, Franklin has often been left in the care of others. Our support system is not perfect by any means, but my family knows him well and about what he's been going through lately. While most of the second generation of children are now living on their own, they remain concerned about Franklin's welfare and look out for him.

At a therapy session where we talk about my leaving Boston for a month or so, Frank tells Dr. L. that he's somewhat upset about this. When the doctor asks him why, my son says it's because I make him feel "safe." This is a good sign, the doctor thinks, in terms of our father-son relationship.

While I'm away, Etta accompanies Frank to the therapy sessions and, when I return to Boston, he greets me at the airport in good spirits. A school report notes his "ability to work with classmates and staff. He is considerate and respectful. He offers support to his peers and they in turn like to work with him in classes."

Hating the ongoing weight gain and excessive fatigue, Frank convinces Dr. L. to let him try acupuncture and wean off two of the antipsychotic medications over a six-week "experiment." The acupuncture sessions are quite intense and ultimately frustrating, because they don't really change anything. He becomes increasingly unstable and relates to me a dream where he has yin and yang symbols tattooed on his back that are affected by a terribly painful sunburn. Frank has long daydreamed about learning to fly and, on his own, goes to see an Air Force recruiter, but is told they won't take him as long as he's on medication and seeing a psychiatrist. He then continues by subway to his next appointment with Dr. L. By early June, he's a mess and agrees to go back on Zyprexa. Dr. L. seeks to comfort Frank, saying how much he respects his attempt to make it without the meds but also being willing to acknowledge that he needs to be on them at this time instead of waiting to be in real trouble as many others do.

My book, *Black Genius*, had been published earlier in the year, and Frank at that time had been a prince at a book party at my editor's apartment. There he and novelist Albert Murray struck up a long conversation, where Murray spoke about how mutual respect and grace are all that keep us from the abyss or, as he termed it, "the blue devils." Now, as Frank returns to the medication regimen, I decide to bring him along to a luncheon event I've been invited to with New York Mayor David Dinkins at the city's National Arts Club. Here, Frank can't handle the crowds. He's having a terrible time. He goes outside for some air. A street musician approaches, asking Frank quietly whether anything's wrong. They sing "Amazing Grace" and other spirituals together. This seems to calm him until I break free.

After I manage to reach Dr. L., we race uptown in a taxi to pick up an emergency prescription. It's been a nightmare. Full of fear-based projections as to what my son was capable of, I realize I don't have as many options as I'd thought. I'd imagined that if I took him out into the world—to dinner or an event—he'd feel better. But the truth was, that's what made *me* feel better. My first line of defense was to try to "fix" things with a good time. What Frank really wanted from me was something else, something internal—attention, care, real love.

Spring brings greater stabilization. Frank has a girlfriend at Beacon High and they have a wonderful time together at the prom. Then comes graduation. The evening ceremony is held in a large auditorium next to the school. I start to cry during the playing of "Pomp and Circumstance," as Frank and nineteen of his classmates walk in wearing their cap-and-gowns. My son receives the school's "Perseverance Award," and a book about Leonardo da Vinci as a gift. At the reception afterward, all the teachers are so proud of Frank.

> Racism is the darkness of the
> mind, the absence of color, a big
> misunderstanding that is unnecessary
> From the soul gives birth to a man
> One is not whole with his ideals
> Unsteady like the sifting sands
> We are made in all colors all shapes
> and sizes, sure as the sun rises and
> sets. The creator is love and love

includes all, together we stand,
divided we fall.

                    —An untitled poem he wrote for the yearbook

That summer, while Frank is working part-time at an auto repair
shop, he takes me aside one evening at home for a talk. Frank says he
doesn't want to hurt me, but brings up my guilt over not being with
him more when he was young and trying to make up for it now.

"You might be right," I say.

"Well, I want to move out on my own," my son informs me.

At first, I'm stunned by his announcement. I stifle my fears, as well
as my tears. "Why?" I ask finally.

"It's something I need to do, now that I've graduated. I've been
thinking about it for a while. I'm old enough, Dad."

I take a deep breath. I wonder, of course, about the periodic separa-
tions between us over the years. While this surely made Frank's life more
unsettled, in the long run might it prove better, allowing him more able
to stand on his own? There is no way to know, but perhaps, in time. . . .

"Do you want me to help you find a place?" I ask him, trying to
hide the quaver in my voice.

"Yes, I would," he says.

With reluctance, Etta is also willing to let him try this.

*I've had my share of emotional devils. Difficult as they are they teach me the
ups and downs of life. Now I am at a halfway house in Cambridge. I have met
most of the 15 or so other people I am living with. They are nice people. I am
opening a new chapter in my life, a chapter of creativity. I want to create a life for
myself that I am satisfied with.*

                    —Franklin's Journal, mid-July 1998,
                    almost two years since his breakdown

The Wellmet Project is a private group home with twelve other
people living there, not including the counselors who work and keep
track of their medications. Franklin will be the youngest resident. The
cost is eight hundred dollars a month, most of which will be covered
by federal SSI disability benefits that, because of his condition, he's
recently been granted. Wellmet is in a large house behind Cambridge
Hospital. Everyone must be out during the day, either working, going
to school, or in a day program. Assigned household chores, Frank must
make one dinner a week.

Only a month later, to my surprise, Etta decides to leave our Boston residence and also move out on her own. I try to talk her out of it and, upon hearing of his mother's plans, Franklin calls them "weird" and initially blames himself. But after a visit to where she's moved, into a friend's sister's home about a mile away from Fort Hill, he seems okay with it. Years later, Etta would write me about her decision: "It was a move of total desperation, one decided in a split second; a split second that was the culmination of many events that forced me to see that I no longer was living a valid life. I could no longer bear to not know, understand, and follow my own mind . . . without continuous input from other people. Franklin's illness and my own feelings of inadequacy in trying to help him propelled the urgency to get my life together. When Franklin was gone, there was nothing to keep me there. I never intended to leave permanently. But after meeting Kamal, I realized that I would not be coming back."

Kenneth Kamal Scott happens to be temporarily staying in an upstairs room of the house where Etta moved. He is a singer, dancer, and actor who'd performed at Harlem's legendary Apollo Theater at age eleven, gone on to the Alvin Ailey company, and rose to star in *The Wiz* on Broadway for four years in the late 1970s. I know him slightly, having interviewed him for my book *Black Genius* about his teacher, Elma Lewis. There is an instant connection between Etta and Kamal. Before long, they would be living together. Kamal would give her voice lessons, they would perform together, and eventually they would get married.

• • •

A fellow living at the Wellmet house gives Franklin driving lessons in his car, which eventually will result in Frank's passing the test to get his license. That's a huge step for him, something he really wanted and pursued. But at the same time, he's having difficulty getting up and out of the house. Before long he gets suspended from Wellmet for failing to follow this rule and comes home for twenty-four hours.

Frank has been even more sedated after agreeing to add a medication called Clozaril, as suggested by Dr. L. awhile back. (The standard procedure, when changing medications, is to simultaneously lower one while slowly increasing the dosage of the other, which avoids going through "withdrawal.") Introduced in the United States in 1990, Clozaril is the only antipsychotic proven effective with treatment-resistant schizophrenia, which is what Dr. L. concluded was the case with Frank. Clozaril is also considered a "last resort" medication, because in a small number of patients (less than 1 percent), it decreases the number of white blood cells—triggering an immune deficiency called agranulocytosis, which can prove fatal. Franklin now needs to have his blood monitored on a weekly basis while on Clozaril.

The days remain difficult. Frank pedals his bicycle for three miles seeking a job as a courier, only to find their office has suddenly moved. And he gets in more hot water for not following house regulations at Wellmet, and is given a month's notice. The program director calls my son a "poor soul" over the phone, and I hate the guy. Then they suspend him for three days for walking around "indecently" in his bathrobe and underwear. Will I have to bring him home? Should I? If Frank is always given an out, will he ever learn about rules in life? But it's agonizing to let him face such consequences, because other choices are so limited. After considerable discussion over what to do, for better or for worse I place a call to the Pine Street Inn. This is a nearby homeless shelter. Any first-timer, I'm told, could simply check in there. Perhaps, just for a night or two. . . .

> Pine Street Inn. It was all guys. . . . There was a man with a severed leg. I wondered if all of his pants legs were sewed up like that. . . . His eyes were oblong but sad and red. There was another man with distinct lines on his forehead. He was a fiery fellow with wrilly eyebrows, a black man with Indian origin. . . . One man broke [open] a package of coffee cakes, and then another one, and we all shared them. The people there ranged from hillbilly longhaired people to short shaved people. There were rustic ones that had almost certainly urinated on themselves, adding to the stench in the building.
>
> There was a lady who helped me to find my bed both nights that I stayed there. . . . She was very kind. On the fourth floor I stayed the first night. There I met Jason and we talked about god and our travels. I said that god comes through spirit, like in dance or singing or enlightened acts. . . . He was twenty-five—we are all in the same boat, as one old man had said in the shower area. I believed him and know now that I could never be that Noah that I believed I could be at age eighteen . . .
>
> —Franklin's Journal

In his verbal description afterward, Frank calls Pine Street Inn "a place full of drunks and people yelling racial insults while about a hundred men slept in adjacent beds in the same big room." At any rate, his "homeless experience" actually seems to leave him in better shape than before. He comes over to the house and makes me a quesadilla lunch, asks if I'll do dishes with him, and volunteers to wash windows. He returns to Wellmet, and begins going regularly to a nearby day program. But by early in the new year, he's being "terminated for failure to meet the program requirements." Wellmet has someone coming soon to take his bed.

I learn about another place called Eikos, a word which means "probable" in ancient Greek; as in "to be expected with some degree of certainty." At a big house out in Newton, Frank meets Eikos's program supervisor, a woman named Holly, and introduces me by saying, "This is my son." She laughs. The director, Dr. B., enters and extends a hand. Frank informs him that the strong handshake crushed his ring. The doctor is unfazed, describing how he'd set up Eikos thirty years ago because he had so many patients who were in and out of hospitals with no place to live and learn to be more independent. Surrounded by Buddhist-type tapestries, Dr. B. asks many questions. Where has he lived? "Everywhere, I'm rather nomadic," Frank says. He describes the various homes that our family has. Throughout the meeting he's articulate and charming, untroubled by the doctor's long silences, which I realize are probably designed to see how Frank will handle such. At the end, Dr. B. says there's an opening in a group home with nine people—including five males in their twenties—a five-minute walk from the main house where he'd go every morning to take his meds. He'd have two counselors and day treatment on the premises. Frank could stay for a thousand dollars a month, but would need to bring his own furnishings. Eikos's facility (unlike Wellmet's) is licensed by the Massachusetts Department of Mental Health (DMH).

Afterward, Frank says to Holly, "That doctor, what's his name—Kevorkian?" and she cracks up laughing once again. Another staffer walks us down the street to a nice old triple-decker where Frank is to have his own room on the second floor among mostly women. He says he feels like he'll be all right here for awhile.

We go together to his weekly appointment with Dr. L., who asks Frank how much of these preparations he's been doing on his own.

"Well, not that much," he responds. The doctor asks Frank to guess how many hours I'd put in on his housing situation during the week. He guesses three, Dr. L. estimates eleven, and I say it's more like twenty, which surprises my son. Dr. L. is tough on me about this; he wants to establish that Dad is no longer the authority figure in the relationship and the importance of Frank standing on his own. "I've got the reins," Frank says.

On his twentieth birthday at the end of January 1999, my son moves into a sunny, spacious room at Eikos with some furniture from home. With Etta, we go to Legal Seafoods to celebrate. I tell Frank and Etta that I've written a strong letter to Wellmet's director complaining about his treatment, and sent copies to state health officials. Frank responds that he doesn't really want me to stick it to the people at Wellmet.

> I hate them, I love them. I live away from them yet I come to see them. They love me but they pressure me. This pisses me off. I can't always express the truth about being pissed off at them or at others in the world. Then it becomes an alien wad of green goo stuck in my sub-conscious. When I scream it out or more often let it be known that I hate something, I am much happier. . . . My mother is a beautiful person but she is tough. My father has an easy streak. Well so does my mother. Within the last few years, although they have gained a few grey hairs they have generally remained young in looks and at heart. My mother gets confused easily—that is if I try to confuse her. I know exactly how to get her goat. My dad is articulate but his not knowing me very well in my early life upset me because I grew up without knowing some essentials of life. Well maybe I was just supposed to grow up on my own.
> —Franklin's Journal, with a section headed *Parents*

• • •

> *I met this woman on the way back from the phlebotomy lab. She was middle aged and cute for her age. We talked briefly about how cool it would be to be in Star Trek. "Beam me up Scottie," I said.*
>
> —Franklin's Journal

It seems that Eikos is much more on top of ensuring that he takes his meds regularly than they were at Wellmet. Frank has landed a part-time job at a Valvoline Jiffy-Lube doing oil changes on cars; they tell him to bring some old clothes. But Etta calls to let me know that he'd had a hard night after his first day in training, during which some fellow who'd been a "gang-banger" told Frank that *he* was one, too. This made Frank paranoid—and he'd decided it was the medications causing his problems.

I meet Frank at Dr. L's office. He immediately brings up that he wants to go off the meds; they are robbing him of his energy. He wants to travel or go to school or get his own place. "I've been listening to everybody's advice forever. I feel like I'm being used." I leave the room for awhile, angry and distraught and not knowing what I could possibly say to affect him. When I return at the end of the session, Frank informs me that he's stopping the medications starting tonight. The doctor explains that he'd told Frank he thought this was a bad idea and he might end up being hospitalized, but that he would nonetheless respect his decision to go cold turkey. With trepidation, I agree that my son shouldn't be forced against his will. When I'm briefly alone with Dr. L., he indicates that while this goes against his professional judgment, he doesn't see any way to overcome Frank's adamancy. The doctor tells me that classically another breakdown would recur somewhere between five and twenty-one days, but there's a "small chance" this won't happen. In the car, Frank tries to reassure me, saying: "This will be good, Dad."

The staff at Eikos are taken aback by the decision, but say that perhaps this is to be expected and that he's in good hands and they'll keep an eye on him. Etta has had long talks with Kamal, whose son had been faced with similar problems—but as Christian Scientists, they'd never put the boy on medication, and he'd turned out all right. In hindsight, as far as Frank is concerned, we agree that this was a big mistake. You can't go off any strong medication suddenly. He was already ungrounded, and there was no place to land.

A few days go by. Frank calls me at 11 o'clock at night and I ask how he's doing. "Oh dad, I had a really hard day, I got so paranoid!" Then he laughs at his joke on me. He's coherent, but clearly moving very fast, telling me all about a TV show on vampire bats and being back into astrology—his fire signs balancing out his "airhead tendencies"—playing some keyboard, planning to write, putting in more hours at Valvoline. I'm on tenterhooks afterward, trying vainly to get some sleep.

As I toss and turn, I consider that you can't preserve a young man's honor by denying his right to choose. I also think about how the medication can be a godsend, but also—certainly the way Franklin sees it—a soul-destroyer: the weight gain, the fuzziness and fogginess.

At his next therapy session, Dr. L. says to him, "It feels good to have your mind back, doesn't it?"

• • •

It is another snowy winter night in Boston. The earth and the cars are white with the soft snow that covers them. I left dinner feeling frustrated. This feeling is an aftershock of going off medications. Yet I felt worse while I was on medications. I am trying to go off of them for good and prove that I can. I work now and this is very stressful . . . I feel really fucking paranoid, angry, resentful at the world . . . I think that since I am getting down that the whole world is getting down. Today I was manic, I let myself go and I went downhill . . . I am writing so that I will feel better . . . I have a strong spirit and I hope that I am strong enough to go off my meds and not self destruct. I don't know what the date is or what is up or down whether one arm is longer than the other whether I will have to lose an eye to see things clearly whether I will have to jump in the train tracks.

I am falling in love again. . . . Why are there so many lovely ladies in Eikos . . . I am easy going and say hello to everyone. Am I too easy going? That's probably what makes me so vulnerable. Time will tell! I do value life but sometimes I am too unbalanced. Hopefully I have written some valuable information after having just gone off meds. I hope I have a good day tomorrow. Trust the world and goodness and have faith. Have good judgment. Work hard at Valvoline, be friendly but don't get out of control. My angry feeling hasn't left even though I just wrote two fucking pages . . .

Did god create language? Who exactly is god? Is he the Zeus of the Greek myths or Neptune, god of the seas. . . . So I take a minute, let myself lose track, and let myself feel, and try not to classify. For who am I to classify. But I look at her, and I see a spark of hope, that's not all obscured by smoking dope. Then she's on the brink of insecurity, unsure of me, my motives. Really she's losing hope and wondering if I can understand how she lives. Yes in chaos and the party life, of youth, and of no worries, of love? oh no that is negated, for the sex and for the mind elated, for escape into a netherland, without a plan but with a man, where she's listening to her new tapes, and the man beside her contemplates a rape, or better yet he just wants sex, but he knows the girl won't let him touch her beautiful chest. So this is just a story wrought in confusion, from a mind momentarily miles away from consistency, but just noticing some lack of love in this so called reality.

—Franklin's Journal

For awhile I've been amazed at how well he's doing. Then one afternoon, Frank calls to say he had to leave his job. He was fine until he started scrubbing the floors but then became angry, paranoid, his eyes rolling back in his head. Would I contact Valvoline and plead his case? I do and ask the assistant manager to be tolerant because my son has gone off his medication; he says they will. But by his next session with Dr. L., Frank has dropped work altogether. Then the following week, he is very manic. The doctor asks if he'd be willing to go back on a mood stabilizer. After an hour of talking, he still refuses. So, reluctantly, he instead gives Frank an anti-anxiety drug to help him sleep (he says he's only getting a couple hours a night). Frank is rapping out poems on the way out the door, exclaiming "Next Friday's 21 days!"— a reference to the "deadline date" for breakdowns to typically recur.

I have to leave town on work and can do with a rest. Dr. L. is reportedly amazed to see how well Frank is doing after a month off the meds. Etta writes that he is "learning more how to simply balance his moods . . . learning to check himself and know better how to handle difficult situations. . . . He's been busy busy . . . writing, talking with everybody playing his keyboard and drum . . . making friends." And he would begin training at a Stop & Shop to work there thirty hours a week.

When I return to Boston, it's late at night and Frank is waiting for me at the house, peeking out the window. He looks great, has lost about twenty-five pounds, and his face is much clearer. I drive him back to Eikos around one in the morning as he talks all the way about girls and particularly a twenty-six-year-old Iranian counselor that he's crazy about. Later I pick him up at Eikos and we go to a nearby Thai restaurant, where Frank beckons some younger kids who are selling walk-for-hunger donations to join us inside. "Gathering his flock," Alice says. Dr. L. is struck by how little paranoia exists.

The professionals call this a "flight into health." It seems too good to be true . . . and it is.

Early in April, two months since his decision to stop taking medication, Franklin shows up at my house a little before 11 p.m. I find him downstairs eating some food. He tells me rather flippantly that he's been fired already from Stop & Shop for being rude to someone. He becomes quite hostile, saying he'd been getting a raw deal all his life while I'd had it easy growing up in a "white world." This raises my ire, but I say nothing. He refuses to reveal more about what happened at work and he's just come over "to get some more money." I hit the roof.

"I just gave you thirty dollars a few days ago, where did *that* go?" It was the last of his monthly money from SSI disability, having just paid Eikos the rent. He says he's leaving Eikos, and that he's sick of the white world. It feels like he's writing me off for good, and I immediately see red. "Then get out of my house," I tell him. And he does.

He goes to his mother's house not far away bad-mouthing me and seeking train fare to head south, which was not forthcoming. He's having ringing in his ears, a sign that a major crash is coming, according to Dr. L.

I call Eikos. The day before, after the counselor who Frank is crazy about told him she has a boyfriend, he'd apparently told her he was going to kill her and himself. Dr. B. had come in to talk to him. He says he doesn't feel Frank needs to be hospitalized, that he's very lucid and aware of what's happening. Boundaries have been discussed with the counselor. Frank says he understands and doesn't want her to feel uncomfortable.

A week passes before I call Frank and say I'll pick him up and drive him to his appointment with Dr. L. "I don't want to see him anymore," he responds. By late morning he's spoken to the doctor, who convinces Franklin to come, given their long history together. The doctor wants the parents there, too, so I pick Etta up on the way. When we get to the office, Dr. L. and Franklin have already been talking for awhile. Frank glances icily at me in the doorway, not even saying hello. Since there is clearly some strain between us, the doctor asks Etta to "take the lead" in talking with him about how we see things. Frank holds her hand briefly. His mother speaks for a little while until Frank interrupts to say he wants to be with "his people." Dr. L. suggests that "his people" are right here in the room, but he doesn't want to hear that. I say nothing, just let it hurt. Who knows what he is talking about or what world he's living in.

Etta finally says she feels he should go back on a mood stabilizer. If that's what she thinks, he's out of here, my son says. Dr. L. then states flatly that he thinks Frank should be placed back in the hospital. My son starts flipping him the finger over and over, then leaps to his feet and bolts out of the room, slamming the door behind him. The doctor goes for the phone. He calls the police and then the EMTs. He asks me to try to get my son back. I take the elevator down to the street, but it's endlessly slow. When I finally get outside, I can't see Frank anywhere on the street. Defeated and heartsick, I return to the elevator.

And as I walk in, he's already there! He's pushed the button for the fifth floor, preparing to go back up.

My heart pounding, I step in and say nothing. When we emerge at the doctor's office, Frank says, "I'm really in your way, aren't I, Dad?" No, Franklin, you're not in my way, that's not the point. He says he just has to go to the bathroom and then he's leaving. In the hallway, Dr. L. emerges with Etta to join us.

Suddenly two cops appear in the outer doorway, along with three EMTs.

"So you're coming to take me away?" Frank says.

"We heard you'd threatened suicide," one of them says.

"I didn't say that! I said I was leaving! You're my father, you'd better defend me!"

"He's right," I tell them. "He didn't threaten suicide."

The question is whether he would accompany the EMT team voluntarily or be forced by the cops. But the EMT men tell us that, once on the street, they can't legally stop him if he runs. Frank says he'll go to the hospital if his mom accompanies him. Standing beside the doctor, I watch them all return to the elevator.

Dr. L. is clearly shaken, too. "Are you all right?" he asks as we sit down again in his office. Though I am shattered, I simply say, "Yes, this was not unexpected." When I raise the question of why my son is so into race again—that I'd thought we'd worked all that out long ago—Dr. L. replies that race is Frank's "fault line." Once he "decompensated" (an increase of symptoms), the break comes along the fault line where his identity questions exist. The doctor adds sadly that he wished that, after all this time, there existed more of a connection between himself and my son. But then again, Franklin *did* agree to come see him and *did* return after running off.

Somehow, despite feeling betrayed, abandoned, and utterly alone, Frank knew that he needed help.

I drive to a hospital emergency room and sit with Etta. Eventually a psychiatrist emerges with some questions and to say there's no need for us to stick around; our son will be moved to another hospital nearby and that this process would take some time, and that they'd let us know.

Notes:

1. Weston La Barre on fatherhood: Ronald Schenk, *Dark Light: The Appearance of Death in Everyday Life,* State University of New York Press, 2001, p. 71.
2. *The 50-Minute Hour:* See "The Jet-Propelled Couch, Part II: Return to Earth," by Robert Mitchell Lindner, *Harper's Magazine*, January 1955, available online at http://harpers.org/archive/1955.

CHAPTER 4

Between Scylla and Charybdis

Sitting thinking of pyramids . . . as the sun sets and sinks into the abyss of the pure blue clouds. Rats scurry down below in the crusty cities and obsolete humans roam about aimlessly believing they own the earth. . . . A boat bobs in the water, Noah's ark of the 21st century. In his boat there is no more AIDS, Cancer, etc. . . . Round saucers fly through the air. Alien life forms free from earthly hindrance. . . . Let's burn the money and make history! You could call this—thoughts and dreams manifested on paper.

Part of a dream—and a paranoid one at that! The python tightens his grip around the young man's neck. This is not a safe place thinks the young man. He struggles and struggles to break free. The beast won't let go.

—Franklin's Journal

BETWEEN A ROCK AND A hard place, the devil and the deep blue sea, Scylla and Charybdis. Those were the mythical sea monsters first described in Homer's *Odyssey*, residing in such proximity that choosing which one to pass by was an insoluble dilemma. There was really no "right way" to set a ship's course. I can think of no better analogy to describe what I went through over (and with) my son throughout much of his twenties. It was all Scylla and Charybdis.

Mid-April 1999, another hospital. . . . Franklin tries to throw a chair at someone and has to be put in restraints. Not having to tenuously keep everything together any longer, Dr. L. says he's just letting it rip. I write in a letter to my son (which I decide not to send):

Right now, there's no way I can help you out of your situation being in that hospital. When Dr. L. called the cops to have you put there, my feeling is that he did it in what he believed was your best interest. This may sound like bullshit to you but I'm saying he felt like if he DIDN'T do that, you were going to end up in some real trouble. He didn't see any other choice. As angry as that has made you, that's the reality from HIS end. And to tell you the honest truth, I don't think he was wrong.

Given that his was considered an emergency hospitalization, they can only keep Franklin for ten days without a court order. Since he's still refusing medication as the deadline approaches, the hospital files to have him committed. A judicial hearing is scheduled on the unit where I see Frank briefly beforehand. I feel like he hates me. He wants only his mother, and Kamal—someone whom Frank felt listened to him—in the hearing room. I wait outside in case I'm needed. The proceeding goes on for more than an hour. The psychiatrists testifying, Etta and Kamal tell me afterward, treated Frank like a "thing." They're enraged. The judge ends up committing him for up to six weeks, forced by the court order to go back on the original antipsychotic (Risperdal) that he'd been prescribed when hospitalized after his first breakdown. Franklin tells your honor that he'll cooperate. In my home office afterward, I break down in tears.

Two days later, I visit him for about fifteen minutes. The hostility is gone. We hug hello and good-bye. A hospital social worker tells me of an "incident"—a bipolar girl with a crush on Frank walked into his room and jumped on top of him. They had their clothes on, I'm told, and were quickly separated. My son starts making 911 calls alleging that the hospital is holding him hostage. In the next day's meeting, with his mother and me, Frank ends it with a series of fuck-yous. I move all his things from Eikos into my basement.

Time passes. He stabilizes, as they say. Toward the end of May, after being hospitalized this time for almost two months, Frank writes retrospectively in his journal:

> The environment was so difficult, they did not let me out for fresh air for a whole month. . . . On the third day I was restrained and then the worst came. I was placed on a room program and for fifteen days. My eyes were dry, my nose stuffed up and they would not treat my cough that was steady as the rain. At one point I wondered if I

would ever talk again. At other times I could barely think and then I said, "all I *see* is darkness in the shadows." My fear of committing a crime began to override everything in my mind. I don't have forever to live and I've barely gotten started. My parents weren't there to help and I felt that god had deserted me and my brain was beginning to desert my body. I had never had an experience so horrible in my life and through it all I began to see through the lies of the mental health system.

Prescribed a mood stabilizer as well as the antipsychotic, Frank is released into a state-run group home in Mattapan, where a contingent of primarily black counselors and male residents think they can help him. Sadness overwhelms me sitting with him in his new room at the home; I tell my son I love him and he's glad to hear it and I cry the entire two-mile drive back to Fort Hill. I'm going to have to leave soon for Alaska for two months of research toward a natural history book about the migration of the gray whales. After I see Frank for the last time, on a basketball court down the street from his new residence, I write: "I felt such a distance in his eyes, as if I no longer entered into his world."

Before I leave Boston, Etta and I go together to see Dr. L. He says that Frank's hands-off attitude toward me isn't necessarily personal, but rather my son's seeking his own identity. The doctor speaks of how much he respected Franklin's openness with him in trying to sort out those difficult questions, but admits how helpless and frustrated he himself felt. "I can only hope," he tells us, "that I planted some seeds that will one day bear fruit."

While I'm away, Frank splits from the group home on a bus with a backpack of personal belongings, bound for Etta's apartment. He makes it, but leaves the backpack behind. He moves in for awhile with his mother. One night after she makes a few simple demands upon him, an argument escalates and he impulsively calls the cops on Etta. When they show up, they realize the situation isn't at all like Franklin described. And he ends up being taken to a psych emergency ward.

By late August, when I return to Boston, Frank has been transferred to the Shattuck hospital. It bills itself as an "extended care facility" with 250-some inpatient beds, said to "deliver compassionate psychiatric care to patients requiring multi-disciplinary treatment." But as Etta remembers, "He really suffered there. Their assessment of a patient was whether someone was compliant in taking their medication and so keeping out of trouble. So it didn't matter if Franklin lay around all day and didn't change his clothes." That fall, Etta goes back to school at Harvard toward a master's degree in education. For several months, pretty much every time she attempts to visit, Frank refuses to see her, apparently blaming her for his situation. He will sometimes agree to see me, but I feel more hopeless than ever. And facing a book deadline, I feel I need to get away, and I leave that winter to write in Mexico.

At the end of January 2000, two friends who helped raise Frank take him to a Boston restaurant to celebrate his turning twenty-one. As he unwraps a necklace I've sent him from the Baja, he tells them: "I'm going to look like an Aztec king in this." One of them writes me: "And he made a stance, backbone straight as an arrow, chin pushed out, fiery look in his eyes—and that's what he looked like all right." He was, she added, "not talking crazy talk all the time, though he does every now and again get going about how he controls the weather; the wind that blows ferociously he can order up or tame. He tells me this on one of the most blustery, wind-howling-smashing days of all and I tell him, 'Okay, Franklin, do something about this wind. I don't mind the wintry snows at all, but the wind like this I despise!' 'Sure,' he says, 'I'll do it.' And who knows, maybe he did."

My friend continues: "In many respects he seems 'better' than ever. But he is so unmotivated in an ever-growing smaller and smaller existence. He's still full of all his many illusions about the things he wants to do eventually—but even those have lost their impact as the dreams. I do worry about him becoming forever one with this institutional life."

Franklin spends more than a year in the Shattuck hospital. He and I see each other only sporadically. Etta visits often, sometimes with Kamal, taking Frank out as much as she can (when he wants). Sometimes they have dinner at the hospital. "It was a terrible, terrible place, only a step above prison," she remembers. "I would beg Franklin to please be careful about what he said. One time he was just about to be discharged when he started talking about hurting himself. As awful as the place was, it was safe and secure, a place that he knew—so he sabotaged his own release on more than one occasion."

It's November 2000 before Frank is released and living in a supervised triple-decker about a mile from me in Jamaica Plain, alongside youth with similar problems. Etta and Kamal are now residing only a few blocks away and see him regularly. He's staying on his medication. He gets a Saturday job at Starbuck's (which doesn't last) and takes a pottery class (which he follows through on). He also works awhile in a grocery store a block from his mother's place.

During one phone call between us, Frank describes having landed a one-day job driving a truck. He'd barely been behind the wheel of a car, let alone a heavy hauler! I'm so nonplussed I can't even think to ask Frank what the cargo was. But he'd driven the truck for some eighty miles around the Boston area—lost for much of the day and exhausted by the time he turned in his keys at the end. But at least he did it . . . and survived!

Through it all, Frank is writing regularly again in a journal.

10/3/01: What is a tree if it is stripped bare. What am I if I seek not to comb my hair. . . .

You dreamed your father was Japanese and your great-grandfather was a Mongolian riding into the sunset on a horse he broke. I dreamed away the violence I dreamed away the thieves. They played with my emotions as they spread their seed. I dreamed I was a movie star but life's already a stage. So take the stage away from me and I'll still have the written page. I dreamed I stop all suffering, I did it in a rage. I dreamed that I was violent, I dreamed I was a sage . . .

So many trials, long laborious trials. Take a minute to examine yourself. . . . Are you hard inside, displaying no emotions? . . . Are you a void inside with nothing filling you but darkness? Are you at peace with yourself. Philosophies seek to answer these questions. Religions seek to comfort and guide us. Could you do it on your own? . . . Aggressiveness is not bad. Nor is suffering or anger. They are emotions and states of being just as Happiness and wholeness. We were made from the earth. The earth erupts, shakes, gets wet, dry. The earth expresses itself regardless. It has been here for billions of years. Why can't we coexist with all our feelings. Why can't we just express our selves. Why can't we just admit the faults in our lives and go on. Dead ends. Projects that take forever and that give me no sense of salvation, no sense of stability. So I spend time now just not paying attention to the hurt and pain. I just try to get by. If I don't succeed, I get back up and try again.

Trying again, Frank wants to enroll at Franklin Technical Institute in Boston's South End and study mechanical engineering. I know how difficult this kind of concentration will be for him, but he's determined, and I co-sign an application for financial aid. Frank writes in a letter to a friend in March 2002: "I will be done with school in a little over a year. This [first] semester I obtained an A in Intro to Calculus, a B- in Sociology, and a C+ in Statics (a type of Physics). I believe I have about five or six gray hairs already. . . . It's funny, when you are little, doing things is like pulling teeth. At twenty-three you are much more confident and patient. It's more like digging holes in a garden. You know the plants will grow. And if they don't there's always next year."

Frank continues, bringing up a theme that will play an increasing role in years to come. "I got a guide to speaking Arabic off the Internet. Since I know some numbers in Swahili, I can compare them . . . the languages have some cross references. . . . I write sometimes for fun and right now I am working on some canvases. I use oil paint. In particular, I am doing a picture from a book of cultures. It is of Mongolians on horses."

There was no way, at the time, to envision the higher significance of what Frank set down in that paragraph. Ten more years would pass before I introduced my son firsthand to Swahili-speaking culture. And longer still before I came upon a book called *The Horse Boy*, the true story of parents who take their severely autistic son to Mongolia for a healing encounter with a shaman, a book that would kindle a quest to do something similar.

By early that fall of 2002, Franklin has managed to complete thirty-one hours toward an associate's degree in mechanical engineering. With the help of a case worker who "thinks the world of Frank," through the Center for Independent Living, he's received a federal housing voucher (called a Section 8) that isn't easy to get without spending months on a waiting list. And, for the first time, he moves into his own apartment, in the Boston suburb of Somerville. Both the realtor and the owner are retired gentlemen who like Frank very much, and his monthly government benefit check will be enough to cover his rent.

However, between the two of us, it feels like things have grown progressively worse. "My relationship with Franklin sank to a nadir this summer," I write in my journal toward the end of September. "I didn't think there was anything I could do anymore, he really resented me and wanted to cut ties and hit the ceiling when I suggested he needed to be on more medication." Hoping that his newfound independence might make a difference, and deciding that the best thing I could do was leave him alone to try it, I head for LA to write.

In November, Etta contacts me. Frank has been arrested twice in one day, first for trying to take someone's motorcycle (the police let him go) and the second time after being found in his underwear trying to do some laundry at MIT. Charged with trespassing, he'd been taken to the Lindemann Mental Health Center, a state facility in downtown Boston.

Frank told the doctors that he'd stopped taking Clozaril a couple of weeks back. The reason? Even though he'd been right on time for an appointment to have his biweekly blood test, the pharmacy said the hospital hadn't yet sent over the results and so refused to give him his medication. In frustration, Frank had walked out—and not returned.

Before his arrest, Etta had sensed something was very wrong. She later writes me: "I searched everywhere for him that night—I was so afraid that he was in trouble. Never found him. Don't think it was meant to be. He had to do what he did. . . . This episode seems to be a desperate cry for help." When she visited him at the hospital, "he was happy to see me, very soft and very vulnerable and needing just to be loved. . . . He talked about the cops taking a print of his hand . . . and of being in a place with terrible vampire people and then being res-cued and brought to the hospital." Now the doctors had him "pretty doped up."

Years later, re-reading my son's writings from those last days before this happened, I would come across this passage:

> The zombies walked around the smoking gray grounds. Trees around them reversed their growing patterns and grew into the dark recesses of the earth. . . . Zombification is undesirable. It means that you exist after spirit and soul is stripped from you.

In the hospital, Etta writes, "Apparently, he became violent . . . throwing his bed out of the room . . . talking about hurting people. So, they have him on constant supervision. He has not been officially charged for anything, but they are evaluating him to see if he is com-petent to stand trial."

I don't hop on a plane and fly back right away. There seems noth-ing I can do for him right now. Besides, his mother is there . . . or so I told myself. Hearing that he only has hospital slippers, I order Franklin some sneakers from City Sports a few blocks from the hospital, and they are kind enough to personally deliver the shoes. As Etta writes, Frank "does seem to have a few guardian angels 'cause there sure are a lot of people looking out for him." His feelings and thoughts seem much closer to the surface, but at the same time he appears to have "let go of something . . . like he just doesn't care anymore."

His mother also writes me: "He is so unsure of how you really feel about him. . . . He is the one thing in your life that you absolutely cannot control, cannot make do what you want and absolutely do not understand. You humor his crazy whims, take him to dinner, buy him stuff and hope that he will be a grateful and loving son. BULLSHIT! You need to do some deep soul searching or you will never have your son's love. And even if we both do change or learn—the resolution may not come in yours or my life time."

Her words sting, and somewhere inside I know there is truth in them, but they also arouse resentment. At this juncture, she and I are clearly estranged as well.

• • •

"I went through an existentially profound moment with your son," the doctor tells me over the phone. She'd asked Frank if he realized why he was in the hospital. Was he mentally ill? Franklin said no. Then why did he feel he was there? She expected a rambling answer, but he simply said: "My chief complaint is loneliness. I am lonely." In that moment, as the doctor put it, he was "so sane."

He's been phoning Fort Hill, where he spent so much time growing up, at least twice a day. A friend there writes to describe how Frank said he was coming to pick up all my filing cabinets and dry them out. There were a couple dozen of these, filled with manila folders concerning the many topics I'd written about. Told that the basement storage area was actually pretty dry, Frank had sighed and said: "I am coming there and I am going to re-cement the basement floor." My friend goes on: "The strange thing is, the basement is getting water-proofed next week and he has no way of knowing that. So, as so often happens with him when he is way out there, he tunes in to the facts."

In our own earlier phone conversations, Franklin at several times mentioned the need to safeguard my vast archive—just as my files were about to be moved out of one basement into another. Another time, he'd raised the question about how I was using old files to rework new material—again, with no idea that I'd just gotten a contract to revise and trim my book about the Kennedy assassination for republication on the fortieth anniversary.

"Alice came to see me," he says, although she is also on the opposite coast.

"How could that be, Frank?" I ask him.

"In spirit," he says.

When Alice and I return to Boston over Christmas, and Frank comes to the house on a day pass from the hospital, there isn't a trace of paranoia. Yet as the new year begins, his delusional thinking escalates . . . or so it seems at the time. Only now am I able to interpret some things my son says in a different context, in a sense a premonitory one. He wants to go to school in Africa and alleges that I won't help him. He also desires to have a crafts-type store selling products from Africa. He asks if I might be an "undercover African." He's changed his name to Kwasi Mifune, or something similar. It will take another decade for the African context to unveil itself.

He tells his case worker that his birth certificate is a fake. He's Japanese and has renamed himself Kitu Sumukuan, which he says means "Come to seek my meek energy." When, on March 19, 2003, Frank is released from the Lindemann hospital and goes back to his apartment, he's decided I'm not his father after I refuse to pay for a plane ticket to China. At the same time, in what seems an encouraging connection to reality, he gives Etta the doctor's report on his health, which clearly states bipolar and schizophrenia, and asks that she keep it somewhere for him.

I'm back on the west coast when Franklin calls and informs me that he now has a genie named Caliph. The genie had come to him one night, when he was alone in the apartment, and offered to grant him three wishes. Frank doesn't want to tell me the outcome, but adds: "You're a genius—you need to be more famous. My genie said that, he makes all the headlines." My son assures me he is taking his medication.

Within days, I find a message from his case worker on my voice mail. Franklin has walked into another hospital and announced, "I'm 108 years old and my feet hurt."

Later, he will explain that he only went to the emergency room because he'd lost his apartment keys. But following an evaluation, he's been admitted to a different facility with an available bed, a small private hospital called the Arbour. I try calling him. "You're not my dad!" he exclaims and hangs up.

By the end of May, Alice and I are again back in Boston. My son still does want to talk to me. He asks if I'm learning languages such as Norwegian. He doesn't know—nor will I, until looking through ancestral records at my brother's home some years later—that my heritage turns out to be one-quarter Norwegian.

The Arbour isn't far from Fort Hill and, when Alice and I stop by in hopes of visiting him, Frank's very glad to see us. His hair is long and in the "rasta" style. He looks taller and thinner than the last time I saw him two months earlier. He shows us a couple of very good architectural-type drawings he's fashioned of ancient dwellings. Frank asks to stand back-to-back and measure our heights, and is pleased to now have a slight advantage. But he still won't acknowledge me as his father. He's decided that it's Eddie, who lives on Fort Hill and has been close to Frank all his life. Eddie and I were born a week apart. Originally from Samoa, he has a biracial son a few months older than Frank, and they'd grown up together.

The next time I visit him Frank speaks about a dream he'd had where a tiny fellow from Jupiter landed on his chest and worked on some physical problems in his body. "What's wrong with *you*, Dick?" my son queries. I ask him to tell me what he sees. He lists off arthritis (which my mother had suffered from), too much drinking, and not enough direction. The last two could be right on the mark.

Alice and I drive over to Franklin's apartment to meet with the landlord. He'd found the heat going full-blast inside and is worried that holding the space for my son isn't going to work out. He hands us a set of keys. The apartment is a holy mess, filled with diagrams posted on the walls like something out of the movie *A Beautiful Mind* and the floor covered with a variety of old engine parts that Frank had apparently gathered off the street. We clean up the place and fill three garbage bags with laundry and head back to our house, feeling quite depressed.

Several combinations of medications have been tried, according to Frank's hospital doctor, and none have resulted in more than a modest improvement. My son still won't take the Clozaril anymore, due to the required blood draws. *Is there any way around the FDA's regulations on that?* I wonder. I'm informed that the blood check requirement was rammed through on a congressional bill awhile back after a couple of people died from the rare side effect of a rapid loss of white blood cells. The only real solution? "Move to Europe," the doctor says with a shrug.

He wants to try a very short course of Electroconvulsive Therapy (ECT) to relieve Frank's acute symptoms. It used to be called "electroshock," and in my mind conjures terrible images from the 1975 movie, *One Flew Over the Cuckoo's Nest.* The doctor assures me that the procedure has come a long way since then, now lasting for only a few seconds while using anesthesia and a muscle relaxant. I make a number of calls about this, including one to Mark Vonnegut, author of *The Eden Express* (a fine memoir about his own experience with mental illness) now a pediatrician in nearby Milton. Mark is also the son of the famous novelist, Kurt Vonnegut Jr. Vonnegut says that ECT had indeed worked for him thirty years ago, "though I won't tell you how pissed off I was at my father for forcing me to do it."

Frank agrees to a trial of ECT, and comes through the first one fine, with maybe six to eight more treatments over the next couple of weeks. After another three sessions, he seems to be in a kind of Zen place . . . way slowed down. At one point when another patient is banging his fist against the wall and yelling "Fuck you!" Frank tells me not to worry: the fellow shouts a lot but is basically harmless. He informs me that he himself is "Gandhi reincarnated." He speaks of wanting to attend an art school in China. Later he will tell Etta that "the monks are calling" him to come to Tibet, and she writes me that his remark doesn't seem like a delusion. "Seeking spiritual fulfillment of some sort seems to be a big part of who he is. Perhaps his therapy will come from an atypical source." (Before coming to Fort Hill, Etta herself had lived in a Buddhist monastery for the better part of a year).

Frank says, toward the end of a visit, that "these shock treatments are working; I feel like I did when I was in high school [before the breakdown happened]. My mind has been deteriorating a long time." I tell him "I love you," as I leave the room. "Likewise," Frank says. It's been quite awhile since we exchanged that sentiment. Soon he's scheduled to be released back to his apartment and to attend a day treatment program.

I attend a pre-release meeting between the hospital and reps from the state Department of Mental Health (DMH). According to the doctor, Franklin's reluctance to take Clozaril is based on his "psychosis" that the blood being drawn is used in experiments, to father children, or by vampires. When Frank wants to know what's transpiring at the meeting, he's allowed to come down. This proves disastrous. Somehow, he believes I'm trying to "finagle a way" to keep him hospitalized. When he finally says "fuck you" to me, I walk out of the room. His outburst ends any chance of being let out in the near future.

Since the Arbour is only for acute care—and costs the insurance company more to keep someone there than an "intermediate care" facility—Frank is asked to sign papers permitting his transfer back to the Shattuck. But this comes amid aggressive hostility throughout the meeting because he is worried about losing his apartment. When Frank storms out of the room calling the social worker a "fat koala bear," the doctor can't stifle a laugh. "Sometimes I think Franklin is the sane one and we are all insane," he says.

On the morning of his transfer when the ambulance shows up, Frank simply gets out of bed, puts on his shoes, and hops onto the stretcher, seeming resigned and very sad. I bring a book of the Dalai Lama's sayings to give him at the Shattuck. Frank thanks me from his bed. He's on four frigging drugs. On the way home, driving near where two of his middle school friends had lived, I'm overwhelmed once again by sadness—so wanting my son to have a life, not knowing if he ever can.

Keeping pretty much to himself, he's restricted to the unit. He says his name is not Franklin Russell, but Mr. Lee (from China). However, rather than attend a court hearing, he signs his own name, authorizing a three-month voluntary commitment. The main hospital therapist, Dr. P., obtains Frank's permission to tell me a few things. Psychoses such as believing that Etta and I are not his parents are very hard to shake and not uncommon. Sometimes patients believe that one of the parents is a double. At least he acknowledges us when we visit. *Thank goodness for small favors.* I think to myself. Dr. P. suggests Etta and I see our son together, and is pleased to learn that he didn't deny his parentage during the visit. "This means that, at some level, he knows it's not true," the doctor says. (Several years later, Elyn Saks—herself diagnosed with schizophrenia, an expert in mental health law, and the author of

The Center Cannot Hold—will tell me that the delusion of being of other parents or nationalities is not unusual.)

When am I moving to Alabama? Frank asks when I next see him. With his assistants from China and Africa, he says, he's going to move all the white people in Boston down there. My son does a drawing for me of what our quarters would look like. What's curious is that this coincides with religious conservatives descending on Alabama to protect a granite Ten Commandments monument that a federal judge had ordered removed from the Capitol rotunda. Has he caught this on the TV news?

A suicide occurs on his unit. Someone had gotten keys to gain access to a window and jumped ten floors to their death. I'm told that, in a meeting with other patients about this, Frank "spoke in a non-psychotic way" about what had happened.

His mother and I take Frank on a pass for lunch and then to his apartment, where he's excited to gather up his CD player and some drawing books. "I'll grant you three wishes," he says to me. "I can read your thoughts, you know, I was doing that all the way in the car."

After a moment, I say: "Okay, I've made a wish, but you have to guess it."

"You want to be happy."

"You're right. That's what I was thinking."

• • •

By September 2003, four months into his latest hospitalization, Franklin has signed a consent form to receive a blood draw and start taking Clozaril again. For a time, he has no problem with staff telling him, "Your father is here." Back and forth we go. Next time: did I know I always made him feel inferior? Then a call on my office phone: "Dad?" I've been Dick Russell for almost six months. He's working on a cartoon with Etta, "I mean my mom." We have a wide-ranging talk. At one point he says, "You repeat the question, to turn it around and make it yours." I concede that his insight might well be true. He brings up his suspicions of the hospital and its vampiric element. "Karma must be fleshed out, expressed," he says. I respond that yes, once things are expressed they often don't seem so big. This impresses him. "After all, I *am* your son," he says.

Back and forth we go. Soon I'm no longer Dad, and then I am again. Many of his latest drawings, all about mathematical formulas and wiring and spaceships, remind me of the true story told in *A Beautiful Mind*. Frank says: "Sometimes here I feel I might die and not come back. I went through a black hole—to a different star every day. I become Spiderman, or whoever—to keep my imagination going."

What is so perplexing—and common among people diagnosed schizophrenic—is how Frank can engage in normal and "psychotic" thinking simultaneously, while seeming indifferent to the dichotomy.

The Shattuck plans to release him in a couple of weeks to return to his place in Somerville, which the owners continue to kindly hold for him. He's been taking his medications regularly. Then, one evening in early October, during a fire drill at the hospital, a nurse finds him in his room. Frank says he's been trying to hurt himself. He's made a small cut on his right wrist. He's used his apartment keys to do it.

The previous winter I'd gone to the Caribbean island of Antigua on a story assignment, and felt Frank would love it. We'd talked about my taking him on a trip there. Now, when I see him next, he says sadly: "Well, I guess we didn't make it to Antigua." He tells me that the hospital has changed its plan; he'll be in the hospital awhile longer. And he's "lost" the apartment keys, which I suspect the hospital has actually confiscated.

Perhaps it's all indicative of Frank's fear of what might happen if he returned to living on his own again, but I'm deeply troubled by the pattern. Every time he's close to departing the hospital, Frank does something to scuttle it. Some part of him doesn't want to leave. The result is, I'm now at odds with the Shattuck administration, in particular Dr. P. Not only is my son not ready for release into the community, he says, but should be put on a waiting list for a supervised group home. That would mean at least another six to eight months before Frank can be discharged from the hospital. On the positive side, the doctor says, his eventual acceptance by a group home is likely, since he's not been a lawbreaker, nor does he have a history of drug abuse.

But simply to get on the waiting list, Dr. P. adds, Frank will first need to give up his Section 8 housing voucher. The doctor knows how difficult those are to get, but he is adamant. "No matter how good he might get on Clozaril," Dr. P. feels it makes no sense for Frank to return to his own apartment. Moving him home again would also be problematic, given "the impact on other parts of your life . . . the burn-out" that parents experience in such circumstances. So the upshot is, "you need to give up degrees of control over your son's life."

On a walk around Jamaica Pond with Alice, she says perhaps there's ultimately only one lesson to learn in life, and that's acceptance.

Yet the language of the medical world grates on me. Yes, Dr. P. says, Frank has moved forward from the truncated language and the trouble he had constructing more than the simplest sentence at the beginning of his latest hospitalization, but he continues to exhibit an inability to sustain logic. According to the doctor, "his illness does not allow him to be free from the vulnerability of psychotic interpreta-tion," hence the unpredictability as to whether he will acknowledge me as his father in the future. "His denial is so dense, he's so invested in not cooperating. . . . He has no clue to having a psychiatric illness, it's simply not a part of him."

Again, looking back, this whole interpretation is suspect. No mat-ter how medically strung out, Franklin seemed consistently able to focus when a real situation demanded his attention—such as the recent suicide at the hospital. His mother particularly noticed this capacity to pay attention in moments requiring alertness. Frank himself no lon-ger expressed any interest in driving (perhaps that long day behind the wheel of a truck had frightened him too much), but while going somewhere with Etta, he would consistently tell her to be careful when he sensed—remarkably accurately—a possibly difficult situation. She trusted his instincts enough to ask Frank to check whether it was okay to change lanes.

Had the medical language not been so negative, might Franklin have come to understand or publicly accept things more readily? It's certainly true that he remained ambivalent about the medication. But was this only about "denial?" Sometimes, he says, the medication *creates* his strange thoughts. On a hospital pass, walking together around the Arboretum, Frank says profoundly: "When I feel guilty about some-thing, it is magnified a thousand times."

He has been asking to return home with me to Fort Hill. But there are no other young people there, and no rooms where some-one isn't already living, and the doctor believes he "doesn't need to be where old things are reinforced." When I explain some of this to Frank, he gets furious, says he'll "start calling Eddie my dad again," then refuses his evening dose of Clozaril three times and loses his off-unit privileges.

Simultaneously, Franklin's delusions become full-blown once more; he's Slim Shady and Tutankhamen. Dr. P. says that clinging to these things provide him an emotional sense of relief because he wants his parents to suffer as he does, but the robustness of such thinking disturbs the doctor because Frank hadn't missed enough medication for there to be "a biological effect." They've now increased his daily dosage of Clozaril, and it will continue to be raised, making him even more sedated.

I can barely make it through my next visit with Frank, who can see the tears in my eyes as he speaks of how long he may need to be in this hospital. For the first time, though, he's open to the group home idea. With Etta I attend one more meeting, intent on fighting for my son to keep his apartment. But I get talked out of it by the DMH representatives. They describe how their places are spacious and supervised round-the-clock, very different than a Wellmet or an Eikos, and how eventually you can get your own place but under their supervision to ensure "medication compliance."

Early in December, the hospital social worker calls. Frank has signed the paperwork giving up his apartment. Realizing how upset he must be at having done this, I go to see him that afternoon. More fixations are evident. He's the reincarnation of Jesse Owens and Bob Marley. He's receiving messages from the radio about a fifth race that will come to pass. He shows me his blueprint to divide up the country into regions based on racial characteristics. Also the intersecting lines of his latest drawings, while designing a spaceship to leave planet earth.

However, when I recall being in the waiting room at the California hospital when he was born, Frank says: "You never told me that before," and adds that he'll have to revise his thinking about his parentage. We're suddenly speaking quite rationally, including my telling him how interesting it is that he keeps returning to the *same* delusions as six months ago. What an imagination he has, if he could only channel this into writing or art—but first he had to realize the difference between illusion and reality. Toward the end, I'm not his father again. It's an endless cycle. "Turning and turning in the widening gyre. . . ."

When they think you're trying to flee the hospital, they oddly call it "trying to elope." That's what was claimed a few months ago when Frank rushed up some steps. While he'd denied any elopement plans, he ended up restricted to the unit. Now, on a very cold night in December, the hospital calls to inform me that Franklin went out on an hour-long independent pass at 4:30, but has not returned. Alice and I get in the car and drive around the hospital vicinity, but to no avail. When I call the unit again, they've received word from another hospital in suburban Norwood. Frank had boarded a bus, seen that hospital out the window, and walked in to tell the staff he wanted to be admitted, because he wasn't getting good treatment at the Shattuck.

By the following morning he's sent back. Frank calls wanting to see me. In his room he shows me computer printouts about the human body and chemical elements, which he wants to use to build a "transporter." He reminds me that, while living in his apartment last spring, an alien from Jupiter had inhabited his body.

Christmas Eve. Another call from the hospital. After an argument about whether the lights should be on or off, his roommate—a big African American guy in his mid-thirties—had jumped on my son in his bed and given him two black eyes. Frank had kept yelling, "Chill! Chill!" but the fellow wouldn't let up. The attacker is now in "the quiet room." Frank gets an eight-hour pass to join his mother and then me. Dropping him off again, I tell him I'm going to give the doctors hell about why they aren't more aware of a possible situation like this. "Thanks, Dad," he says. I'm in tears much of the rest of the night. The next day, Frank doesn't want to press charges, but I convince him to fill out a complaint form. He's given his own room. After the terrible reality of getting beat up, he doesn't appear at all psychotic.

As we walk together around the grounds, Franklin's allusions to the *Star Wars* movies are quite remarkable; he remembers all the characters, while juxtaposing them to himself. But I suggest he not repeat such things to his doctor, if he wants to get out soon. He says he won't, because the doctor—like the other patients—is a robot.

Who am I to say he's wrong? I'm up against the terrifying realization that my son has been on the verge of being lost to an often inhuman system. Yet, through it all, miraculously enough, his spirit remains strong.

There is the rule and the exception to it. In the mental health system sometimes people that could be assets to society are turned into so called crazy people. Probably the grouping together of them by the system is many times a mistake.

Extreme talent can be taken as out of the ordinary. Instead of being cultivated it is commonly rejected. Instead of molding our young into people with lives of meaning, they are often labeled and put into mental institutions. These places of "stable" environments provide almost no opportunity for growth or change for the better.

—Franklin's Journal, a year earlier

CHAPTER 5

· · ·

Battling the System

. . . Marketing is moving us steadily from what was the practice of medicine to a healthcare products limited market, and indeed not just a market but the creation of a new healthcare universe—a universe where the focus has shifted from medicine, in which progress occurred slowly but patients benefited, to a healthcare products market in which science and progress have become marketing terms and where benefits accrue to companies even while patients suffer harm.

—David Healy, *Pharmageddon*[1]

IN JANUARY 2004, SEVEN MONTHS into Franklin's latest hospitalization, a group home in Cambridge has an opening. Several staff from Aberdeen House come to the Shattuck for what proves to be a successful first meeting. Shortly thereafter, I pick Franklin up at the hospital and we drive to visit the privately owned "rehabilitation services" residence that accepts SSI disability insurance. It's a triple-decker in a quiet neighborhood near Mount Auburn Street. Frank is very polite and straightforward, and plans are made for him to come to dinner there the following week. The eight residents have quite a bit of freedom to come and go, although the staff wants to know approximately when they plan on returning. A sign in the bathroom endears me to the place: "God grant me the senility to forget the people I never liked in the first place."

With Alice and Eddie helping, everything is moved out of Frank's apartment in an hour-and-a-half and stored in our basement at home. He comes over on his twenty-fifth birthday, and we spend several hours together in our woodshop, where he wants to build a boat. He's gathered some old boards and meticulously puts the wooden frame together, concentrating on sawing and drilling. I find it fascinating to observe it all come together from a design maintained in his head. Having dinner at our home for the first time in quite awhile, Frank is relaxed and makes everyone laugh. He says he couldn't really figure out why I hung around down there in the woodshop all that time: "Was he going to write a book about it or something?"

On February 11, 2004, my son is discharged from the Shattuck, I pray for the last time. He's referring to Etta as "mom" and me as "dad." Settling into Aberdeen House, he's getting out and around, doing considerable Asian-type artwork, taking his medication regularly, and seeing a new therapist once a week. This is as much as I could hope for.

But before long, old patterns begin reasserting themselves: going off his medication for a week, disappearing for two days, found by the police wandering around Northeastern University with a Wiffle bat and turning lights on and off. Hospitalized briefly, he's set for discharge when he throws a chair at someone on the unit. This time I let Frank handle getting out on his own . . . and he does. But the racial issue has resurfaced. Back at Aberdeen House, he refuses to come downstairs to see his mother, and says that my hands are "too white" and his real birth certificate would show that he's Bruce Lee.

It seems a never-ending spiral, about which there is little to be done. In my diary I write, with frustration if not bitterness: "He made a choice about six months ago, I believe, to live in a fantasy world of his own creation where he is all-powerful and doesn't have to listen to anyone and can basically say whatever he wants."

What is behind a situation is a mystery. We are left searching for reasons that things are the way they are....Clarity and cloudy times come and leave. Points are made and life proceeds.

—Franklin's Journal

• • •

Jung, in one of his more extensive explorations of psychosis, described the compensatory role of delusions in attempting to rescue the personality from a patho-

logical one-sidedness; also he saw in delusions the attempt of the pathological complex to destroy itself.

—John Weir Perry, *The Far Side of Madness*[2]

In the mid-1990s, my family had discovered the writings of James Hillman. He was the founder of what came to be called archetypal psychology, which emphasized the importance of myth, imagination, and aesthetics. We found a strong resonance in Hillman's twenty-some published works, as well as benchmarks toward meeting life's challenges. Alice, far more psychologically attuned than I was, would point out passages for me to read and contemplate in an anthology called *A Blue Fire*. I devoured Hillman's best-selling *The Soul's Code*, whose "acorn-and-oak" theory raised the intriguing possibility that we "choose" our parents in order to fulfill our destinies.

Then, in 1998, two years after Franklin's breakdown, I was personally introduced to Dr. Hillman by a mutual friend who sold him organic vegetables at a Connecticut farmer's market. We eventually exchanged visits to one another's homes. In the summer of 2004, he asked if I was interested in being his authorized biographer, and I accepted. By that time, Hillman, twenty-one years my senior, served at times for me in a mentoring role—especially when it came to my relationship with Franklin. Early on, I wrote down a single line that penetrated deep into my psyche: "Even your solicitude is confining to him," Hillman said.

On the same day in June 2003 that Franklin went back into a hospital, Alice and I had gone to see Hillman and his wife at their rambling colonial-style farmhouse in Thompson, Connecticut. He'd immediately tuned in to my sadness. "So you've been having a hard time with your son," he said. I brought him up-to-date. Hillman had been a practicing therapist for forty years and had broad experience with mental illnesses. He proceeded to speak of how, as years went by, the intensity of schizophrenia lessened—but the personality diminished at the same time. Basically, he meant that people afflicted with the disease often don't grow emotionally beyond their first breakdown. Hillman didn't necessarily buy into schizophrenia being strictly genetic. He spoke of how mysterious the disease is; that doctors don't really know what causes it or what medications will work best, coupled with the fact that it strikes most all of its victims in their late teens to early twenties. He seemed to be indicating that there is a soul choice involved by the individual so afflicted.

Later, in terms of Franklin's unwillingness to take certain medications, Hillman said it is important to "respect resistance"—that maybe he knows something we don't. And during the back-and-forth with his Shattuck Hospital doctor over whether Frank could hang onto his federal housing voucher, Hillman told me that his formerly being able to live independently had marked real progress, but it's always one step forward and a half-step back.

"How old is Franklin?" Hillman asked when I saw him on another occasion. At that point, Frank had moved into Aberdeen House but been temporarily hospitalized once again. When I told Hillman my son was twenty-five, he reiterated that schizophrenia "tends to calm down" with age but "a contained environment is good." The disease is cyclical, he went on, and then said to my surprise: "Regression is crucial for recovery. Falling into nothingness, being useless and dirty." I noted that that was one plus side of being hospitalized. "Yes," Hillman continued, "they let you be a lump—that's the good thing about psychiatric care." That same day, I returned home to a message from Franklin at the hospital: he wanted me to come see him . . . and also to return to Aberdeen House.

• • •

By the end of September 2004, Frank is back in the group home, but the repetitive cycle is taking its toll on me. On a trip to interview Hillman for the biography, I decide to raise the big question with which I've been wrestling. This concerns my son's delusions, which persist despite taking his medications. I explain that one fantasy is that I'm not his father, even though Frank concedes sometimes that I did raise him. He clearly doesn't want to be who he is. He takes on substitute identities as the reincarnation of Tutankhamen or Bruce Lee.

So what do I do in the face of this? Do I accept the delusions? Do I challenge them over time? Or do I simply listen and try to figure out what my son might really be expressing underneath?

My tape recorder is running as Hillman responds: "You listed the choices already. 'I *am* your father' is one way to do it. Another way is, you enter the delusion with him. The main aim is to maintain a conversation, I would think, to keep connected with him. He's testing you. I don't mean in an oppositional way, but just unconditional acceptance of whatever. Because you really can't change anything. The tendency is to treat everything as if it's acute, but you need to accept the fact that a chronic condition is different. You have to realize that it's Chronos, the god of time; you don't look for improvement. It's really walking along with. It's accompanying. Without any end in sight. Accepting what is, and just going along. And talking with him. Also about things you want to talk to *him* about—this is a very important part—about what *you've* been doing or thinking. Maybe he doesn't want to hear it, but that doesn't matter. The point is that you're not there out of guilt and fatherhood and all that, but you're talking to him as a human being. Your normalcy is helpful. Because nobody he talks to is normal, they all talk to him about being a sick person."

I interject that I'd like to be able to tell my son: "When you took this particular medication, you were able to go to school. Or that maybe we could write a book together someday, but we can't do it if you are delusional." But then Frank immediately starts arguing with me.

Hillman continues: "Well, again, you probably have to re-constellate the relationship. *Not* in terms of where you're trying to help him. And not trying to *get* anywhere with him. Simply, 'You know where I was today? I went to Connecticut. . . .' You let go of his being a 'sick man.' Then you may find he tells you things that he doesn't talk about otherwise. You don't know what is going to come out, but it's almost as if you've abandoned being the responsible father. Because you can't move him. Okay, so that's over with. Make him feel that you really want to see him and tell him things. You say, 'This guy drove by and I thought: *I wish Frank had seen that car.* What do you think of that kind of car?' He might go into a delusion about the car, but it *doesn't matter*—you've approached him differently from the therapeutic."

I interject again, "And differently from my expectations of Franklin."

"Exactly. It's something that's not your world, and not his world, like in the sense of writing a book together. Or his world without his medicines, hospitals, and all that shit. It becomes like sitting in a bar together side by side, talking about the day."

Yes, I reply, he says he'd like to write *his* book, not with me.

"Exactly. This whole thing with the therapy—he's been innoculated, he doesn't want that, it *drives* you crazy. That's the last person I would want to see. I used to ask people, what does going crazy mean to you? Does it mean you're gonna lay around with your clothes off, go shoot somebody? The other question is: Where do *you* want to be? On an island? With no phone? Curled up in a room in the dark? Who do *you* want to talk to? People don't want to see therapists, they really don't. They want to go to a bar, find a lover. All I mean is . . . I think the most useful thing is to get around all that clinical area that, in a way, he draws you into—the delusions."

Does it do any good, I wonder, for me to try to figure out where the delusions come from? Hillman shakes his head. "Very mysterious," he says.

• • •

Reasoning with people about their delusions is like trying to bail out the ocean with a bucket.

—E. Fuller Torrey, *Surviving Schizophrenia*[3]

The mystery doesn't go away. But after Hillman's sage advice, the usual way I approach my son assuredly does change—and *that* changes *everything* . . . at least between the two of us. I take Frank to one of his favorite restaurants, Chef Chow's. We're perusing our menus. When the waiter comes over, Frank starts speaking to him in invented Chinese. The poor fellow looks quite nonplussed. Ordinarily I would cringe and perhaps even mutter an apology on my son's behalf. When I instead say nothing, Franklin doesn't skip a beat. He continues speaking to the waiter, this time in English, while pointing across the table in my direction. "Oh don't worry," Frank says, "he can't understand, because it's Mandarin. He [meaning me] only speaks Cantonese." When the waiter nods and quickly disappears from sight, I start to laugh. And laugh. Frank has what we used to call in the Midwest, "a big shit-eating grin" spread wide across his face. And I just keep laughing.

I begin to think about why so-called "normal thought" at the beginnings of conversations often turn "delusional" without any seeming provocation. Maybe, I consider, it's so that he'll have something new and interesting to say. When it comes to generalized anxiety, you will hear people talk without taking a breath, just because the act of talking prevents the uncomfortable silence that feeds into their anxiety. Whether serious or gibberish, talking takes the mind off what causes someone's worries. I wouldn't be surprised if it's the same with Franklin. While speaking seeming gibberish may make me uncomfortable, he perhaps sees it as "breaking the ice" and lightening the mood. By my accepting that, he becomes more comfortable with me, not feeling as though he's constantly being judged.

One day Frank calls and asks me to write down the "stories" he is telling. At another Asian restaurant, he says he's Mongolian and indeed, with his wild braided hair that day, he does look the part. Frank enjoys that I jot down his heritage. (A friend suggests that Frank's idea of being Asian makes sense, because he needs that quiet, meditative sensibility.)

I write in my diary: "My new approach is to just let him riff, don't try to stop or contradict him, even do some whole new languages with him. I just go with his delusions and don't try to respond, except subtly. Ever since I have stopped trying to correct his insanity, we get along fine." Hillman tells me, when I report having turned a new leaf with my son, that it's good to "show your *own* insanity" and to not put myself in the position of being an adviser on his illness. "The less you have to do with his treatment, the better," he emphasizes.

After all, I consider, in the course of numerous hospitalizations, Frank has been around doctors from morning till night, watching and judging every move he makes. It's not unlike having a large pimple or a big stain on your shirt, where you think everyone sees it and is silently disapproving. With my simply being his father, the last thing Frank would want to do is dismiss me, as he sees I'm not doing what everyone else is doing—and simply accepting him for who he is.

While I'm back in LA for a bit, the Aberdeen House staff report that Frank is doing so much better, always coming to get his meds, calling staff by their first names, and hanging out with others in the house. He tied a fellow's tie for him. He catches himself when he brings up bizarre subjects and is sometimes embarrassed about it.

My friend Eddie rings me up. He's taken Frank bowling along with his son. What had ensued still has Eddie shaking his head. "First Frank takes a long time to select his shoes and then the right ball. We divide up into teams and he's talking to everyone in the place, giving instruction like he's been doing this for years. Everybody's paying close attention. By the time Frank actually gets up to the lane, he's holding the bowling ball almost at the floor, and the whole place seems to be watching. Franklin stops, stands there at the line—and just drops the ball. You could've heard the clunk in the parking lot. The ball starts bouncing down the lane toward the pins, *very* slowly. I don't know how long it takes, seems like almost a minute. Finally the ball touches the first pin, and I figure that's about it. But damned if all ten pins don't fall, one tumbling into another. Frank gets a strike! And everybody in the whole damn bowling alley starts cheering! We gave him high-fives!"

Then 2005 dawns. During one phone conversation, I decide to write down Frank's thoughts to see if I can decipher any pattern. When he was growing up, he says, "you wanted me to be your kid so bad, you tried to control me. But you are one of my sons. . . . You must start using your own Confucian way. You're half Chinese and half African. . . . A secret society, with codes, want you to be involved. It's GPID—Generic Practice of Independent Discussion. . . . When are you coming back here?" He wants to create a spaceship that will hold six people, and I can be one of them on board. My code-breaking has failed, but I'm pleased to be included in Frank's launch.

At intervals throughout this year, I write down a series of dreams about my son. In the first, I'm going fishing with Budd Schulberg (a writer who, in daily life, I've recently spent some time with), and Franklin is coming along. He is blind and, when I introduce them, Schulberg is surprised at this. Once on the boat, Frank can nonetheless figure out how to tie the line onto his fishing rod, which is something I cannot do. (In truth, I've never been able to figure that out.)

Next I dream of hanging out with a black man, telling him about Franklin being so delusional. The response is something like, "Oh, we were counting on him to tell our story." Then the fellow hands me a pair of castanets, along with another unusual musical instrument.

In a third dream, I'm working with Franklin—who seems younger in years—delivering groceries and wine to various customers. We arrive at an apartment complex, where two women are waiting inside a door on the first floor. One isn't satisfied with her order. While I try to reason with her, Franklin disappears and I must catch up with him. We return to the same building with more goods for the ladies.

I then begin to traverse some stairs which, to my surprise, lead right into a swimming pool. I'm fully clothed, but my shoes get wet and I can tell the pool is quite warm. So I tell Frank that I want to get my bathing suit and go in. As I depart, I notice a couple floating around in the pool, gazing lovingly into each other's eyes.

Accompanying these shifts in my own psyche, the psychic side of Franklin's nature seems to be coming more to the fore. Frank doesn't know that, given his often-expressed interest in the East and meditative practice, I've come across a possible group-type place for him to live in India and mentioned this to Etta. When I raise with Frank that perhaps he should get his passport renewed, he says yes, he's been thinking about going to New Delhi. Another time I call Frank from the airport, on the way to an environmental conference. He immediately tunes in that I am traveling and begins discussing his own upcoming imagined wanderings, as well as recalling the true story of how the Indians on the Lakota Sioux reservation presented us gifts on a trip we made to South Dakota when he was twelve. Yet another time, the first person mentioned by Franklin is my old friend Hugh Kaufman of the Environmental Protection Agency—who Frank has no idea I've just seen in Washington.

There is another curious crossover between the two of us. For many years I'd studied the Kennedy era and published two books on the assassination of President Kennedy. Part of the dedication of my first, which came out in 1992, was "to my son Franklin." In the course of my more recent environmental writing, I'd become friends with Robert Kennedy Jr., stayed at his home and gone sailing with him from the family compound in Hyannisport. One day in the car, Franklin asks, did I know *I* was Robert Kennedy? He says *he* is, sometimes, and John Kennedy at other times, but that he and I also shift occasionally between those identities. He mentions the year Robert Kennedy was assassinated, 1968, and says that the fellow they arrested (Sirhan Sirhan) was the wrong man. I don't believe I've ever told Frank of research indicating that the fatal shot had come from behind, not the front where Sirhan Sirhan was firing from.

The Kennedy linkages could, of course, be simply delusional allusions to a subject my son knew was of great interest to me, both personally and professionally. Could it even be that Frank was making himself into people I study, as a way to get closer to me? Yet I could find no explanation, logical or illogical, for something else he brings up, connected to James Hillman. This was prefaced a few visits earlier by Franklin asking, "Are you still doing a book on a psychiatrist?" I told him I was. "Did he write *The Soul's Code*?" Yes, he did. Then on a drive back to his house, Frank announces emphatically that my real birthday is April 12. As far as I know, Frank doesn't do online research, and would have no other way of knowing that is actually Hillman's birthday. "You're an Aries, with Neptune in Cancer," my son goes on. Frank is knowledgeable about astrological signs, and while these particular aspects are not in my own birth chart, both are true of Hillman's from 1926.

"Who knows where Franklin's mind goes on its amazing wanderings?" I write in my journal.

• • •

A rock is a rock. As hard as we try it can't be destroyed easily. People on the other hand are fragile. Easily swayed this way and that, we lose track of what we are. We lose track of our souls and our bodies.

—Franklin's Journal

During this period, Etta and Kamal move to New York, where he has landed a job teaching at the city's New School and she secures a music instructor position at a Brooklyn middle school. They've kept a one-room apartment in Boston so as to have a place when wanting to visit Frank.

Meantime, something initially discussed as a necessity by the doctors at Shattuck has come to pass. A female lawyer in Cambridge has been appointed as a guardian for Frank. In Massachusetts, when a court determines that an adult is incapacitated and requires someone to make medical decisions on their behalf, it's known as an Outpatient Rogers Guardianship. The guardianship order compels Franklin to take medication. But since he is once again rejecting Clozaril due to the bi-weekly blood draw also required, he is now back on Zyprexa as well as Depakote. And Franklin has begun to gain tremendous weight. The group home staff aren't sure if the cause is the medications or is related to inactivity, since it's winter and Frank rarely emerges from his room.

A physical exam reveals that his heart rate is more than twice of what it should be. Frank's eyes are rolling back in his head again, a sign of paranoia that hasn't happened in a few years, which often seems to arise out of nowhere but he says happens when he becomes fearful. "I have some health problems, you know," he confides. When I drop him back at his house, Frank shakes hands and says, "Thank you."

Next time we're together I take him to the gym, where he enjoys the pool, whirlpool, sauna, and some weight lifting. This will hopefully increase his endorphins and get him moving, also perhaps help with Frank's mood swings. He agrees to stop by the Cambridge YMCA and start a membership. To my great relief, his heart rate soon falls dramatically, but his cholesterol level is high—which means yet another medication to try to lower it.

Etta takes him to a holistic doctor, who prescribes several vitamins that might alleviate the side effects of the medication. Indeed, once Frank starts taking them, he looks and feels so much better. But then, incredibly, the house takes his vitamins away because they've not been officially prescribed by his psychiatrist. Score another round for the bureaucracy of the mental health system! I complain, but then Frank says he doesn't want to take the vitamins anyway because he has trouble swallowing them.

I have a dream about desperately going to some agency for him with assorted paperwork, trying to persuade them to offer my son more help.

Though he continues to gain weight, the DMH psychiatrist doesn't appear inclined to change a thing, he's simply eating too much, the "authorities" believe. I'm left in the dark about vast weight increases observed in other people taking high doses of the "atypical" antipsychotic drug, Zyprexa. Over less than six months, Frank balloons up to nearly three hundred pounds.

In June 2006, learning from staff at Aberdeen House that he's spending considerable time alone again and sleeping in the basement area, I see Frank for several hours. He's insistent about wanting to go off his meds, see a Chinese doctor, and join the Army.

A couple of weeks later, I return a call from his mother. Etta has learned that Franklin's been diagnosed with adult-onset diabetes and has been prescribed medication. She's terrified; her family history includes members dying from complications of diabetes. Still in a state of shock, I call Frank. He greets me with, "Ah, my long-lost son!" He really doesn't want to talk about the diabetes. Instead, China remains much on his mind. He'd like to attend a school there to study acupuncture. He wants us to form "a Chinese Network for Indignant Indigenous Personages—a *Large* Business Association." He adds: "I don't want to live in halfway houses all my life. If I went to school in China, I could live a lavish life"—a pause—"of a fool." It's one of those jokes that we both know is not funny.

His by-the-book DMH therapist, due to the diabetes diagnosis, finally decides to shift him to two different medications that don't have the same weight gain side effects. But the gradual weaning off from Zyprexa doesn't prove easy. The substituted medication, a relatively new antipsychotic called Abilify, is more commonly prescribed for curbing mania in mood disorders and as an added "helper drug" for schizophrenia. Frank is spending more time isolated, where he's invented "seafood chambers for Japanese farmers" and created a "five pattern repeater naturalization beam." Over a lunch, he tells me: "The only filthy fish left to catch is the gefilte fish." The line cracks me up and I write it down. A rare moment of humor these days.

• • •

It is just un-stinkin'-believable. It is the best drug for gaining weight I've ever seen.
—UCLA psychiatrist Dr. William Wirshing, discussing a study of Zyprexa prior to its 1996 approval by the FDA, indicating that taking ten milligrams of the medication was equivalent to ingesting 1,500 extra calories *per day*.[4]

That December of 2006, I'm in Baja working on a new book when I have a queasy feeling about Frank. Checking my voicemail, I learn from Aberdeen House that he's been refusing to take his meds for two weeks, punched a staff officer's door, and ran off for twenty-four hours. He then had to be taken under a Section 12 (police and ambulance) to the psych emergency ward at Cambridge Hospital, the site of his first admission just over a decade earlier. He'd introduced himself at the hospital as C. G. Ming. That's what a nurse put on his wristband. She wasn't sure *who* he really was; he was denying that his name was ever Franklin. Later, I will contemplate the similarity of Frank's chosen name to C.G. Jung. As Frank knows, I've begun working with James

Hillman on his biography—and Jung was influential in Hillman's thought process. Perhaps, once again, my son is overlapping boundaries of his life with mine.

Making slow progress—"not up to baseline yet," as the phrase goes—he's been taken off Abilify and put back on Zyprexa. Later that same month, perusing an online edition of the *New York Times*, I come across a front-page article about Zyprexa. It begins:

> The drug maker Eli Lilly has engaged in a decade-long effort to play down the health risks of Zyprexa, its best-selling medication for schizophrenia, according to hundreds of internal Lilly documents and e-mail messages among top company managers. The documents, given to the *Times* by a lawyer representing mentally ill patients, show that Lilly executives kept important information from doctors about Zyprexa's links to obesity and its tendency to raise blood sugar—both known risk factors for diabetes.

The company had told its sales representatives to play down such data with doctors, including the fact that some patients had reported gaining a hundred pounds or more. The documents revealed that Eli Llly had been concerned about these side effects since 1999, which I recall was the year Frank was first prescribed the drug. Today, Zyprexa was by far the pharmaceutical company's top selling product, hitting some $4.2 billion in revenues in 2005, and being prescribed to about two million people worldwide. Also in 2005, the company had agreed to pay $750 million to settle class action lawsuits by 8,000 people, and thousands more claims were still pending.[5]

I'm outraged. The image of my son, almost a hundred pounds heavier than he'd been before taking this medication, rises up before me. *They knew all along, the bastards!* The drug company had plenty of evidence! Prescribing physicians had the wool pulled over their eyes, or had blinders on and went along with the program. I set out on an intense Internet search for a class action suit in which to involve Franklin. Several United States law firms seem to be pursuing this case.

It would be another six years before I learned more about the background of the Zyprexa story in a book called *Pharmageddon*. Author David Healy recounted:

The first generation of antipsychotics ran into problems in the 1970s with million-dollar legal settlements against their manufacturers for a disfiguring neurological side effect of treatment—tardive dyskinesia [a disorder resulting in involuntary, repetitive body movements]. This led to a period of almost twenty years when no new antipsychotic came on the market. The only antipsychotic that did not cause this problem was clozapine [Clozaril was the brand name], but clozapine had been withdrawn in 1975 because it was associated with a higher rate of mortality than other antipsychotics. The way forward seemed to lie in producing a safe clozapine.

One way to do so was "to make minor adjustments to the clozapine molecule. Tweaking a molecule risks producing a compound with all the hazards and none of the benefits of the parent. This is what Lilly did: in 1974 the company produced a series of compounds that were all abandoned because of toxicity." The company was in serious financial trouble, facing potential takeover. . . . On April 29, 1982, they opted to move forward with a compound from the original series that by definition was not novel—olanzapine, later branded as Zyprexa. To make Zyprexa commercially viable, they needed a new patent, which meant demonstrating some benefit not found with other antipsychotics. In 1991, the only novelty presented in the company's new patent application, which was approved, was a study in dogs in which Zyprexa produced less elevation of blood cholesterol levels than another never-marketed drug.

> Zyprexa has since turned out to be one of the drugs most likely in all of medicine to increase cholesterol levels in man. . . . There was arguably a better case to be made for patenting it to raise cholesterol than to treat psychosis. . . . There was no basis to think this drug was any more effective than dozens of others and a lot of reasons to think it was more problematic for patients, but the marketing power that came with its patented status enabled Lily to hype its benefits and conceal its hazards and steer doctors to write enough Zyprexa prescriptions to save the company.[6]

When I call Franklin in January, he's back in the group home and no longer being prescribed Zyprexa. "I think you're in some trouble and need a lawyer," he says. I tell him I'm looking for a lawyer all right—to sue the drug company that makes Zyprexa.

The Mental Health System in the U.S.

In this time, in this era, this 2000 period of time, people seem to assume that they know reality and others do not. Doctors believe they are fully knowledgeable of the scientific area. These doctors go around diagnosing people of this disease and that. Many times they steal lives and get paid for it. I resisted treatment in my young years.

—Franklin's Journal

· · ·

Back on Abilify, Franklin initially seems to be doing better, despite running into some policemen in a park who were looking for a burglary suspect and stopped him because he appeared to be behaving oddly. His name, Frank told them, was Marvin Yang (Master Yang had been his Kung Fu teacher as a teenager). The cops came to Aberdeen House asking if Yang lived there, "but once they described him we knew they were talking about Franklin, so luckily it was all set straight," I'm told by the staff.

In January 2007, I'm still away when Frank undergoes another brief hospitalization after a series of incidents at his house: binge eating, forgetting to turn off the gas on the stove, flipping out at the staff for "being racist" concerning taking his medication. When he returns to his house, he's been prescribed three different meds—but not Zyprexa. I find a law firm in New Orleans that's organizing a new class action suit against Eli Lilly and learn how to get my son involved.

This is followed by a very positive dream: Franklin's lost considerable weight and looks great and addresses me as Dad.

And then comes an email from Etta about her most recent visit with him—in fact, off Zyprexa, he's fairly rapidly dropped sixty pounds!

One step forward, half a step back. Frank has developed strange skin blotches on his face. The doctors think the discoloration is due to being outside too much in the cold weather. But he's been behaving very oddly at the house—going into the bathroom and leaving the water on for an hour but never getting in the shower, flushing Brillo Pads down the toilet. He's suddenly obsessed with cleanliness, always leaving windows open in the house. Staff are now performing an hourly check of the premises. Etta is terribly worried—"you wouldn't believe how he looks!"—and says there *has* to be some other living situation we can find for him.

As Etta has been urging for a long time, I start to think seriously about alternative treatment possibilities. I get in touch with a psychic healer in New Mexico who turns out to have a son with a similar diagnosis. He tunes in to the possibility that Franklin may have a food allergy, but knows of no alternative living places. I have another dream; this one of traditional healers somewhere in mainland Mexico who might have a cure for schizophrenia. Another dream has me finding Clozaril in Baja that Frank could take without getting the required blood test—something that in actuality I'd been looking into.

Several years earlier, I'd also been in touch briefly with a place in rural New Jersey called Earth House, which looked like an excellent place for young people in their twenties, but was also prohibitively expensive. Now I call my brother for the first time in ages. Two years younger, Bob is a commercial real estate developer out west and has done very well financially. But we have vastly different lifestyles and outlooks, and have not been close since our childhood. He and Franklin have never met, although Frank has spent some time with Bob's eldest son when he once visited our Kansas farm. To my pleasant surprise, if I need monetary assistance finding Frank a better living situation, Bob says he'll be more than willing to help.

Frank, after allegedly threatening someone at his house for the third time in recent months, is shipped out to Cambridge Hospital again. At first he refuses to receive any visitors and is adamant that he won't return to the group home. I'm about to fly east when an email comes from Etta: Frank has agreed to take a small dose of Clozaril, and has emerged from his isolation to play the piano. It feels like a miracle. Or at least a window; and one that I know may not stay open for long. Etta has contacted Earth House. The cost is $20,000 for three months, and most people stay for up to nine months. But if my brother could come through with assistance, we might be able to swing it.

End of May 2007: Etta and I meet with the doctors and the social worker at Cambridge Hospital. Franklin is staying on the Clozaril and doing much better and the diabetes doesn't currently seem to be manifesting. We all agree that he needs a change of scenery.

His primary physician here is originally from Bangalore—a place in India with a youth facility for schizophrenia that I'd previously looked into—and I tell her about Frank's interest in the East and my idea. She doesn't discourage me altogether, but emphasizes that psychiatrists in India generally are not all that good, and also that Bangalore is very chaotic and I ought to surely check things out first. When I see Frank in his room, once again somehow in tune, he immediately starts talking about how he'd like to go to India. But he is also open to hearing about Earth House.

For years Franklin had periodically brought up the subject of his Uncle Bob and expressing a desire to see him. Now I fly to San Francisco to attend my niece's wedding, whom I haven't seen since my mother's funeral eighteen years before. Here a large gathering is on-hand for a lavish affair. I don't know what to expect. But over a long breakfast with Bob, I'm amazed to find that our political views have converged somewhat. Maybe because of how bad things have gotten in the country, we agree, we're able to laugh about our differences.

The wedding is done in the round, with bride and groom under a canopy in the middle. I'm impressed with my brother's sincerity and ability to articulate and entertain in his impromptu speech. After a Sunday brunch the next day, he and I sit down privately to talk about Franklin. Following some up-and-down times, Bob says, he's had a hugely successful year. If Franklin wants to go to Earth House, he will pay for at least the first three months.

"We're still brothers, even though we didn't seem to be for a long time," Bob says.

Be the anchor of my boat in rough seas.

—Franklin's Journal

Notes:

1. Quote on marketing of medicine: David Healy, *Pharmageddon*, University of California Press, 2012, p. 11.
2. Jung quote: Perry, *The Far Side of Madness*, p. 37.
3. Torrey on delusions: *Surviving Schizophrenia*, p. 55.
4. Dr. William Wirshing is quoted in "Bitter Pill," by Ben Wallace-Wells, in *Rolling Stone*'s article on Zyprexa, February 5, 2009.

5. The *New York Times* series by Alex Berenson began appearing on December 17, 2006.
6. Zyprexa and Clozaril: *Pharmageddon*, pp. 31–32.

. . .

CHAPTER 6

An Oasis Called Earth House

But the brilliance, the versatility of madness is akin to the resourcefulness of water seeping through, over and under a dike. It requires the united front of many people to work against it.

—F. Scott Fitzgerald, *Tender Is the Night*[1]

IT SEEMS, TOO, THAT THE often strained relationship between Frank's mother and me is changing; that we are much more on the same page about him. Etta writes to his psychiatrist about the alternative program that we've found: "I was very afraid these past six months that we might lose him. I've never been so terrified in my entire life, nor has his father. Franklin's decision to take the Clozaril is the biggest turnaround in years . . . I think he finally understands that he is in trouble and must accept some guidance."

Earth House is a little more than an hour's drive down the Jersey Turnpike from New York, and Etta goes there with Kamal for a visit. She writes me: "The whole atmosphere of the place is very calm and feels good. No hysteria—no emergency or hospital feeling. Everyone is quite occupied with various studies and projects all day so you don't see people just aimlessly wandering around. The students seemed to be all about Franklin's age." The teacher of yoga and drama is an African American man who'd been there since Earth House's beginnings over thirty years before; in a wonderful coincidence, his brother was among the cast of *The Wiz* when Kamal starred in the production on Broadway.

The clinical program director, Deborah, informs us that Frank can go right from the hospital for admission in the near future. She speaks to Franklin over the phone and reports that he sounds apprehensive but that's not out of the ordinary. My brother says he'll wire funds for the initial three months and would pay for a whole year if necessary. Without Bob, I'd never have been able to afford sending Frank to Earth House.

Following a big meeting at the hospital—including the woman in charge of the Department of Mental Health for the entire city—Frank tells his mother how kind everyone here has been to him. "I'm going to miss this place," he says. A girl walks into his room, says "Thanks for everything, Franklin," and departs. Frank looks at me a bit later and says: "I'm taller than you now."

He and I pick up all his belongings at Aberdeen House and commence the long haul to Somerset, New Jersey, and an overnight at a Ramada Inn. It's a pretty quiet trip, with Frank asking occasional questions: "How are you? Are you happy these days?" We both express that we are. But at a lunch stop en route, it's hard for me to watch him eat. While he does use utensils, he will disgorge food that he doesn't like and often devours his meal more like an animal. Alice will tell me later that any semblance of table manners is one of the first things to go from being institutionalized.

That night in the hotel, I sleep for twelve hours—and Frank for fourteen. We get lost in the morning trying to find Earth House amid the Jersey hinterlands, but still arrive just ahead of Etta and Kamal. It's in a peaceful rural setting not far from Rutgers and Princeton; a converted eighteenth-century farmhouse located on six wooded acres above the Delaware and Raritan Canal. There are no fences, no locks on the doors, or any seclusion rooms. Behind the main office, across a small brook, is a larger wood-frame house that serves as a common area, living quarters for the "students" (as they're referred to), as well as a kitchen and dining room.

In a conference room, Deborah gives us the scoop. The food is organic, a modified vegetarian diet that may include fish or chicken, but no red meat or pork. No junk foods, stimulants, refined or highly processed products. The current group of thirteen young adults (eleven males and two females) share meals at a communal table and do everything else together as well: group therapy, yoga, tai chi, chores, and outings. The curricular emphasis is on arts and crafts, writing and literature, dance and drama. There are almost forty hours of activities weekly, including about fifteen hours of exercise. And there are some thirty staff who are in-and-out, including a medication therapist and an orthomolecular physician.

The latter is particularly intriguing. Rosalind LaRoche, a niece of the actress Rosalind Russell, was a recovered schizophrenic who received enough money from her investment in the hit Broadway musical *Man of La Mancha* to purchase the land and farmhouse that became Earth House in 1971. As its founder/director, LaRoche was also the first person to be trained in the new field of orthomolecular medicine. This was an attempt to normalize brain chemistry through individually prescribed regimens of vitamins, minerals, and amino acids. Biochemical testing of many of the early Earth House students revealed abnormal levels of toxic metals such as lead, mercury, copper, cadmium, and aluminum. Others were found to have had cerebral allergies. The Earth House program didn't emphasize the orthomolecular approach at the expense of standard psychotropic medications—Franklin would stay on Clozaril—but the hope was that his dosage would decrease (the hospital had him up to a highly sedating 600 milligrams daily). Most of the other students had multiple diagnoses and had been hospitalized, some for as long as ten years or more. Here, most of them wind up getting jobs. Tragically, so few could afford a place like Earth House.

Filling out the forms, Franklin denies his parentage and his name, inserting some exotic AKA, but Deborah doesn't bat an eye. A young psychology graduate from Rutgers comes to help Frank unpack, and will be with him constantly for the first several days of adjustment. By the time we depart, he appears to be feeling very relaxed.

I basically let him settle in without regular phone calls. Early reports are that most of the other students are higher functioning and have some trouble handling his delusions, such as talking about vampires. Alice reassures me that, in a new situation like this, he would push the delusions as far as he can because that's the only form of conversation he knows; however, because he wants to stay there, he'll back off.

Twice I dream about Frank being happy and very friendly at Earth House. Deborah tells me that, while he continues to retreat to his room, "he does have a feeling of freedom here." Susannah, Frank's tai chi/creative movement instructor, finds him "a joy, sweet personality, very gentle nature," despite that "his reality orientation is pretty non-existent." However, "he does some of the exercises his own way" and she is "coaxing him in." He gets along with everyone and "invited me to become part of his tribal council," she says.

Etta and Kamal go to see him on a Sunday and she comes away elated about the visit. He looks better than since his days growing up on Fort Hill, and the delusions only persist when he's with more than one person, like a kind of defense mechanism. Kamal asks, "How's your Dad?" Frank responds, "Dick?" And he shares his food with the two of them.

Earth House Progress Notes for July: In art, "he added Indian arrow designs to our Georgia O'Keefe Southwestern study. He has also done sketches of abstract shapes and designs, not always connected to the assignment of the day." In Taiji/Creative Movement/Oigong: "Franklin enjoys performing, asking if he can do his martial arts forms."

I touch base with Dr. Bonnet, his orthomolecular doctor, who says Frank's urine shows that he has a metabolic disorder called pyroluria, which causes a severe deficiency of pyridoxine (vitamin B6) and zinc under conditions of stress. Franklin shows deficiencies of both critical nutrients. Pyroluria was first identified in the late 1950s through tests with patients in a psychiatric hospital, and is relatively common among about 70 percent of schizophrenics, as well as 70 percent of those plagued with depression, 50 percent of those with autism, 40 percent of alcoholics, and 30 percent of individuals struggling with ADHD. It might take some time, but the doctor would try to remedy Frank's condition with supplements.

By August, Earth House is calling me that Frank is refusing to get out of bed and Deborah wants me to intervene. He's insulting when I speak with him on the phone, says he doesn't know who I am and wants to return to the hospital and would punch me in the nose if he saw me. But after our conversation, he *does* get out of bed and join the others. That same day, the New Orleans law firm filing the Zyprexa class action calls: they've reached a settlement with Eli Lilly that's likely to net Franklin some thousands of dollars, since he contracted diabetes at such a young age.

In late August, more than two months since his arrival, I drive to Earth House from Boston. Frank is wearing a Harlem Globetrotters

T-shirt and glad to see me. As we pass by the waterway that meanders through the property, Frank points and says: "Stream of consciousness." Over lunch I try drawing him out about his life now and whether he likes being at Earth House. He says he doesn't really, but offers no further explanation and says it's better than the hospital or the group home. He's tentatively agreed that I can be his father, though not to say so in public. On the way back, we stop at a mall to get him a new computer, his first laptop.

But I can sense the anger in him seething right below the surface. He brings up that he needs a new Social Security card that accurately reflects his birth date—he's centuries older than 1979—as well as a new driver's license. I can't always follow James Hillman's advice. I get tough in response: "You need to use those cards because that's who you *are!*" His rage comes to the surface. I don't know him, I'm a vampire, and so is he. "So you're going to treat me like shit at the end of our visit?" I ask coolly. No, he won't, Frank responds. Back at the house, when one of the young ladies says to me, "You have a nice son," he insists this isn't the case. But he invites me to sit down and watch an MTV program with everyone, which I do.

I leave feeling very discouraged. Expectation has reared its hopeful head; I'd thought the delusions would have lessened somewhat by now. Spending the night in New York on the way back, I meet with my playwright friend, Arthur Kopit, who's been doing research into psychosis for a new script. The delusions offer a kind of comfort zone, Arthur says insightfully. Frank's afraid of what life would be like without them—because then he would be back in a real world that, at twenty-eight, wouldn't measure up to the image of who he is in his fantasies. Whether someone is paranoid psychotic, as Franklin used to be, or grandiose as now, both are dream states; one is terrifying and the other is self-gratifying.

Reflecting that night, I set down some further thoughts: There is a particular helplessness—even hopelessness—that comes with rejection. Now it is reversed, it is he rejecting me as he no doubt so often felt I had him. It is I who am left with the disappointment. In delusions, he is all-powerful: God, Father, Son. He has wealth and is able to dispense it. "Here is the bank account code," he says. But, as his own transcendent hero, he is also more sealed off from the rest of humanity. With no personal past, he is a timeless, ageless figure. Christ and Vampire, all in one eternal Now. Latent possibilities—and hidden sufferings—all are kept at bay, blocked, subordinated. And challenges to this state of being are often resisted angrily, even volcanically: A "Do Not Disturb" sign at the gates of the fantasyland of his life.

• • •

Starved for affection, I look around. Icebergs float in my eyes. My expression of words is complicated. To some sophisticated.

—Franklin's Journal

"You ought to see him holding court with the other students; he does things, goes places, takes hikes," I'm told by Deborah, several months into his time at Earth House. Going to visit him, Etta can't believe how much more weight he has lost, and observes "no fantastic stories or references to supersized dreams. The Franklin that we have known for the past ten years is no longer the same person. He is conducting himself in the world differently."

Even on a bad day—Frank refusing to take his medication and wanting to return to the safety net of the hospital—after another phone call when "you don't know me and you're not my father," he willingly goes downstairs for his meds. The venting is followed by an acceptance; he actually *is* hearing me. He's allowed to stay back from the day's outing and just get some sleep.

My brother pays for another three months at Earth House. He's taking care of my son, as he had our father in his advancing years. Beyond whatever judgments I had about him over the years, we have reconnected and Bob is helping Franklin in ways I didn't think were possible.

Toward the end of October, Etta and I attend a meeting with Frank, Deborah, and another counselor. It's an intense ninety minutes, the first time we've challenged certain delusions that he hangs onto with a maddening consistency. Though he complains about being ganged up on, we all continue the "reality checks," and eventually Etta and I are acknowledged his parents. Deborah tells my son he's doing well here for the most part, but needs to "step it up." A poignant moment ensues: Etta gives Frank a photo album that she's assembled of his early years, and he concentrates on the pictures for a long time.

When Alice and I go see him in November, Franklin bounds up the steps and a big smile crosses his face when he sees her. He's so different, it's rather astounding. And he's down to around 220 pounds, 80 less than two and a half years ago! After doing a height comparison with me, he tells Alice, "My dad's a pretty good-looking guy." He wants to go clothes shopping and is very quiet on the way, which surprises Alice as she's accustomed to his chattering on. At one point, Frank does tell her that being at Earth House is "like being in prison." But when Alice and I talk later, she doesn't see this as a bad thing— after having minimum accountability all these years, he finally had some structure in his life and of course would feel that as confining. I feel more hopeful about him than in a long time.

Earth House mails me Frank's Progress Notes for November. Particularly in art classes, he's avidly participating: a Native American design "using symbols and glyphs from many tribes," an excellent rendering of "a medieval duel on horses," and "his original abstract drawings are complex and creative."

Then, one night early in December, my brother calls. He's had a line of credit called and is temporarily unable to help Franklin beyond this six months at Earth House, and then not until probably springtime. "Oh no, oh no," Etta keeps repeating when I inform her. I'm at a loss. This couldn't happen at a worse time. Deborah says Frank was incredible in a play production there, is doing very well in therapy sessions, and is scarcely delusional. Frank had asked recently whether he'd be able to stay there and, when told they thought so, exclaimed "Good!"

After Franklin's recent success, 2008 dawns. With some financial aid from my extended family's construction business and my publisher agreeing to assist by providing the full advance upfront for my next book, I'm able to keep Franklin at Earth House awhile longer. He starts working part-time at a gas station, cleaning up each night for a couple of hours, five days a week. But by

Earth House Progress Notes for February: "His 'Reality to Abstract' transition started with a colored drawing of the Earth with its layers and outer crust. It ended with a non-objective drawing of a circle divided into pie-shaped segments with decorative shapes surrounding it. He is happiest when left alone to do his own work at his own pace."

February he's lost the job because he's simply too disorganized to handle it.

When I visit Frank that month and we take a booth at a crowded restaurant, he asks to switch places so he can watch the door. Are you nervous? I ask. No, he's just picking up on all the vibrations, "all the families," he says. We eat in silence. After some clothes shopping, we go to a Starbucks, where I bring up the question of his beginning to consider what he wants to do after Earth House. "How much longer do I have?" he asks. "Three months?" I hope so, I tell him. He goes silent.

"How have you been?" he asks me for a second time.

"Do you mean spiritually or physically?"

"Both," he says.

"I've been very sad since my cat died."

When I'd arrived that day, a black-and-white cat was on the prowl outside the Earth House office. It reminded me so much of Dexter, Alice's and my cat at home who coincidentally entered my life around the time of Franklin's teenage breakdown. After suffering from diabetes for some time, Dexter had to be put down and I'd buried him in the backyard. Frank knew Dexter and was sorry to hear this, then asks how another family cat named Jake is doing. I am forced to tell him that Jake had passed awhile back.

Back at Earth House, all the other students have gone on an outing. Frank is living in the downstairs of a cottage, and the door is open. He says he's very tired and wants to take a nap. Fine, I say, I'll read for awhile in the hall. Sudden snow flurries commence outside. I'm sitting in a chair with my book, not far from my son's room, when I hear someone talking and wonder where it's coming from. Then I realize it must be Franklin talking in his sleep. I walk to his slightly ajar door and listen. I can make out the words: "John F. Kennedy . . . brothers and sisters . . . you have a lot of potential." It's as if he's reporting to someone about our earlier conversation. While I hadn't mentioned Kennedy, I did speak to Frank about his potential and my wish that he could do something he enjoys.

I'm already somewhat spooked by his sleep-talk when, sitting down again, I notice a stuffed black-and-white cat from a toy store perched on a white blanket on a nearby dresser. I get up and press a hand onto the cat's back, as if to pet it. "Meow . . . meow . . . meow . . ." it squeaks back loudly. I'm startled, and I don't know how to make the godawful sound stop. Mercifully, it ceases after the sixth meow. More shaken than before, I hear Frank starting to talk again inside his room. I peek in the door. He's lying on the bed on his back, knees up in the air, hands folded across his chest. I detect the phrase, "mother and father," and the tone feels almost religious. But this monologue ends quickly. Outside, the snow flurry also stops as immediately as it began.

I stand there, alone in the empty hallway, trying to catch my breath. I feel caught—dare I say—between dimensions.

> Then the young hero said one day to the cat, "Why are you a cat?" And she said, "Don't ask me yet. Ask me some other time. I hate to live in the world. Let's go together to your father." Again she took her whip and made a sound with the whip in all three directions and the fiery carriage came, so they arrived at his home in it.
>
> —From the Romanian fairy tale, *The Cat*[2]

• • •

> Live my life for God. Is that odd.
> Going for the streams of gold. My heart isn't cold.
> Fishermen cast into the ocean. A life filled with emotion.
> Each man has strength inside. Send me love to live by.
> Beautiful are the rays of sun. Find the reason start to run.
> Rectify your complex life. Love your kids and love your wife.
> When conflict comes your way, be like a tree bending but not breaking.
> Believe in yourself every morning. Move your soul with earnest yearning.
> —Franklin's Journal, ten years earlier

I'm losing sleep exploring different possibilities for my son to remain at Earth House. I place a call to Deborah. After discussing the money situation and the inability of my brother to continue to help, I'm clearly anxious about Frank's future. The program director finally says she has something to tell me. She sounds very serious and I steel myself for bad news.

"There is someone who wants to donate for Franklin for the next year and a half," Deborah says.

I can hardly believe my ears. She proceeds to relate an amazing story. After Frank lost his gas station job, at a group meeting he began talking about how he wants to join the military (a recurring theme with him, perhaps because of the discipline and focus it would require?). An Earth House staffer who'd been in the Coast Guard said the military wouldn't take people who have been diagnosed with a mental illness. At which point, Franklin made an eloquent and moving plea. "Please don't throw me out," he said. He loved being at Earth House and wanted to stay forever and didn't want to go back to a group home in Massachusetts. Deborah says it brought tears to her eyes.

Afterward, a female student came up to her. She felt "very connected" to Franklin, she said; her family was "loaded" and she wanted to ask her sister, who handled her trust fund, to pay for Frank to remain.

"That's incredible," I say, in a whisper.

It's not definite yet, Deborah continues, and Franklin can never know. I should keep it confidential and only tell Etta. "This was like a gift from God," Deborah adds.

"My father is coming to see me today," Frank says to a counselor prior to my March visit. She tells me that he's not yet changed the black jeans I got him a few weeks ago, and perhaps I could suggest that it's time for him to do some laundry. "You're the man!" he exclaims when we say good-bye that afternoon. His blood sugar is in the normal range and his blood pressure is good, too.

Then the roof falls in again.

A board of trustees that ultimately controls the girl's finances has turned down her request on my son's behalf. When I arrive at Earth House early on a Sunday afternoon and go to look for Frank in his room, a freckle-faced, auburn-haired girl informs me that he's moved back to the bigger house. I ask her name. "Lisa," she says. I nod and introduce myself. "I'm so sorry it didn't work out," she says. I know you tried, I say. "I learned a lesson," she says. I look at her quizzically. "That I don't have as much control over my money as I thought I did," she adds. I say I know she acted from the heart, and how much I appreciated it. "I just hope he finds a place where he will be happy," she says, and her tone breaks my own heart. "I'm trying to work it out," I stammer in response, "for him to stay here another three months." How I will be able to do that, I haven't a clue.

At lunch that day with Frank, he says that, after Earth House, he'd like to take a welding course and perhaps move to "a warm climate" like the Navajo reservation in Arizona. Incredibly, my son is down to a 34 waist size; our weights are now the same. His hair is wild and he's growing something of a beard. He speaks of living in the sixth dimension, and of my need to "consult the leprechaun" before making an upcoming research trip to Ireland on the Hillman biography. (In 2005, on my initial such trip with Alice in the company of Hillman and his wife, while driving toward Donegal through one remarkable stretch of western Ireland, we were all certain that the "little people" lived under the wispy-branched trees. But Frank knew nothing of this.) He writes out some symbols in Chinese that he calls "the language of trees." He's soon stringing words and themes together so fast that there's no way I can keep up. I simply laugh. He smiles.

After picking up a headset and a book on welding, Frank says as we drive back: "These last nine years, I've been in a self-imposed prison." What do you mean? I ask. "Since I had my breakdown. Which has meant I've had a lot of time alone." A little later, he adds something he's never said before: "Thank you for your commitment." Would I like to come up to his room? We do, but his rather large roommate is sound asleep. "Want to go play some basketball?" he asks. How could I say no?

On the way out, as we pass a tall fellow about his age, Frank thrusts his arm out in his direction. The young man jumps, seemingly afraid Frank might be planning to strike him, but instead my son exclaims, "Hugs!" And that's what they exchange. We find a ball with just enough air and Frank suggests we drive to a nearby park. We take turns shooting hoops for about twenty minutes. "I'm really grateful to have parents who care," he says as we pull into Earth House again. For me, another internal *wow*. Finally it's time to say good-bye. "Well, this was really fun," I say as he gets out of the car. "It really was," he says. Watching him walk down the path back toward his house, I couldn't have been happier. Franklin is always the unexpected, my biggest unknown in life. And how far he has come!

But time is closing in on us again. At the end of April, Frank shaves all his hair off. At my request, Deborah calls Lisa's sister about funding my son for a short

> Earth House Progress Notes for March: "He excels at reading Shakespeare with alertness and comprehension…he is the reigning ping-pong champion in the class!" When Etta visits him, he introduces her to several people as his mother. She writes me: "He was so happy to see me and gave me a big hug—a real one. First time for that in a very long time."

while longer. The answer is an emphatic no: "This would affect Lisa adversely." Deborah says it's all about greed, and suggests I give my brother one more try. I do, but he says he's had to close two of his offices. It's due to lenders and hedge fund people, a foreign realm to me. Everyone he knows is scared, Bob says. The financial debacle of 2008 is closing in, too, less than a half-year into the future.

I'm forced to turn back to the state mental health system in Massachusetts. In a long talk with a woman from the DMH, she speaks of the tragedy of having to be wealthy to get good care. No new money has come into the department for a decade. Currently there are no spots available in group homes. The "homeless shelter transition" isn't quite as bad as I'd imagined, but Frank would be rooming with up to eight men while waiting for something else to open up. No way I'll do that to him. But if he moves home with me, that erases his name from the priority list for housing altogether.

Several of my closest friends on Fort Hill—all of whom have set aside trust funds for their own children—agree to pool resources and foot the bill at Earth House for Frank for another three months.

> The World has Yet to be Really Built: One man can build something based on his individual capacity and capability. A group is a vehicle from which the combined efforts of people can bring a goal into fruition.
> —Franklin's Journal

Before long, though, the Earth House psychiatrist tells me that Franklin's delusions have worsened over the past month or so. We discuss how anxious he is about his future. When I see Frank next, he asks about everyone on Fort Hill and says he's realized he was always moving too fast and "took up too much space" to live there. Etta doesn't want to bring him to her home in Brooklyn, because the neighborhood is far too dangerous. For a time the Earth House team looks into ways that Frank might remain in the area, perhaps sharing an apartment with another young man who'd left the program or even with a staff member. None of this, however, pans out.

Earth House Progress Notes for June: "Occasionally, just when he seems so withdrawn, he will come out with the most profound and/or insightful observation. He is a complex individual."

Options are again running out when a wealthy friend in Cambridge says she will loan me $25,000, which I can pay back over time with the anticipated royalties from my latest book.

He has now been there for more than a year when I pass the road sign—"You are entering the Township of Franklin"—and shortly thereafter pull into the Earth House

> Earth House Progress Notes for August: "His section of the Diego Rivera [mural project] included a large bunch of Jalapeno peppers in bright tropical colors."

parking lot. Very glad to see me, my son reports he is "too old" to go off his medication in the future. "I'll never get as high again, no matter how bad a medication I'm on," he says. It's an interesting juxtaposition of phrase, and I believe him.

At a meeting that Etta and I attend, officials from the DMH say an opening is expected soon in a small group home near Somerville's Union Square. There's a questionnaire that Frank is required to fill out. "What is your disability?" is the first question. He writes down in block letters, "Paranoid schizophrenic." I bring up his leaving Earth House in the relatively near future. "Nothing is forever," Frank says.

Once again he discusses his interest in welding. Of course he says he knows how to do it already, but wouldn't want to find a welding job without a "refresher" unless it was "psychoclysmic." I raise my eyebrows. "Cataclysmic?" I ask. "No, that means destructive," Frank responds with a chuckle, adding that the word he'd just invented means "outside yourself."

As we pull into an Italian place for coffee, Frank looks at me and asks: "Your boys?" The next day, I mention this at home to my friend Melinda. She has known and loved Franklin since he was a baby, and in some ways identified with him. She believes that the Mafia image often referenced by Franklin is "protective"—choosing a type of family where he's included in something so secure and powerful that he can never lose. All of his fantasy images describe a need, she points out. And it's up to me to learn how to translate that language and speak to him from there.

Accompanied by Kamal and Etta, we visit Frank simultaneously. He plays the piano for us. When Etta praises the fact that I still have all my hair, our son suggests that I get a Mohawk cut. The four of us laugh together. Etta emails me afterward: "It was a great visit. Very reassuring.

I love the way Franklin is with you. I think that you really help him to have a good sense of his manhood. Seeing the two of you together was so clear—how much a young man needs his father. I tend to 'mother' him too much and will have to learn to let go more. He looks great—this has been some year for him."

After Etta departs early that afternoon, Frank and I are driving along when I recall the story he'd once told me, about the genie who came to him that night a few years back while he was living alone in Somerville. "Oh yeah, he was from Jupiter!" he exclaims. He "actually looked kind of like a hornet" and was no taller than the dashboard. He then mentions the different time zone that he himself lives in, where forty years can be packed into a single day—and that our approaches are really from two different dimensions. He adds, in terms of his future, that he knows I've been working very hard for him. Yes, I sure have, I say. "Well, I've been working hard for you, too," he says. And I don't doubt that he's right.

When the bureaucracy at the Somerville Housing Authority delays Frank's moving back to the Boston area, he shrugs and says only, "That's the price of the pudding." And the fact is: nobody wants him to leave Earth House. The director offers to let Frank remain another month for half-price. But when it seems there will be a room in Somerville ready for him as of early October, it feels like time to stop postponing the inevitable.

Through generosity I can never truly repay, Franklin spent sixteen months at Earth House that had changed his life. I get there shortly before 10 a.m. and Deborah gives me a big hug. Etta arrives shortly thereafter. Franklin is packed up and ready to load his things into my car. First, though, the staff and about a half-dozen other students all gather in a circle off the dining area. His drama teacher recalls seeing "the least and the most" that Franklin could be, and the impromptu acting performance he'd given while wading in the water one day, and how good he was at reading Shakespeare aloud. Each student speaks to Frank about what he's meant to their lives, of his insights and how he's helped them at key times. Lisa is in tears. She coaches Frank not to get "too analytical," and says how much she will miss him. He, in turn, warmly addresses each of them.

As the farewell ceremony draws to a close and he's presented with a Certificate of Achievement, one of the students says: "You *are* Earth House, Franklin." His mother and I are, of course, moved to tears as well. And faced once again with the agonizing question: where does he, where do we, go from here?

> If you are trying to cross a river, you take a boat. If you have no boat you either make one or swim. If you can't swim then grab onto a log. If there are no logs then swing from a vine. If you do not succeed then try again. If you do not succeed a second time then ask your neighbor how you will cross the river. If he does not know then ask someone else. If the whole world doesn't know how to cross that river then you will either have to give up or invent a new way. You invent because you need. You need because you desire.
>
> —Franklin's Journal

Notes:

1. "But the brilliance....": Fitzgerald quote: cited in Edwin Fuller Torrey, *The Invisible Plague: The Rise of Mental Illness from 1750 to the Present*, p. 293.
2. "Then the young hero said one day to the cat....": Marie-Louise von Franz, *The Cat: A Tale of Feminine Redemption*, Inner City Books, 1999, p. 19.

CHAPTER 7

• • •

Back to Boston

*If you are deep as a person, it is sort of like living with your feet in mud for
four hours each day. The other part of the day is spent in cleaning the feet off.*
—Franklin's Journal

T HE CLOSER WE GET TO Boston, the more agitated Frank becomes.
He's been plucking pieces of hair on both sides of his face for
awhile and, when we walk in the door on Fort Hill a little before
5 p.m., his eyes are starting to roll up in his head. But he's very
happy to see Alice and Eddie. The next morning I drive him to his
new house just up the street from the Somerville police headquar-
ters at Union Square. The other three men on his floor seem pretty
low-functioning; one has lived there for nineteen years. I go to get
Frank some furnishings while he does grocery shopping with one of
the staff members, while another sorts his large number of vitamins
from Earth House.

I realize this will not be an easy transition after the full days and
energy of Earth House, but I've enrolled him for some free computer
and gym classes at Boston University's free Center for Psychiatric
Rehabilitation. Reluctantly, Frank agrees to see his former DMH
therapist. She is very impressed with his weight loss; he speaks of
being on Clozaril now as making an "atomic difference" inside him.
Afterward the doctor tells me privately that it's so vital to compensate
for the glaring deficiencies of the health care system by doing what
I'm doing.

But when he sees another doctor for a physical, she takes him off all but four of the nineteen vitamins he'd been taking while at Earth House. Apparently Frank told her that he didn't need them anymore. At a nearby restaurant, Frank becomes immediately defensive when I mention my concern that he not slip back to how he'd been functioning prior to Earth House. He's testy in response, saying he's actually working very hard. Later he decides his name isn't really Frank (again!) and, when I drop him off, is talking about being a gun-runner and a gang-banger. I drive home pissed-off, frustrated, wondering if my son is simply going to return to his old ways.

On the way to his class at BU, he starts singing, quite beautifully, in a made-up Asian language. It's the first time I've heard him sing in some time. Later we drive to the Carpenters Union Apprenticeship Building, where Frank fills out an application. He's thrilled and tempers all kinds of wild thoughts that follow, saying he doesn't know why he's talking so much and he shouldn't be.

He wants to have lunch at old familiar places, including a Thai restaurant near where he lived at Eikos almost a decade earlier. He likes the place "because it's dingy." Had I ever been to China? he asks. No, but I describe having recently watched the movie *Mongol*. He's seen it, too. "The Year of the Snake," he adds. The snake motif will arise on several occasions over the coming months. Frank will tell me that he'd been headmaster at a school where they served snakes for lunch. What kind? I ask. "Red snake and a yellow-tailed basket snake," he responds, quickly and specifically. Another time after I'd been away for a couple of months, I return to find that he's painted snake-eyes on his bedroom windows, for fear the hydra was going to come after him. "You know, Adam and Eve, the snake," he says.

The Asian theme is another that persists. At Franklin's favorite restaurant, Fugakyu, he talks to the Japanese proprietor about the beauty of the bamboo shades. A cute waitress now recognizes us and remembers that Frank probably wants a Sapporo or a Kirin beer as well as a fork to accompany the chopsticks. "There's only a thin line between a person and a pagoda," my son informs her, then explains to me that it's difficult being both Chinese and Japanese because people expect you to serve them fish when what you wanted was to give them technology. He's talking about learning how to weld again, which he maintains he did in Japan but needs to brush up on. Instead, early in 2009,

Frank starts taking pottery classes near his house. One day, after filling out some local Housing Authority forms using rectangular block
Chinese-style characters, he tells me he "didn't think it was something
I should be reprimanded for." Not that I had, but the forms would
require a fresh start.

A month after his return to Boston, I ask whether Frank misses
Earth House. Yes, some: "I got a lot out of that place." We decide to
drive to New Jersey the next Sunday for a visit, about a five-hour trip
in sparse traffic. His friend Lisa is there and I take the three of us to
lunch. She tells a story about one of the Earth House students who
recently ran off in a car his parents gave him and drove all the way to
California, where he cracked up the vehicle in the desert and it was
nine days before someone found him, dehydrated but alive.

"Do you have displaced anger?" she asks Franklin. Yes, does she?
Lisa is not sure. She gives Frank some advice, to keep his spine lim-
bered up. When we drop her off (he doesn't want Lisa accompanying
us to do some clothes shopping), Frank says to me: "She's a sweet girl."
It warms my heart to see him like this with someone. He thanks me
for bringing him on this trip. But on the way home, we get as far as
Connecticut when it starts to grow dark and he begins picking at his
face and says that something in the car is trying to suck his blood. I
hadn't known him to experience this kind of psychotic episode in a
long while, but he seems okay by the time we get back to his house in
Somerville. However, this marks the last time he will see Lisa. By the
following summer, she will have returned to her family's horse ranch
down south. My suggestions that Frank call her sometime are met with
a shrug.

"I know what it is now about people in Boston: they come here
to pass away," Frank says. Right after our visit to Earth House, he calls
to say he can't handle going to classes at the BU Center anymore. He
wants to stay home and write. I argue with him about the exercise
he's been getting, but finally say that it's his decision and I can't force
him to go. Nor does he want to come for Thanksgiving on Fort Hill,
feeling that the adults still treat him like a child and don't know his
"real" age. Next time we're at lunch, he does a drawing for me of my
"totem animal"—a barracuda!

His interview for an apprenticeship comes up with the Carpenters
Union. Several hundred other guys are there for the same thing, and

the wait is long. I stand outside in the cold until he's done. Afterward, Frank says the interview went well. He'd told them that sometimes he's Zen and sometimes he isn't, "which seemed to surprise them." A letter comes a week later from the Union, saying he'd not passed his interview but to realize that only 10 percent of applicants do. He doesn't seem to mind. At least he'd followed what his heart was set on.

• • •

Martha, of the DMH Community Treatment Team, is an older woman who's known and liked Frank for a long time. They continue to meet once a week, going for a bite or simply to drive around. Martha says he has seemed more reality-based; sometimes he'll make an outrageous comment, but then drop it. "There is good and bad in this change," she suggests, because he's also very quiet and seemingly struggling to find anything to say when he doesn't have his delusions to fall back on; he seems to be "reorganizing his brain."

Frank and I sit down for lunch at the Thai place when he looks across the table at me and asks: "What do you do when you feel bad?" I'm surprised at such a personal question. I respond that sometimes I just live with the feeling and accept it, other times I try to do something to change it, like taking a walk. He then confides that he's had a lot of anger inside him and also feels a lack of direction in his life. He recalls how difficult it can be sometimes to ride the waves, remembering a time years ago when he was visiting in Baja where he almost drowned. He asks, "What's the most pain you can feel, do you think?" In terms of physical pain, I answer, probably to be in an accident, but there's also emotional pain like heartbreak. He nods in agreement and then changes the subject. Did I know of a place called Pangaea, he wonders, where the continent of Europe was once joined to the Americas?

Even if Frank's jump to talking about Pangaea is inscrutable, for him to speak openly about his feelings and ask questions like this feels like a big step. My friend Melinda writes me in an email: "He is like a very rare butterfly, on a test run to see if his species can survive here. . . . I believe that one thing that happens in him is somehow there's a hole in his personal consciousness, which was—like, before birth—replaced by a huge flow of mass consciousness. It took him getting old enough to where he would actually approach the world on his own, for this bizarre combination to take effect, and really consume him—or, like a tidal river created by a flood rain, drag him under and sweep him out to sea. I think he's just starting to wash up on the sand now; barely breathing, but somehow he lived, survived the ordeal. All cheers to him."

> *How could you simply explain a life. Laughing and carrying on. That is too simple. Working and sleeping. Far too surface. Satisfying and full. That would be a dream. Dreary and worrisome. That is more like it. Then you need to add in the quality of time. That is what it really amounts to. Time and energy. It is all up to an individual how to spend their time. How to use their mind. How to mix and mingle. How to stand alone.*
>
> —Franklin's Journal

• • •

I don't know if my son's unusual sense of humor simply rubs off on me or whether he brings my own *out* of me. Maybe a little of both. He says he works for Genzyme now, seeking to cross a human and a kangaroo; he laughs when I say that would make people into fine jumpers. He recalls: "When I was younger, I would say things to you that were out of order. Definitely hospital-ready." And I crack up laughing. He says a new computer has been devised that fits in your brain and extends life ten times. That's pretty far-out, I say, or is it far-in? Passing along the Charles River, he notes it now contains the Loch Ness monster. Oh really? "Yes, I put it there," he says. I hope it doesn't knock over the crew race that's going on, I say. He doesn't do so many illegal things for the Mafia anymore, he says. Well, you're older and wiser, I suggest.

We seem to be connecting on new levels, including my corny jokes. Frank greets me with a hug. After I ask what he's doing these days, he replies, "typing." He mentions that nobody really knows what he—or I—go through, suffering over all the rewrites. He now thanks me on a regular basis, a big change. Drawing Asian-style symbols in my notebook, he glances up and says: "See if I can do it without tampering with your energy."

I'm away briefly when Etta writes that she'd seen Frank and "at several points he gave me his arm (to help me walk down the stairs!). It was the best time that I have had with him in a very long time." On another visit, he rubs her shoulders because her neck hurts. His new social worker, Mike, also relates to me a story about Frank's empathic nature, when my son accompanied him to the post office to mail a letter to a colleague whose wife had died.

He's reaching out in other ways, some of them surprising and amusing. Over lunch at an Applebee's one day, a couple pass by our table and express how good Frank's spinach and artichoke dip with nachos looks. "Have some," my son says. It's such a sincere gesture that the fellow replies, "This is very impolite, but . . ." and dips right in. "Not a problem," Frank says. Another time, Frank accompanies a couple from our family taking a dog for its shots. When the veterinarian appears, my son asks whether he's got any wolves for sale. Thankfully the vet treats Frank's question as perfectly plausible, engaging in further discussion as to where wolves customarily reside in Brookline Village.

He's getting exercise "but not enough," Frank says. So he goes on a three-mile walkathon with others from his house, a fundraising event for the National Alliance for the Mentally Ill. Not only is he getting out of his room more, he goes to a dinner and dance with others from his house. Regularly he sits in the downstairs office and draws and hangs out with staff, as well as a woman who has a thrift store next door. He's learned how to cope with his down times: "If everything's going right, what's the point?" Frank postulates one day.

One summer day, we hop in the car together and drive to Philadelphia to visit his relatives on Etta's side. Checking into a hotel, Franklin flops down on the bed and exclaims: "This is fantastic! We made it and we're happy!" Etta and Kamal are already there, and soon her mother and two sisters arrive. One of them, Carol, who has long had difficulties similar to Frank's, hangs out with him alone in our room for a bit. "God is good," she responds when I ask how she's doing. That night, Carol explains that she'd been a go-go dancer before she found Jesus, and can't go in restaurants where they serve alcohol or play a certain kind of music. So she decides to wait outside. Franklin, in particular, understands.

At almost eighty-six, Etta's mother is sharp as a tack and loves to laugh, and Frank rises to the occasion. The banter is wonderful, starting with my son expressing that he hopes the parmesan cheese served in a fancy bowl "comes from cows." Etta's other sister, Jerri, had stayed with us for awhile on Fort Hill in the mid-1990s, and Frank is thrilled to see her again. It means a great deal to him—and to them—having family together like this. At breakfast the next day, he calls Etta "mom" and, after first describing Fort Hill to me as "your family," he corrects the phrase to "our family."

Even his "delusions" seem to be taking on a more related character. Alice has had a hip replacement early in 2010; asking about how she's recovering, Frank makes a drawing of a motorized device that she could attach to improve her speed. He's concerned about the environment and tells me about a new fuel he's invented (hydrogen mixed with acetylene creating a new form of propane), as well as several cars including the Afro Beacon, Toyota Spurt, and Deluge, the last running on a combination of steam and electric. Not knowing that two family members are consuming wheat grass as part of a cleansing raw food diet, Frank says he's gotten into growing the gluten-free product.[1]

Frank gets talking about different kinds of clocks for different parts of the world, including the Sun Dial for American Indians and the beetle clock in one unnamed country (perhaps Germany, where the VW beetle clocks came from, I learn online). This is all in the context of a discussion about time, and my wanting things done "facilitatively." That was the same word that a psychiatrist friend had just used in a conversation with me. Somehow, Frank picks such fragments out of thin air . . . or the unconscious.

His experiencing periodic problems with his eyes rolling upward, Frank says, coincide with someone on the street doing "white magic" by waving their arms in a certain way. I tell him that I wouldn't rule that out.

• • •

A restructuring of providers contracted by the Department of Mental Health has occurred. Until now, Cascap, Inc., a nonprofit that provides affordable community housing for adults diagnosed with mental illness, has been in charge of Frank's place in Somerville. Now the larger Vinfen human services corporation is taking on the oversight. There are no plans to move anyone. A new program director will take over, but other staff will remain. One of the worst things about such changes, in terms of consistency for residents, is the ongoing turnover. So many times I've seen Franklin's frustration when someone leaves whom he's just gotten to know and trust. Now, at a meeting with the new "management," Franklin says he's concerned about "vampire types" in the mental health system, and recounts an incident where he'd been hospitalized by one such type after a fight at Aberdeen House.

What is it about the vampire metaphor, which often appears with individuals diagnosed as schizophrenic? One website, titled "The Facts About Vampires," notes in a section on their psychology that "they live alone or in small groups; they are forever hunted by the peoples from which they arose—including people they might have known personally.... They also have an understanding that they are different. It is not surprising that vampires often show signs of deep psychosis, experience mood swings, and gross personality changes. It is for the hunter to understand these rival pressures and find consequent weaknesses that can be exposed." So it seems that perhaps the persistent metaphor may be part of a "reverse psychology."

As has happened numerous times in Franklin's life when he's going through a change, it's accompanied by differentiation in hairstyles. My journal entries from this post-Earth House period find his hair "upfront braided," "back to bushy Afro," "one whole side of his head shaved—did it himself—beneath the wildly curling hair above," and "long hair tied in back like Eddie does, with a couple of upward curls in front."

Sometime later, I will come across a study by several psychiatrists in the Netherlands, which reported "manipulation of the physical appearance" as having "a special place in the phenomenology of schizophrenia," with "drastic changes in hairstyle" associated with the "disorganized type" that Franklin often exhibited. In numerous instances, hospitalized schizophrenic patients "were found to have shaved their heads or cut their hair just before or during admission," the patients later maintaining that "the radical changes in their appearance were made in an attempt to maintain identity ..."[2]

• • •

As we drive along, Frank points out a couple of buildings that he's constructed "with Edward." When Frank calls Eddie to invite him to visit, and Ed responds "well, maybe I'll come with your dad," Frank responds: "Oh no! I can't handle both of you at the same time!" I guess oversight, whether by parent or mentor, only goes so far.

What the therapists might call his "reality orientation" is assuredly different since Earth House—even when it comes to his psychiatrist, of whom Frank astutely states: "She doesn't believe what I say, or even *pretend* she does." As we pass through a very confusing rotary, Frank keeps his wits about him and locates the address we're looking for—where I would undoubtedly have gotten lost. Inside an REI store, he seeks a needle and thread for sewing a pair of pants—another practicality where I'd surely strike out. Given his progress, Frank is now allowed to inventory his own medications.

Sometimes, though, reality can bring unanticipated reactions. Etta and Kamal have decided to get married in a private ceremony. When she visits Frank over Christmas and informs him, at first he's very pleased. But then he becomes terribly sad—"I wish I had somebody; I have nobody"—and can't shake it, though he's in better spirits the next day. Yet this, to me, is actually a positive response. There is nothing delusional about it, and perhaps the honesty of the feeling can itself lead to a difference in his situation. This is true as well when, on another visit, Frank tells his mother "I feel like I'm ready for the home." He's pretty clearly referring to a nursing home for the elderly; living with all these older and more dysfunctional men, while keeping to himself more often in his room, can't be helping to maintain a positive attitude. When I next see him, Frank is unusually indecisive about where he wants to go. At Applebee's, he wants to leave right away because the overhead light distracts his eyes. I speak to his doctor; yes, being on 500 milligrams of Clozaril can be a contributing factor. The lethargic effects of the medication remain a terrible reality, too.

Yet, all in all, I dare to believe that he's "better"—perhaps, as he grows older, coming more into his own. I don't feel as concerned about leaving him as I once did. Frank himself seems able to take comings and goings more in stride. I'm soon to head west, and he asks whether I'll be coming back in mid-September, and I say that I'm planning on it. Frank responds: "Planning! Well, don't rush into it. I learned that from you—and from life." He asks if I'd help him clean his room, which is a mess after the house was struck by a bedbug infestation and everything had to be moved around. "One thing at a time, Franklin," he says, suddenly referring to himself in the third person. "You're not four years old anymore, you're thirty-one!"

• • •

I'd been in New York over the previous weekend. James Hillman is very ill, with a diagnosis of lung cancer, and in a hospital for treatment there. I'd spent several days visiting him and going over questions regarding the latest chapters toward my finishing his biography.

Now, when I bring up the trip with Frank, he responds: "Oh right. He wrote *The Human Genome*."

I pause for a moment before replying: "Well, no, actually he wrote *The Soul's Code*."

"That's what I *mean*!" my son exclaims.

I start to laugh, despite the sad situation surrounding Hillman's illness. "You're way out ahead of me, as usual, Franklin," I say. "Sometimes," he responds. At his house, he gives me a complicated triple handshake good-bye, and I happily manage to keep up.

Another time, returning from a quick trip to the Cape, Frank recalls once reading Hillman's *The Soul's Code* with an older family member and suggests that the title of another of James Hillman's books was *Gentleman Jim*. "That's probably what a lot of people think of him as," I say with a chuckle. Later, telling Hillman these two stories, he finds them wonderfully amusing. "That makes my day," he says.

Frank and I are talking more personally than I can remember. He asks twice about Alice and wonders whether we're going to have a baby. "Well, Frank, I think we might be a little too old for that," I say. But it's a poignant moment; I remember him bringing up when younger that he wanted a brother or sister. He had no direct blood relations, except for cousins. Now, when I say I hoped he didn't think being raised among so many other kids was too bad, Frank replies: "Oh no, it was a good way to have grown up"—even though one older boy had once gone after him with an ax and another had tried to get him to stick his hand in an electric socket. The things a parent never knew about!

Again I express regret for having been absent so often during his early years, but you can't bring back the past. He agrees. "You traded adventure for a lot of knowledge," he says without judgment. Does he mean "adventure" in terms of raising him? Does he mean I traded knowledge of him for the adventure of the lifestyle I chose, but he said it backward? I still puzzle over that statement.

• • •

Discovery and discovery, unity, understanding, understanding, intuition, inexplicable, indisturbable, inextinguishable. . . .

—Franklin's Journal

Etta and Kamal are planning a move to Baltimore, to a better neighborhood where the rent is half of what they're paying in New York. Frank seems okay with this, although it's going to mean a longer distance between them. At the same time, with Frank's okay, Etta and I are designated as his co-guardians, along with the current female lawyer in Cambridge. This means that his doctors will be able to speak freely about Frank with us.

I dream about being with Franklin, Etta, and Kamal, all jammed into a room of a seedy hotel, where Frank pokes fun at my somewhat rotund stomach. There are other dreams as well, during the long months when my psychological mentor James Hillman is fighting for life. In another, Frank has asked me to look in his mouth. At first I didn't notice, then am startled to realize that he's had all his teeth pulled out. *How is he going to eat? How could he get to a dentist immediately to get false teeth? How could he have withstood the pain?*

In another dream, Frank is in an Earth House–type of school with other young people and appears in a play that I've come to see, although it's not clear whether he's actually learned his lines.

In yet another dream, I'm at a clinic meeting with some doctors, who tell me of their determination that not only was a misplaced gene causing Franklin's schizophrenia, but also something alive, like a bug. Frank has come to the same conclusion and told the doctors about it. I realize that I need to look into doing something about this right away. At which time a small car pulls up alongside me. Franklin is driving and Etta is in the passenger's seat, a bit frightened it seems but none the worse for wear.

• • •

That fall, I make a research trip to Europe for the Hillman biography, ending up in the archives of a place called Eranos. The word *eranos* comes from the ancient Greek, meaning a "picnic" or "spiritual feast," where guests are presented a gift in the form of a song or poem or improvised speech. For more than thirty years, the annual Eranos conferences had taken place in the little town of Ascona, overlooking the Swiss portion of Lake Maggiore facing the Italian Alps. Initially organized by Carl Jung, these gatherings had drawn many of the twentieth century's leading thinkers: philosophers, theologians, anthropologists, ethnologists, and mythologists. Hillman delivered psychological lectures here between 1966 and 1987.

The librarian tells me candidly that sometimes overnight guests have a difficult time sleeping. It's no coincidence that Jung had once placed a stone monument in an Eranos garden with a carved Greek inscription *Genio Loci Ignoto*, meaning "to the unknown spirit of the place." There are presences here, sometimes spectral ones. Many visitors can't handle it, and simply leave.

I'm spending the night in Casa Gabriella, where either Jung or Hillman or perhaps both once stayed, in a room with a balcony overlooking the lake. I soak in the majestic view for a long time. A half-moon, with one bright star to its left, is the last image I remember before reluctantly going to bed, at which point the dreams begin. Many, many dreams. . . . Franklin appears in two of them. He's voluntarily back in the grim corridors of Shattuck Hospital and I'm calling Etta to tell her. Then, with my son present, I am talking with some professors. My task, they tell me, is to unlock a secret about mental illness that he carries.

In the middle of the night, I awaken in an incredible state of vertigo, something I don't recall ever experiencing before. The dizziness is so extreme that I'm not sure if I can stand and walk to the bathroom or whether this might be a prolonged condition. How much time goes by that night before the sensation passes, I have no idea.

The next day I take a train through the Alps with a Jungian analyst, Christa Robinson, who'd been involved with Eranos for some years. I end up telling her about Franklin. She's worked with a number of schizophrenics. They live in the soul world, she says, out of time. When she wants to know whether a rumor might be true that a clinic patient wants to commit suicide, she doesn't ask the other doctors. She asks the schizophrenics, because they're much more attuned.

• • •

When a mind is scattered it will not be able to translate the feelings from the heart. The heart is important. If you are aware of how to contact it in its pure form you will avoid chaos.

—Franklin's Journal

As the months go by, I experience too many psychic interactions with Franklin for these to be simply coincidences. So many, indeed, that I almost cease to be dumbfounded . . . but not quite.

"Have you watched any good TV lately?" Franklin asks.

"Yes, there was a pretty good movie I saw."

State of Play. He gives the title before I can verbalize it. But no, he hadn't seen it.

On the way to pick up Frank, I pass by the Elephant Walk restaurant, a very nice place with French-Cambodian fare. Somehow, despite my son's affinity for Asian, I've never taken him there. I think I should sometime. He's waiting for me outside his house. "Where would you like to go?" I ask. "How about the Elephant Walk?" he responds.

"That's just what I've been *thinking*!" I say. Franklin chuckles heartily.

On the Mass Turnpike, I've just been thinking about Miguel, a young man in our family, when Frank points to a passing vehicle. "I sold Miguel one of those," he says.

"What's your favorite book?" Frank asks. I've been reading a biography of Henry Miller, one of my favorite writers. *Tropic of Capricorn*, Frank responds for me. That was the first Miller book that I'd ever read.

"Franklin, you're amazing, do you have a direct path into my brain?"

No, he says, but often he feels things.

When I jot down something he says in my notebook, he glances at me saying: "For the book we're doing, eh?" This book had not even been conceived back then.

If in my eyes he is somebody special, that's what counts, he says. He sure as hell is. And our burgeoning relationship is soon to take an unforeseen and remarkable turn.

Far to the south-east, Kilimanjaro was humped and crouched along its 19,000-foot summit, under a far greater burden of snow. I thought what an artist Africa is in the way it displays its great mountains. The greatest of them are never jumbled together as they are in Switzerland, the Himalayas or the Caucasus. They are set in great open spaces and around them are immense plains, rolling uplands and blue lakes like seas, so that they can see and be seen and take their proper place in the tremendous physical drama of Africa.

—Laurens van der Post, *Venture to the Interior*

Notes:

1. Consumption of wheat grass dates back to ancient Egyptians, who allegedly found sacred the young leafy blades of wheat, prizing them for their positive impact on health and vitality.
2. "Schizophrenia and Changes in Physical Appearance": *Journal of Clinical Psychiatry 59:4,* April 1998.

PART 2

. . .

Africa

Africa is mystic; it is wild; it is a sweltering inferno; it is a photographer's paradise, a hunter's Valhalla, an escapist's Utopia. It is what you will, and it withstands all interpretations. It is the last vestige of a dead world or the cradle of a shiny new one. To a lot of people, as to myself, it is just "home." It is all these things but one thing—it is never dull.
—Beryl Markham, *West with the Night*, 1942

CHAPTER 8

• • •

Foreshadowings

I am the drummer, this is my song. I am so full of music that I wouldn't steer you wrong....

So gather round people as I compose beautiful sounds. It will make your head spin, 'round and 'round. Up and down!
—Franklin's Journal, circa 1997, titled "The Drummer"

MORE THAN FORTY YEARS EARLIER, I had ended up in Africa when there seemed no place else to go. Raised in the suburbs of Minneapolis, Chicago, and Kansas City, my adolescence had been consumed with watching and writing about sports. In college, I'd awakened to larger realities of the late 1960s—the Vietnam War, the civil rights movement, close friends becoming hippies. Before I graduated from the University of Kansas, I'd landed my dream job as a reporter on the staff of *Sports Illustrated* in New York. But I ended up staying there less than a year. My interests had broadened; I wanted to explore and write about the radical changes going on in the world. I quit the magazine and ended up traveling overseas for a year and a half with a backpack and a portable typewriter, the first six months exploring various "hip scenes" in Europe.

During one memorable night in Paris, I traveled somewhere else. It was late November 1970, and I was twenty-three. I'd been gathering research for an article about the American Students and Artists Center, a European haven for outstanding black cultural talent. In the context of this I met Elsa, originally from Kenya and regarded among the finest African dancers in the "City of Light." After I watched one of her classes, we talked for about four hours one afternoon. The subjects ranged from the differences between black Americans and black Africans to the initiation rites of the Maasai tribe, to which Elsa belonged. "When you dance," I said, "you look to me like you go into a trance." She nodded and said not many people noticed that. By the time we parted company, she'd invited me to a private voodoo séance. I was told to meet her Friday night in an alley just to the side of the Moulin Rouge.

Elsa hadn't shown by our appointed rendezvous hour of 11 p.m., so I worked my way down a deserted alley until I came to two red doors with a yellow light shining from within. A letter box was barely visible. "Voudou," it said. The doors were not locked and I entered into a surprisingly large space, with about twenty-five people eating and drinking at a number of tables. I was greeted by two young black girls wearing long blue dresses, each with a tunic around their head. They took me across the room to meet a beautiful older woman, dressed completely in white. "*Je suis un ami de Elsa?*" I said. "Yes," she replied. "Elsa phoned ahead and told us to expect you. She will be here soon." The woman, I would learn later, was Matilda, the ceremony's high priestess. Two men were pounding conga drums as I was led to a table.

It was not long before Elsa arrived with several friends. Briefly, Matilda explained what we were about to witness. She had made the practice of voodoo ritual her life's work. It was a right, bestowed upon her by the spirits. She was Haitian and so were all of the girls in blue, who ranged in age from thirteen to seventeen and had also been trained in the art.

The taller of the two drummers was to act as "medium" for the ceremony. He accompanied Matilda wherever she went. Although some type of ceremony was conducted here every night, this particular one was rare, occurring only a few times a year. Tonight, six people, all white, would be initiated into the voodoo religion. All had been to Haiti and studied the practice for some time, and Matilda had deemed them ready. After the ceremony, they would go into seclusion for forty-eight hours. When they emerged, they would have been granted a power previously unknown to them. Sometimes, as with Elsa, this power had always been within them and was only accentuated after initiation. For others, it was an entirely new experience.

Only as time passed and the initiates mingled again with humanity would they realize what this particular power was. And they would not talk about it.

The message of whichever spirit might visit the séance tonight would be transmitted through the dance. It would be impossible for the dancers to lose the rhythm of the drum since the causal chain found the spirit possessing the drummer (medium), who in turn possessed the drum, which in turn possessed a certain dancer. The origins of the dance could be found in Dahomey, West Africa, as part of a ritual involving snake worship. Through the centuries the tradition had made its way to Haiti. The snake would be a central part of the ceremony. Elsa warned that I might go into a trance myself and, if it happened, should not fight it but just relax and wait; she would try to help me.

The guests all assembled in the center to dance with the Haitian girls and each other. There was much falling down, bumping of asses, laughing and sweating—the object being to make everyone relaxed. The Haitians then went through a short dance ritual exhorting all of us to finish our meals so the ceremony could begin. Shortly before 1:30 a.m., the medium walked to the center circle with a bowl of white chalk. The guests assembled outside the circle on straw chairs. Slowly, the medium began placing designs of four bisected lines along each corner of the room. Then he went into the middle and constructed an incredibly intricate design, which took about an hour. He finished with two snakes, male and female, on each side of the inner design. Elsa told me that the medium had had no idea of the design's context before he began. It was a product of his own knowledge combined with a spirit instructing him where to work. The bisected lines were crucial. If anyone stepped on one, it was a bad omen.

I sought more information, but Elsa only stared blankly at the chalk design. "I know I should help you," she said slowly. "But I . . . cannot . . . think . . . in English . . . right . . . now." She was entering a trance, and could no longer communicate. At last the medium returned to his drum. It was after 2 a.m. Lights were extinguished and candles were lit. The medium began to play. I would never forget the rhythm. *Ba-da-dada-dada-dadadadadada, bada-dada-dadada-dadada-dadada.* Over and over, the other drum blending with it. I began to feel very strange. Chanting and writhing to the music, the blue-clad assistants and the high priestess descended from some stairs behind the drummer. Matilda then stood before the drummer and raised a bottle of rum to her lips. Three times she spewed the rum from her mouth, a clean spray that wafted visibly into the air. Walking around the circle, she repeated this ritual twice more.

Afterward, I could not bring back all the details of the ceremony. I recalled a pumpkin being placed hard on my head. I remembered seeds being scattered and falling at my feet. The initiates, two women and four men, were blindfolded and led upstairs. The dancing continued. After fifteen minutes the initiates were led down again, now wearing white robes. Matilda took a forked piece of wood and lit it from the blazing rum-fire in a bowl. As she leaned to light the first end, I felt a chill ripple through me. Elsa had told me earlier, before she left this realm, that a sudden chill was indication of a new spirit, perhaps even one with whom I was already familiar, entering the room.

Now the initiates were led into the center and began dancing ecstatically around the fire. One fellow seemed particularly lost in it all. He had not struck me as a good dancer earlier in the evening; now he was shaking his upper body in a frenzied rhythm, which echoed that of the girls. Soon the six were seated in front of the drummer. One by one, when Matilda deemed them ready, they were led into the center again. She walked each through various symbolic steps, then a white sheet was thrust over their heads and they were left holding an outstretched candle. The guests assembled and kissed each one on both sheeted cheeks. For the last time, the initiates were led away, to enter their period of confinement.

Most of the guests left about this time. I, too, was tired. Elsa came out of her trance and departed with her friends. For some reason I stayed on. Perhaps ten people remained when, the clock approaching 3 a.m., the drummer-medium (who had not ceased playing) began to induce an ecstatic urge in the Haitian girls. Each of them writhed around the circle, in perfect time with the drum. Matilda was dancing also. Suddenly, she seemed seized with a violent convulsion. Thrown backward, she almost fell, regaining her balance as her tunic flew off— revealing beautiful black braids caressing her shoulders. Now another girl began to feel a similar sensation, only stronger. A strange agony came over her features. She seemed to cry, "Let me go!" Round and round she went, occasionally falling against one of the seated guests for support. I looked into Matilda's eyes. They showed a look of genuine concern. Something was going wrong and there was nothing false about it.

As the drum would echo a more powerful note, the medium would cry out. The girl would go absolutely mad, alone in the circle now, her friends watching in silence. She would cringe and flail, orgiastically, convulsively, falling against tables, keeping her balance only through the aid of outstretched hands. She was clearly possessed. Now another girl felt the same urge, though her movements were different. Matilda vanished momentarily. The same wild movements continued, ten minutes passing, twenty, thirty. The two girls remaining on their feet, my eyes mesmerized by them. Words could not describe the intensity of their expressions. Finally, exhausted, the second girl fell and was attended by her friends. Still the first "possessed" continued, oblivious to anything and everything. She would not, could not, stop. And then a spirit seized a third girl. The medium uttered a chilling cry. I saw the girl's upper body constrict and her face grimace in great pain.

She, too, entered the circle. She leaped toward a pillar and began ascending it. Matilda ran toward her. She beckoned me and another man, who must have weighed at least 200 pounds, to help try to pull the girl off the pillar. The girl's strength was unearthly. The three of us could scarcely contain her. At last we managed to free her and she floated away from us, her eyes incandescent. No training in the world could prepare a dancer for what I was witnessing. It was spontaneous, violent, all too real.

They tried various remedies and chants. Finally, they set a bowl of rum aflame in mid-circle. Matilda took me and the other remaining guests by the hand and led us toward it. The two possessed girls looked at us and knelt by the bowl, but seemed not to see us. Then one of them took my hand, staring right through me. My heart pounded fiercely. She placed her hand in the fire and came up with a flaming palm and set my own hand ablaze. I felt warmth but no pain. She did the same with my other hand, then rapidly rubbed my arms. A third time she set her hand on fire, this time going to my head and running the flames through my hair and down onto my face. She raised my arms into the air, looked at me for a long moment, and moved to the next guest.

The possession seemed to last an eternity. I went into my own type of trance. There would be many details I couldn't remember, a long passage of time that remained a complete blank. Then, within a five-minute span, both girls collapsed. The first to be possessed was the last to fall, and only after whirling out of the circle and toward the candles on the back row. She lay on her back there for some minutes, moving all the while. When both girls had collapsed, the demons apparently exorcised, the first possessed seemed to be having a difficult time re-entering this world. She could only mutter incoherently; slapping her face did not help. Again Matilda gathered the guests. She went to each of us, placing her upraised palms against ours, and finally to the still-mumbling girl, passing the knowledge of our hands to hers. Soon she seemed all right. The drumming stopped.

"There were three spirits here tonight," the high priestess's husband told me. "One was the spirit of war, which possessed the first girl. The other two are very old spirits and I cannot remember seeing them in many years. Two of them came on the same night. It is very strange."

In a daze, I walked to the door, hailed a cab, and rode in silence through the 4:30 a.m. Paris streets, back to the apartment where I was staying. The drum yet resounded as I tried to sleep. In some subterranean part of me, its echo has remained since 1970.

> The club was wild. There were people from all nationalities . . . dancing every which way. . . . The lights were low. The club was in full calamity and action. . . . And there was a soft grind signifying the motion of the people. The emotions were evidently charged and a kind of natural Afrodesiac permeated the atmosphere. . . . As they touched hands, the music faded into another song. The fast rhythm of the record made them move into a dance. The girl shifted into a frenzy and her skin began to shine. He became her slave as she told him how to position her body and dance with her. Then the record skipped and scratched. She left him alone as she disappeared into a screen of darkness.
>
> —Franklin's Journal, early 2000s

• • •

From Paris, I'd moved on to Algiers in search of Eldridge Cleaver and Timothy Leary, who'd gone into exile there. But the Black Panthers wanted nothing to do with me, and Leary, with whom I spent a couple of hours in a sidewalk café, was still mouthing the same platitudes from his LSD-guru days at Harvard. This marked the nadir of a young Midwesterner's search for meaning among the revolutionary and hippie movements that I'd been exploring overseas.

With a photographer friend from Kansas, I'd headed south across the great Sahara Desert. For an arduous six weeks, we hitchhiked some 4,000 miles to Accra, on the West African coast. En route we passed through Dahomey, where voodoo originated. Over the course of two months in Ghana, we spent time with Ashanti royalty and a former prime minister and an African medicine man.

Long after this, at some point during those first years after suffering his breakdown, Franklin had written the outline of a novel. In it, he said:

> On his world travels he dances with an African witch doctor in a village in Ghana. People are around smiling as this half black half white man of the people dances with their tribe. They are poor for Western standards but they are living like they always have off the fat of the land and with love and little greed. At another incidence he is warned of a lion that would appear and is possibly dangerous like a ghost in the darkness. He is unafraid but for that time decides just to stay safe and stayed in the village for that night. That night the lion was heard outside the village as it ravaged a hyena.

What is curious is the composite nature of the description. For I had done just that in the course of my "world travels"—journeyed to a small village near Mampong in central Ghana where the "witch doctor" (though I referred to him as "fetish priest" or "medicine man") had beckoned me into a circle to dance with him. My traveling companion had taken a picture of me as a bearded twenty-three-year-old, one leg off the ground, arms outstretched, eyes intent on the much older African man facing me clad only in a loincloth, while a younger man stood playing a large drum and the other villagers looked on from behind us. Franklin knew the photograph, as I kept it framed on my office wall. Yet, of course, I was not a "half black half white man of the people" from my son's imagined profile; that would have been him.

Franklin then—and later—had personally expressed a keen interest in seeing Africa. In a journal he kept while at Beacon High School in the late '90s, he wrote: "There are many possibilities for my future in traveling . . . I could go to Africa—Ghana, or Uganda with my mom's friends or with the people at the African store in Porter Square, or with the program that I was informed about one day from a lady on the street."

There are numerous other references from my own journals. From October 1996, when my son was first in the hospital: "On Halloween, Frank puts on costume of an African chief." From December 1998: "For Xmas, I get Frank a shirt/pants African outfit that he wanted." From January 2003, again when he was in the hospital: "He wants to do a craft-type store selling products from Africa, and other countries, with profits going back to those countries." From that same month: "He wants to go to school in Africa [but says] I won't help him. 'This is why I didn't talk to you today.'" And: "Franklin was asking if I wasn't an 'undercover African.'"

Could he have been harkening to what happened to me that morning with the medicine man in central Ghana, some eight years before he was born? Might all this have been a foreshadowing of a journey we would one day make together?

· · ·

April 1971: Somehow my photographer friend Steve and I have heard that a local "fetish priest" is planning a sunrise ceremony in a nearby village. So, shortly before dawn, we embark on a three-mile hike down an old dirt road toward Anansu. When we arrive, people are emerging from thatch-roofed houses and assembling in a small court-yard. Three men sit behind cowhide drums, while a fourth holds two large round castanets. Behind them a group of women chant quietly, while two old men in leopard-skin cloths sit huddled against a wall. These, we learn, are the medicine man's advisers, without whom he may make no independent decisions and through whom all visitors must pass.

A schoolboy, who alone among the villagers speaks good English, brings us to be introduced. I bow stiffly and they each smile back. The boy nods toward a far corner. There, immobile amid paint-daubed dolls and other "fetish" ornaments, waits the medicine man. Bosom-for Kwase Sekyere invites us to share a "hot drink" of schnapps, and through the boy translator speaks of his calling.

"All of his ancestors were priests. By profession he himself was a mechanic in the capital city. But in one of his dreams, he felt possession by the spirit. It called to him. This spirit was near to Odango, the chief spirit, and he is called fetish. The main purpose is to stop evils that might harm a person. If you are in trouble and you wish to know the cause, he will be able to tell you why you came, even before you tell him yourself. For many years he learned the secrets of the forest. People walk miles from other villages for the curing power of his herbs."

At certain seasons, on days long ago ordained by the ancestors, the wood-carved fetish dolls decorate all sides of the village compound and animals are slaughtered for a feast. And on Fridays—like this one— the medicine man always conducts an offering to the gods. Now his apprentice walks into the center of the courtyard. The medicine man thrusts his fist toward the sky and pours some drink on the ground. "This means Odango is here," the boy whispers in my ear. Weaving to the drum rhythms, the apprentice's mouth makes a chuffing sound. Several men gather behind him as he appears to lose control of his movements. Abruptly, the drumming stops. Still the apprentice paces, slower and slower, back and forth across the courtyard. The priest sheds his robe, down to a decorated loincloth, and kneels to pray as the apprentice grabs an egg from a bucket and puts it on the ground. "The priest can look at this and see what is coming," the boy says.

The apprentice returns to his normal state and walks to the corner to sit down. "Odango is gone," the boy says. But one of the drummers continues to pound forth a beat, and the villagers have begun pointing in my direction. "The drum is calling you," the boy continues. "Me?" I say, pointing to my chest. "You," he repeats, as the women renew their chant.

I had long been considered the least graceful of dancers. The Jitterbug mystified me and the Twist was the bane of my adolescent existence. A sixties dance called The Jerk always seemed more up my alley. So it is with some reluctance, but apparently no choice, that I agree to take off my shoes and socks as the drumbeat intensifies. Feeling tight and embarrassed, I move warily toward the center circle, where I find myself alone. Oddly, I feel a mysterious force surge through my body, urging me round and round. My arms feel detached, my legs begin moving as if to some inner command as my feet whip against the cool earth. I feel caught up in a vortex of motion. I close my eyes. When I look up again, the medicine man has joined me and our hands are weaving an intricate tapestry in the air. The ground seems to vibrate beneath my feet, like an earthquake might be about to happen. The closer I come to the drum, the more intense my dancing becomes. All of my concepts spin and drown in a wave of energy. At last, out of breath, I fall away and collapse beside my friend Steve.

"Russell!" he exclaims. "You were great!"

But the medicine man is only warming up. "When the spirit comes to him, he puts on his dress," says the boy who speaks English. The medicine man now dons a dark burlap robe, with two sacred talismans (beads and a horn) draped around his neck. He moves onto a goatskin, clutching a hatchet-like tool called an "akonti." A conical helmet, stained with sacrifices of sheep and fowl, is placed upon his head. The women chant a droning but mesmeric melody and slowly the medicine man falls into a trance. His neck arches to one side, his mouth gapes, his arms jerk, he dances as if over coals. Round and round he goes, intoning the forces that govern the land—Odango, Breswa, Cancomia, Paga, Botuo—as the pair of talisman around his neck leap to the soaring rhythm.

"Sometimes this will last three days," our translator says quietly. "Now the spirit Paga has taken him."

He's been eating kola nuts; mild stimulants that grow wild in the forest, which suddenly begin spewing from the medicine man's mouth, etching his chest in a grotesque stream of juice. Finally, with a deafening cry, he thrusts an arm toward the heavens and falls into the arms of several of the villagers, who cradle him and continue their chant.

Twenty minutes pass while Bosomfor Kwasi Sekyere is taken elsewhere to recover. Then we are invited into his private quarters, bare but for a mat, a wooden chair, and a wall lined with herbs and small medicine bottles. The medicine man has stripped down to a loincloth wreathed with shiny cowrie shells. He taps the floor with a long stick no wider than a string bean. Three times it makes a *shh-hhh* against the earth. "The gun of the spirit," the boy says. From his shelves he reaches for a vial of licorice-looking powder. Pouring some into a glass of water, he stirs it with his finger, drinks half, and then passes it to my friend and me. It is colorless and tasteless. Then he sprinkles some herbs onto my palm, and instructs me to lick them off. They contain a piquant sensation, like inhaling a meadow of sage.

Uncorking another bottle, the priest pours a final libation onto the ground outside.

"What is he doing now?" I ask.

"He is praying that, as you are here, nothing evil will happen to you. If anybody thinks evil of you, he will go away. So that you may have a safe journey, too. That is why you take his medicine. You have left your family and, when you go back to them, you will still be alive."

"And does he see any danger for me during the rest of my journey?"

"No, unless you contrast [contradict] the god."

Later, I wrote: "For the first time, I felt the power which the Anglo-Saxon so fears and admires in the black man. A raw, vital, earthy force. Screaming of blood and birth and harmony and uniqueness. Nature. The African, curing his ills with jungle herbs and tilling his field with oxen, lived near the heart of things. . . . What Bosomfor Sekyere symbolizes is the need to explore an inner world before we presume real knowledge of the outer."

> The dance the dance that goes on, and on, and on. All the way from Africa, and the Caribbean, and bells from China. The dance that renews the spirit.
>
> —Franklin's Journal, from a piece dated "5/6/96"

• • •

My friend Steve had gone home not long after our visit to the medicine man's village. I'd flown on alone to Kenya, where I contracted and recovered from malaria, smoked a *bhangi* pipe with pygmies deep in the Congo rainforest, and then found myself spending several days at the foot of Mount Kilimanjaro, in the land of the Maasai.

I'd never previously imagined traveling for almost a year in Africa and, while it was a life-altering experience in many ways, afterward I never thought I'd go back. Yet there was something Franklin wrote when he was seventeen, a quarter-century later in 1996, the same year he would soon have his first "psychotic episode." I'd come across his piece not long after that happened, and saved it in a folder labeled "Frank's Writing." He wrote part of this in the first person. Another part was in the third person, as if he was on the outside looking in.

> Where do I fit as an African American European in this chaotic mix of a world. This question, and how I look have always followed me

like a gloomy ghost. In the shadow of what is tormenting—from where, from what, and how did I get here arises. Constantly I imagine myself in the societies of the past. For example the Harlem Renaissance. The Industrial Revolution. Etc. What part would I have played back then. . . . The question of race has always followed me even when I was young and I first realized I was different. All I wanted to be was black. There was no in between for me. I recognized something in the black culture that I adored. What is it? It is a beauty that left an eternal quest for it. Yet somehow I never felt I measured up . . .

What is it like to be black? What is it like to be half black and half white? No matter how much we don't want it to matter it does matter. It is like one half of you is dancing to the drums of mother Africa, and the other singing in the choirs of classical European music. That's a lot of rhythm in one person.

What is it like to live in a tribe? All of the people share common ancestry, and common skin color. Wouldn't there be less competition. Wouldn't that be the definition of a perfect world?

The character could be a time traveler that travels from place to place trying to find somewhere to fit in.

Is it conceivable that, in Africa, half his lifetime later, he might find that missing "somewhere to fit in?"

CHAPTER 9

• • •

What the Doctor Ordered

We carry with us the wonders we seek without us: there is all Africa and her prodigies in us.

—Sir Thomas Browne, *Religio Medici,* 1642

D URING THE YEARS SINCE FRANKLIN moved out, Dr. Reiner always dropped by Fort Hill for dinner on the same night. "Thursdays with Larry," we call the ritual. A short, bespectacled, balding gentleman with a white mustache and kind blue eyes, Larry had been the pediatrician for Frank and many of our family's children who grew up in Boston. Now in his mid-seventies, he maintains a small practice in nearby Brookline.

Dr. Reiner had grown up in East Africa, as the only son of missionary parents. His first languages were African dialects, including Swahili, which he still speaks fluently. He continues to make annual pilgrimages back to Tanzania, customarily bringing friends or family along in the winter months to witness the wildlife migration across the Serengeti Plain. He would return after a month with new stories and remarkable photographs, several of which grace our walls. Larry has often expressed the desire that some of us accompany him on the trip.

In late September 2011, we are sitting across from each other at our dinner table, when he mentions that a couple who've been planning to come along next January have bowed out. Aileane Doherty, his twenty-six-year-old former office assistant, is still going—but traveling with less than four people made the trip prohibitively costly. Larry fixes his eyes on mine. Might I be interested in joining him and bring-ing Franklin along?

I knew that he was aware of my son's difficulties (Larry's son Marshall had been a psychiatric resident at one of the hospitals where Franklin spent time), and this is not the first time that he's expressed the idea that the trip might be good for Frank. Years earlier, when Franklin was released from his first hospitalization, he and I had talked of making a trip to West Africa, where some of his mother's ances-tors came from—but it had never seemed like more than a dream. Yet, surprising myself, I respond to Larry that I will be seeing Franklin the next day and will broach the subject. Money for the trip would have to come out of the trust fund I'd been starting to build for his future. It's known as a "supplemental needs" trust, available for personal expenses that his government benefits didn't cover. So the decision will ulti-mately be Frank's.

A few days later, we are having a beer together at the Bang-kok Bistro, waiting for one of the daily luncheon specials. I explain about Dr. Reiner inviting us to join him. Franklin remains silent for a moment, studying my face. Then he asks, "How would we pay for it?" I reply that I'd need to use his trust, and that it would cost about five thousand dollars apiece. My son says nothing and I drop the subject.

We're driving back to his house when Frank says: "So, you want to go to Africa, huh?"

"Well, I want to go with *you* to Africa," I reply. "I've been to Africa."

Now, as I make the turn into the Target parking lot so my son can pick up a sketch pad, I tell him of a time in Kenya when I'd spent the night in a tent and been afraid to get up to pee as I listened to animals prowl around outside. At least one of these was distinctly a lion. Franklin goes silent and I inwardly chastise myself for telling that particular story. "Yeah, I saw this movie on TV," he says finally, "where a couple who are traveling in Africa get mauled to death by a lion."

"Well, we won't be staying in those kinds of primitive surround-ings like I did then," I tell him. "These will be nice lodges. With some excellent food. Dr. Reiner has been there many times." Franklin simply nods. End of conversation.

I don't want to push it. If he has reservations about making the trip, I certainly don't want to foist it upon him; that could be disas-trous. It seems a long shot, at best. Since he was very young, we've never lived as intimately on a daily basis as this would require. Larry is identified in Frank's mind as the doc who once stuck booster shots in his arm and behind. And Franklin is often uncomfortable around young women close to his age, as our other traveling companion would be. Nor has he ever been in the proximity of wild animals, except in a zoo. Could he really be ready for an experience this intense? Could I?

Still, since his youth, Franklin had always been fascinated by other cultures. He'd written a detailed third-grade paper on China. He'd been to Spain with his middle school class and spent a number of months during different summers in Baja. Mexico, he'd told me, was his favorite place growing up. When he was twelve or thirteen, I'd also taken him to an environmental session of the United Nations in New York, and I'd rarely seen Frank as excited as he listened to various translations on a headset.

My diary entries of recent years reflected a metaphorical, multi-cultural reality for some of Frank's descriptions of Etta and me. From January 2004, in the course of a hospitalization: "When I mention his mother coming next Sunday, he says, 'My mother? My parents are from Tibet and Africa.' She is not the same Etta, nor am I the same Dick Russell who he knew 2,000 years ago." From January 2005: "Franklin said to me: 'You've been a wonderful father but you must start using your own Confucian way. . . . You're half Chinese and half African.'" Opposite sides of the globe, but in his psyche, the opposites attract.

When, at my impetus, we recently stopped by the post office to renew his passport, Frank had said he wanted to change his name to Simon. Why did you choose that one? I asked. "Because it's a combination of Sun and Moon," Frank replied. Oh, of course, I must be pretty dense not to have guessed that! I'd responded. I thought later about the other metaphoric meanings implied: night and day . . . white and black. On the passport application, he decided to stick with being Franklin. And shortly thereafter, he'd said to me: "We both like to travel, don't we. You're a good traveling companion."

A week after I bring up the possible Africa trip, I take my son out to lunch again. He seems to be contemplating something. On the way back I casually mention that I'd be seeing Dr. Reiner again this week and, if Frank wanted, I could ask for more specifics about what kind of accommodations we'd be in. He doesn't miss a beat.

"When are we going?" My son says it declaratively, not as a question.
"January 13."

"Great!" he exclaims.

His so-enthusiastic answer, itself a rarity, takes me by surprise. I press back hard against the driver's seat. My hands grip the steering wheel so tightly, I wonder if he notices. He picks up on things like that. "Great!" I echo.

When I tell Dr. Hillman this story, the psychologist smiles and makes a striking observation. Even if something goes wrong, Hillman says, and we can't make the trip and it would be such a disappointment, it is still Franklin's initial reaction that counts—because it is outside the literal. It's in the realm of being able to *imagine* going.

I call Larry to tell him that Franklin is truly interested, and the doctor is very pleased, saying we could finalize plans soon. And, as Hillman had suggested, the fact that my son could imagine making the trip seems to shift something around inside his psyche. He wants to get all of his old stuff out of a U-Haul storage place, where I've been paying monthly fees for several years. "I don't want you to have to do that anymore," he says. It takes awhile—and some heavy lifting—to put everything into a van. "I had a good time, did you?" Frank asks as we unload everything once more into a corner of his house's basement.

Next time I see him we stop at the post office to pick up some visa forms for traveling in Tanzania and drop these off at Dr. Reiner's. He says he'll take care of the details.

• • •

I get a call a few weeks later while staying in Los Angeles from Erin, the supervisor at Franklin's house. Feeling suicidal, he had called her into his room to say that he needed to go to the hospital. He'd been seeing corpses in the carpet at his house. He was also hearing voices, including those of numerous dead people, and began talking of how the hospital staff could "decease him," and how he could be cremated and people could use the ashes. This came out of the blue to both me and the group home staff. Erin says they've been monitoring Franklin's medication, and he'd assuredly been taking it. Now he'll need to go through medical clearance at nearby Cambridge Hospital, which will see where they can find my son a bed.

The timing couldn't have been more eerie. Only a few days before this, James Hillman had died from complications of lung cancer. Alice and I had attended his burial ceremony in Connecticut. It was only the end of October, but it had snowed the entire time. I hadn't yet seen Frank to tell him about it. I'd just been describing the day to friends when Frank's house informed me of his suddenly obsessive thoughts about death.

A hospital social worker calls the next afternoon. Frank has finally slept, started eating, and has become calm and cooperative. He's told the social worker that he cuts meat at the grocery store, is 70 percent Chinese, and lived with his wife in China. She finds it noteworthy that these delusions were not outlandish or bizarre. Indeed, I think to myself, they are simply indicative of Franklin's attunement to a different reality.

I reach Franklin on the phone and he thanks me for checking in. Later Erin calls from his house to tell me that he's so much better, very talkative, "as if yesterday never happened." In the evening, Etta phones. She'd taken a bus to Boston and, when she showed up at the hospital, Franklin couldn't believe she'd come all the way from Baltimore. "He was very sweet," Etta says. She feels that he looked better than the last several times she'd seen him, and was jovial and unguarded, saying he could sneak out and meet her downstairs.

But I don't know what to do about Africa. Maybe, even probably, the thought of making a trip like this was simply too much for Franklin. Africa would be raw reality, up-and-at-it every morning as we moved from one place to another, toward and then across the vast Serengeti Plain. One thing I know: Franklin does enjoy being in motion, inside a vehicle. Oftentimes when we go out he asks if we could just drive around.

When I contact Larry to tell him that Franklin has been hospitalized, he says "oh, no," but we'd just have to wait and see what transpired. The next time I speak to Frank, he is feeling better. Is there anything he wants to talk about? I ask. "We're going January 13th, right?" he says without hesitation. "Yes, we are," I say.

A friend suggests that I check with Dr. Reiner about contingency plans in case something like this happens while we are over in Africa. Larry says it won't be a concern; that there are Western-trained doctors at Arusha, our first destination in Tanzania and one in a nearby town.

After spending a week in the hospital, Franklin returns to his house. Answering his cell phone, his voice sounds clear. "I feel a whole lot better," he says He adds that sometimes when he gets talking fast, he forgets what he's said, and he apologizes for that. I tell him how good he sounds and that sometimes you just need a break. He agrees.

By the middle of November, Franklin has been to a follow-up transitional day program at the hospital and is taking his medication in the presence of the staff at his house. As the holidays approach, he's out-and-around his neighborhood every day, which is a good sign. And he remains excited about Africa. While I get the required yellow fever preventative shot, as well as some anti-malaria pills, Frank ends up being inoculated as well against hepatitis-A, typhoid, polio, tetanus/diptheria, and the flu.

The staff at his house is shocked when, shortly after receiving the shots for our trip, he also has two of his wisdom teeth extracted! They'd had no idea, knowing only that he was at the dentist for a surprising number of hours. But according to Erin, he'd made his own way back on public transportation and handled the whole thing remarkably well. I remember Franklin saying that getting rid of the uncomfortable wisdom teeth was something he wanted to do, and now it seems he was "taking care of business" on his own. Maybe this is part of his ritual of preparation for our trip.

Over Christmas, he takes a train by himself—another first in many years—to see his mom in Baltimore. "We really had a great visit," Etta emails me afterward. "He has changed quite a bit. After the first few hours, there was no strangeness and we all had a really warm, relaxed few days. . . . When he couldn't sleep, I gave him a sleeping pill (after checking whether he could take it with his medications). He slept like a baby and felt great the next day. He was very concerned about his hygiene the entire time he was here and took three long showers. At one point he asked Kamal for some deodorant and then if he could use his cologne. . . . Franklin took the plane back and a taxi from the airport and got home by 2:00, in great spirits. . . . He's really into this trip to Africa with you."

These are all extremely positive developments, much more than I could lately have anticipated. What worries me, as our Friday the 13th departure date looms closer, is the timing on taking his Clozaril medication, given two long airplane flights (we'd change planes in Amsterdam) and the eight-hour time difference between Boston and Tanzania. But his psychiatrist says it's not really a concern precisely when Franklin takes his medication. He recommends just taking the morning and evening doses according to whatever time it is at our location. This sets my mind at ease . . . but only somewhat.

Etta makes a day-trip to see Franklin in the week leading up to our departure. They do some clothes and luggage shopping—"lime green . . . tried to get him to choose something else but he stuck with that," she writes me. "Found him a small dop kit and a money belt. He is still in a bit of a fragile place. Really wants to go on this trip, but is a bit afraid. He got very tired yesterday afternoon after we'd been out a while and he said, 'I don't know if I can do this.' To which I replied—it's okay to be worried but it's all of this getting ready that is the hardest part."

I sure hope she's right. A couple of days before our scheduled departure, Frank and I go shopping, too. He picks out an inexpensive Panasonic camera with a long zoom lens that takes both pictures and video. He asks if I'll help him pack. I can't remember seeing him this excited in years. That night, Larry comes by my place for dinner with the flight information. He's told our other traveling companion, Aileane, about Franklin having a mental illness, which she doesn't have a problem with. Larry lists off the various places we'll be heading, and as he does so, I realize that this is the least-planned adventure I've embarked upon since my youthful hitchhiking days. And, as I did then, I'm just going to let it unfold.

Franklin calls in the morning to make sure I have his passport, which I do, and wondering what time I'll be coming by. We'll stop to pick up Dr. Reiner in the afternoon and fly out that night. "O-kayyy, boss," Frank says.

> *He had never dreamed of going to such far away places. . . . But when he joined the "One World Club," he knew he was to fill the dream that Martin Luther King spoke about. His life was to become an adventure that was inexplicable.*
> —Franklin's Journal while at Beacon High School, late '90s

• • •

Over the phone, my literary agent wishes me well and says: "He will know you love him. But more than that, it is an adventurous love." I consider that, having faith in Franklin to take an "adventure"—or to imagine him as "adventurous"—and therefore to take him seriously as an adult with a life that's about something I might never be able to really understand, he can and will come through.

On a chilly afternoon in mid-January 2012, as Eddie drives us to Boston's Logan Airport, Franklin sits in the backseat looking out the window. "If you paint clouds," he finally says to me, "it's hard not to get dew on your pencil."

In the front seat, Dr. Reiner is excitedly anticipating our first stop, Mount Kilimanjaro, where his family had lived in the foothills shortly after the Japanese bombed Pearl Harbor in 1941. As a boy, Larry would draw back the curtains of his bedroom window and gaze upon the tallest mountain in Africa, with the biggest land rise of any mountain anywhere, from 3,000 to 19,600 feet, greater even than Mount Everest.

Aileane Doherty shows up soon after we arrive at the airline ticket counter. Neither Franklin nor I have met her, but Larry is sure we'll enjoy each other's company. She is currently attending nursing school in Boston, a red-haired, freckle-faced, attractive young lady of Irish descent. Franklin, on being introduced to Aileane, gestures at Larry and informs her that "he used to look in my larynx." Frank then removes his cap, points to his bushy Afro, and says to the doctor, "I want to be bald like you." Franklin proceeds to show him a book that he's had me purchase at a newsstand to read on the plane. It's titled *What Color Is Your Brain?*

The first leg of the trip is an all-night haul. I carry Franklin's medication, pill-strips dated and marked "morning" and "night," stashed in my carry-on. I'd been worried that the two long flights might make him agitated, and his psychiatrist had also prescribed Atavan in case he was. Although he doesn't want anything to eat, Franklin does sleep most of the way across the Atlantic. The occasional turbulence seems to pose no problems for him.

After a brief layover in Amsterdam, we're set to board another nine-hour flight to the Kilimanjaro International Airport. "You know, when I hitchhiked around this region about forty years ago, they didn't even *have* an airport," I tell our traveling companions.

"When I came here seventy years ago, they didn't even have a *road*," Larry responds. Frank looks at him quizzically. The doctor goes on to relate how he was only three when the fundamentalist African Inland Mission enlisted his parents to leave Illinois, take a freighter across the Atlantic, and make their way to what was then the British protectorate of Tanganyika Territory. From a railway station, they'd traveled with their goods by Conestoga-like bullock cart, fording a river on the last leg. "I still have pictures of my mother being carried across and uphill on a palanquin," Larry says.

"What's a palanquin?" Frank asks.

"It's the kind of thing you see in the old movies being used to transport Indian rajahs, an enclosed litter held by poles on the shoulders of four bearers. Altogether the trip took us three months."

"And now we're flying there in less than a day," Frank marvels.

Warming up to his audience, the doctor goes on: "The mission station—at the southern tip of Lake Victoria—was this incredibly big, thatch-roofed house with thick walls that were supposed to keep everything cool, with a big veranda all around. But it had no electricity and no running water. When we eventually did get a car, we'd take the battery and hook it up to a shortwave radio to get our news. It took like three months to get a message of the fastest sort back to the United States. My father's father got sick and died before word of it ever reached us."

Larry's father was assigned to train future Christian preachers from among the twenty or twenty-five African families living at the mission station. It was no easy task. The Sukuma, largest of the country's 120 different ethnic groups, still believed in spirit possession. Larry learned their Bantu language from his friends. "I considered myself a Sukuma kid. I thought of the white folks as 'they,' and the black folks as 'we,'" he says.

I notice Franklin nodding, appreciatively it appears. Larry goes on to recount how he felt when, at seven, like all the other children of white colonialists, he was sent off to a segregated boarding school run by the Anglican Church. "The school had about sixty students in the five grades," he says, "and I felt really out of place among all these white kids." Then, at fifteen, he'd left East Africa and returned to his grandmother's home in Illinois to enroll in high school. "It was quite a culture shock. The other kids called me 'the jungle bunny.' But I had enough intriguing tales to tell that they seemed to enjoy my company."

The jungle bunny. That, sadly but ironically, is how some of my own high school classmates in suburban Kansas City had referred to African Americans—of whom there were none in my graduating class of 800-some students. I say nothing about this, but I imagine that Franklin has probably heard the phrase before.

Our plane is packed with more than two hundred tourists, for this is the height of their tourist season. We'll be landing not far from Mweka, Larry says, where his mother taught English and which later became the African College of Wildlife Management. That's the same school where Ernest Hemingway's son, Patrick, was teaching when I once stayed at his house in the foothills of Mount Kilimanjaro. What a small world! The memory returns as Frank and I find our seats on the plane a few rows behind Larry and Aileane.

• • •

In June 1971, when I first entered the land of the Maasai, I was in my "Hemingway period." I'd heard that Patrick, born while his father was writing *A Farewell to Arms*, lived there and taught African students vehicle mechanics and statistics. I'd sent a letter ahead asking if I might perhaps pay him a visit, ostensibly to talk about game conservation. I hitched a ride up a dirt road that seemed to climb forever past blooming mimosas and acacias and a sisal plantation, the mountain obscured by the curving road and the density of the trees. Patrick's house was the last before the road became a tangle of bush paths where Kilimanjaro began.

What I remembered now was a conversation we had one afternoon about first mental illness and then about the Maasai. Ultimately, Patrick felt that there was no other choice but the one his father had made in 1961—to kill himself. "If I had been in his shoes," he'd said matter-of-factly, "I'd have done the same thing. He would have been committed to an institution, there is no question." His words came slowly, pensively. "My father was always absolutely heartless when it came to mental illness. He would say it was the fault of some weakness on the individual's part. Then, when it began to happen to him . . ." He didn't have to complete the sentence.

Ernest Hemingway was surely suffering from manic-depression, and it was this—coupled with aging and the effect of alcohol on his liver, according to Patrick—that led to his suicide. His son disdained critics who preferred instead to cite his father's "abnormal" dislike for his mother. There was nothing Freudian about it, he said.

Patrick then began to talk about his definition of abnormal, as it applied to all the restrictions that Western society placed on any natural outlets needed to cope with adolescence and all the physical changes taking place. Adolescence was equally as important as childhood in framing one's character. He recalled for me his traumatic teenaged years in Key West, Havana, and at a Catholic boys school in Florida. The fishing and hunting. The loneliness. The emotional breakdowns. Denial, always denial, while the body urged new needs on the soul. Sexual needs. The need to encounter danger.

Of all the systems he knew of, Patrick continued, the Maasai best suited their environment to the needs of their young. They are a proud pastoral people, he explained, wanderers over vast areas of Kenya and northern Tanzania. Their men are tall and lean, with stretched pierced earlobes that accentuate the chiseled slopes of long faces. Their women shave their heads with the naming of a first child and drape their bodies in colorful burlap garments.

The Maasai believe in total education. When a boy is twelve, he enters his years of initiation with other males of his age group. At a ceremony he watches as his elders mix the blood of a slaughtered bullock with the warm milk of a cow. Sharing the others' fear, he drinks deeply and then dances for four consecutive days. Another year passes. The physical tests grow more arduous. Bare-hand grappling with the largest horned bullock. A circumcision ceremony. The boy becomes a warrior. He builds his own *manyatta* of branches and mud. He takes a woman to his bed. He carries a spear for the first time. And if a tribal war seems imminent, he may be one of nine spies—one for every orifice in the human body—sent to scout the enemy's territory. Then the young warriors—and they alone—would attack the rival tribe.

Finally, at the twilight of adolescence, a Maasai settles into the adult way of raising cattle and family. Death is not feared, but an accepted part of life. The Maasai don't run from it or build monuments to it. Sometimes the body is even placed outside on the ground, sustenance for the scavengers of the night. The system wouldn't work in *our* world, Patrick Hemingway had told me. But this doesn't mean you can't admire it. Because for the Maasai, it is the perfect system.

Now, just over forty years later, my son and I will soon be in Maasai country together. The tribe had long been of special interest to Franklin. In the late nineties, after his breakdown and before finishing

high school, he had written poignantly: "Africa, the cradle of civilization, where 'Lucy' was found, is in a rapid state of decline. . . . Africans
struggle to find food. The bushmen are pushed from place to place and
left homeless and isolated. The Maasai wear watches and T-shirts where
they once wore beautiful bracelets and complicated tribal outfits."

The Maasai speak Swahili, and Frank had more than once mentioned wanting to learn the language. In March 2002, he wrote in
a letter: "I got a guide to speaking Arabic off the Internet. Since I
know some numbers in Swahili, I can compare them. The areas that
speak the languages are side by side and the languages have some
cross references."

An excerpt from my travel journal, 1971:
They certainly are a distinctive people. Riding the bus this morning
from Moshi, after leaving Patrick Hemingway's home, numerous Maasai stood at roadside or sauntered on or off the bus. One old man was
particularly fascinating, his earlobes stretched below his cheeks, his eyes
hard and a wooden staff supporting his brown-cloaked body. He was
as intrigued by me as I was by him, and stared at me for the first five
minutes after he got on the bus.

An excerpt about Franklin from my diary, June 2008:
He was not delusional except for saying to me in the car that I'd once
been a Maasai warrior.

I close my eyes. It will be night when we land at Kilimanjaro.

CHAPTER 10

• • •

Africa Beckoning

Though we've not been here long it seems like a lifetime. Africa has a way of imposing its own time scale, reducing our busy Western lives to its own pace, its own stately rhythm. In Africa the concept of the eternal seems much more meaningful. It also allows you more time to take things in. Events become clearer and impressions sharper and memories more indelible.

—Michael Palin, while filming the documentary *Michael Palin's Hemingway Adventure*, about Hemingway in Africa.

OUR PLANE TOUCHES DOWN AROUND 9 p.m., after nearly twenty-four hours in transit. Franklin finds it odd that they take your fingerprints at Tanzanian customs—later he would specifically recall them taking a photograph of four fingers of one hand, though not his thumb—but he gets through the waiting line without issue. Outside in the parking lot, we are greeted by an African driver for Serengeti Select Safaris, a company that Larry has used for many years. Stephan Lucamay, who will be our guide for the next two weeks, loads our luggage into the back of a Land Rover. He will turn out to be of the Maasai, and the same age as Franklin.

It's only a few miles from the airport to the KIA Lodge, situated on a secluded hill amid the savanna. While we'd thought there would be a full day to recover from the long trip, Stephan informs us that we'll be setting off first thing the next morning. Larry and Aileane are to share a cottage down a cobbled path from the thatched brick cottage where Franklin and I stay, which has a single large bed under a mosquito-net canopy. It's so warm that there's no need for covers. Sprawled alongside me, my son is soon fast asleep and snoring; I pop a sleeping pill.

When we're woken by bird calls, we go outside to find Mount Kilimanjaro shrouded in mist. It's long been known as the roof of Africa, a place of mythic power. Menelik I, the ancient Ethiopian king, said to have been born to the Queen of Sheba and the biblical Solomon, reputedly fell ill and died after ascending Kilimanjaro and was buried in the snowy craters with Solomon's ring on his finger. According to legend, whoever may find Menelik's corpse and remove the ring shall be given Solomon's wisdom.

Franklin and I have coffee by the swimming pool amid tropical gardens with birds and lizards. He's enthralled by a panoramic vista that offers Mount Meru, the Blue Mountains, and the Maasai Plains. Amid the lovely trees with red flowers and hanging pods of seed, Stephan stops by to inform us that they are called *nandi*. By 9 a.m., we have gathered our box lunches from the hotel and are on our way, a two-hour trip to our first game-drive destination at Arusha National Park. Larry sits in the front seat, while Aileane, Franklin, and I crowd into the back, our luggage stacked behind us. Setting out, Stephan explains that Tanzanians drive on the left side because, back in the day, British colonists used their right hand to make their horses move.

Although Stephan speaks fluent English, Dr. Reiner smiles and commences talking with him in the Swahili tongue he learned as a boy. Our guide, of course, is curious why and how Larry learned the language. "Well, I was trilingual by the time I was four," the doctor says with more than a touch of pride. "English, Swahili, and Sukuma." He goes on to explain about his missionary parents being dispatched to Tanzania, then adds: "If we hadn't come here, I doubt very much that I'd be a doctor now."

Larry relates how, when he was about five, a blind leper woman would come to beg at the mission station. She sat on one side of the house looking for a handout, and Larry's mother usually gave her something. As the boy sat and spoke with her one day, Larry recalled the family's house servant asking her, "Who is this person you're talking to?" The woman replied, "Oh, this is one of the *waneje*," a word referring to the local Sukuma children. The servant said, "No, this is a *mzungu* you're talking to." The woman said, "Ah! No white boy could speak Wasukuma language this way." The servant said: "You put one hand under his mouth and the other hand on his head and see what his hair is like, and then maybe you'll believe this boy is a *mzungu*." She touched the boy's straight hair and gasped.

The blind leper woman came more than once to visit with Larry. Hers was a form of leprosy that had eaten away her nose, as well as most of her fingers and toes. Larry asked his father why they couldn't give the woman a new nose. He wanted to glue her fingers and toes back on, and couldn't understand why "it doesn't work that way," as his father told him. Around the same time, an African man came to the house carrying his big toe in a jar. He'd hacked it off with a hoe while he was gardening. Larry was sure *this* appendage could be reattached.

"From that point on, there was nothing else I wanted to do with my life—except be someone who could glue toes back on and take care of people with no noses," Larry recalls as we turn onto a paved road. In childhood, he says, he also contracted his share of African diseases, including malaria at least once a year, the parasitic disease bilharzia and, at nine, blackwater fever, which in those days proved fatal in nine out of ten victims. Somehow he survived, an experience that he believed also contributed to his later interest in medicine.

"I remember some of those shots you gave me," Frank says, "and I survived those, too."

Everyone in the car laughs. The trip seems to be starting out on a positive note. Frank, however, is more interested in Stephan, and asks about his tribal heritage.

"I am Maasai, but I look different from other Maasais," Stephan says, "because my mom died when I was five and the second mom took care of me and she didn't want to do anything to my body."

We haven't yet encountered other Maasai, so I whisper to Frank that he's talking about doing anything decorative (such as beaded earlobes and hair braided in red ochre.)

"What happened to your mom?" Frank asks.

"She was killed," Stephan says. "In a car crash." He pauses, then goes on: "She was going to visit her family at the border between Tanzania and Kenya, and on the way she had the accident."

"That is so common," Larry says, shaking his head.

"I don't remember even her face because there were no cameras at the time," Stephan says.

Frank says nothing, but looks pensive, and I wonder whether he's thinking of Etta. After a pause, he asks Stephan, "Do you have any brothers and sisters?"

"Yes, between the two moms, ten sisters and three brothers," he replies. He goes on that his Maasai name is Enga Ng Wo, which means rainbow, because one had appeared on the day he was born. As a boy, Stephan wore no shoes for years while walking six miles each way to a government school. He would go all day without having lunch. His father wanted him to stay home and help tend the cattle, but a couple from Minnesota that he met by chance paid for his higher education to attend the African College of Wildlife Management.

It's a serendipitous moment for Larry, whose mother had once been an English instructor at the college, and for me as well, having visited Patrick Hemingway when he taught there. Stephan appreciates the mutual connection and goes on to inform us that his training hadn't been easy. The culmination was not unlike an Outward Bound experience, except in the middle of the bush. You got dropped off without a tent, or any food—you had to know what to forage for—got provided a gun but only to scare off any animals, not to shoot them. You had to create a makeshift hut for sleeping and find your way back on foot, no matter how long it took.

"Nowadays I live in Arusha town with my father, because it is close to where I work," Stephan says. Now in his eighties, his father still walks six miles to market and had only once been in a hospital, "when one time it was difficult for him to mark territory."

"Like a dog," Franklin says. Stephan smiles and says, "Yes, does anyone need to do that?" So far, we're all just fine.

"In Maasai tribe, if you have only one wife then you're not a real man," Stephan continues, turning to face Frank, "you must have five or six." My son grins and asks how many wives *he* has. Stephan reveals, somewhat sheepishly, that he has only one, and they are now separated. Franklin seems relieved to hear this. One wife seems like plenty to him.

Dr. Reiner wonders, "Is there any tribe where a woman has many husbands?"

"In Tanzania, men are polygamous but also women," according to Stephan. "Most people must carry firewood to cook their food, and if you need something hot, you must have like three sons to haul your pot. So even woman can have boyfriend. One for shopping, one for labor, one like a husband. Always in Tanzania, women work very hard, do everything. Men are just lazy, sitting down, eating, talking. You see a man like that"—his forefinger points toward the roadside—"helping his wife collect water? That's a good man." Frank smiles again.

As he drives, Stephan points out the two kinds of banana trees—one for cooking into plantain and the other to make a home-brewed gin. He also talks about another of the local tribes, which cuts down trees to make charcoal. "Which is not good, because the indigenous trees we have, like acacia, grow very slow. Once you cut one, you never get another back. If there are no trees, life will be difficult. But they need somehow to be taught about that."

I ask Stephan if he's observed many changes in the ecosystem in recent years. It's already been distinctly noticeable that Mount Kilimanjaro is no longer snowcapped. "I see lot of change," he replies. "Like rainy season, previous time you can tell exactly when the rain comes, February all the way to May. My father always knew, but nowadays he can't tell. And you can see our lakes get pretty dry. Like Lake Manyara, last year the water was evaporated up to 95 percent. We are not getting rain to have enough crops, so we have to pack everything up frozen, use a lot of chemicals to keep foods. Previously time, you can just go to a farm and there were so many fruits, you couldn't even fit them in your car."

• • •

There is so much to see in this world. There are so many ways to get over pain and achieve happiness.

—Franklin's Journal, early 2000s

We approach the gated entry to Arusha National Park. Stephan tells us that once inside, "nobody is allowed to get out and mark territory, because there could be Cape buffalo and you can't see them coming." The national park is on the eastern edge of the Great Rift Valley, which was formed by a volcanic explosion twenty million years ago and stretches more than five thousand miles all the way from Turkey to the mouth of Mozambique's Zambezi River. This was once Maasai land—"a really good place for Maasai," Stephan says, "because they always use local medicine and there is a lot in this park. Like this tree with the sharp thorns that you see here—it is called *Oloisuki*—you pick the roots, you can fix stomach pain. This tree is also our perfume, Maasai perfume. When you are going to get married, you rub some on your body. And over there is a quinine tree, used to treat malaria. For local medicine, the Maasai always make tea."

"Do they have St. John's Wort?" Franklin asks.

Stephan, never having heard of this herbal remedy for depression, does not respond directly but instead points to our right. "Look, do you see the giraffe? There's another one lying down. You can tell male from female. Most people look underneath, but if you just look at the top of their horn, the females have hair and the males are bald."

It is immediately apparent that Stephan's ability to spot game while maneuvering winding dirt roads is uncanny. He and Franklin also seem to have established a definite rapport. Later, when I ask how Frank would describe him, he speaks of Stephan's "youthful, strong" presence. Stephan is good-looking and well-built, but very soft-spoken. He can surely tell from some of Franklin's remarks that he's at least unusual, but he treats my son like a regular person, engaging him in conversation no matter where it might meander. Stephan's acceptance seems more than a polite response; rather an approach very different than the Western.

Part of this attitude may have to do with what is described by Paul R. Linde in his 1994 book, *Of Spirits and Madness: An American Psychiatrist in Africa.* "Major mental illness cuts across all cultures," Linde writes. "Amazingly enough, or maybe not, acutely psychotic people in Zimbabwe appear very similar to those in San Francisco. . . . They suffer from disorganized thoughts, delusions, and hallucinations. The content of the symptoms, however, is very much different . . . Zimbabweans do not report hearing auditory hallucinations of Jesus Christ, rather they report hearing those of their ancestor spirits. They are not paranoid about the FBI, rather they are paranoid about witches and sorcerers."[1]

"Do they have snakes in this jungle?" Franklin asks now.

"You have green mamba, spitting cobra, puff adder," Stephan turns again to tell him. "All venomous." He makes a joke about our having an open roof, so the snakes could use their tails to flip up and into our car. Larry remembers a time when his father accidentally ran over a snake on his motorcycle, which then "reared its head and bit him." Frank doesn't find any of this very amusing.

According to Stephan, only in this particular park might we glimpse the handsome black-and-white colobus monkeys amid the high forest canopy. One reason for their scarcity is poaching, but much of their habitat has been deforested as well. The monkeys are instantly recognizable, with bushy white tails and long flowing hair encasing their bodies in a white mantle. They live in family troops, speaking in choruses of guttural calls as they swing through the trees. Sure enough, it isn't long before we spot some, feeding on fresh leaves and leaping acrobatically across the branches.

We also pass troops of olive baboons, the mothers carrying their young jockey-style on their backs close to their tails. It's mating season, and Franklin is interested in the red butts, revealing that some of the females are in heat. Later, when I ask my son to tell me his favorite animal so far, he says: "Baboons. I really get a kick out of the way they scoot."

Toward the end of our first game drive, a poignant moment occurs. The terrain has shifted from rainforest to savanna when, at Larry's request, Stephan pulls over and parks the Land Rover shortly before noon. A plaque states that we've reached Mikindu Point, named after the wild date palms that grow precariously along the wall of the pear-shaped Ngurdoto Crater. A product of volcanic eruption, the crater rises for 4,840 feet and stretches 1.6 miles from rim to rim. It's an ideal place for water buffalo, Stephan says, with good grazing, permanent water, and mud wallows. Because of the damp, misty atmosphere, orchids, ferns, and lichens proliferate in the crater.

Standing at the crater's edge, the doctor tells us: "This is where I want my ashes scattered. I have the tree picked out."

"I hope you have this in your will," Aileane says. He shrugs his shoulders. "No, but everybody who knows me knows about it," Larry replies.

"Why this spot?" I ask.

"I don't know," says Larry, "I guess because it's off-limits to man. There's no road down into it." Stephan notes that the pink flamingoes, currently at Lake Manyara and the Ngorongoro Crater, migrate to here during October and November. The doctor smiles at the thought. "I'll show you the tree," he continues, passing binoculars first to Aileane. "See that one down there all by itself, near the small isolated clump of trees? See the Cape buffalo standing there? That's the place."

Then he adds quietly, "This is my homeland."

Heading onward, our group discusses the visit we'll pay in a few days to the Oldupai Gorge, where fossil excavations uncovered early hominids providing crucial evidence of human evolution. "Lucy," whose several hundred pieces of skeletal remains are an estimated 3.2 million years old, was found not far away in Ethiopia. Franklin turns to me and says: "We've got to make sure we wear the right thing to pay homage to her."

Stephan begins briefing us about the elephants we will soon be encountering. "When you see elephants, they always have a leader who takes them where there is water. You know, when males are old enough, like twenty, they always leave their group and go to find another group. That way they don't need to mix their genes, very smart. When one elephant dies, the others surround it. They say elephants can keep memory for twenty years. If you do anything bad to them, they will remember you. Their eyesight and hearing are very poor, but their memory is good."

Franklin glances down at my tape machine and says, "Maybe when we reach the elephants, we can record how they scream. They scream when they're mating, right?"

"Sometimes, yeah," says Stephan. "Other animals scream like lions."

"Are there any jackals in here?" my son asks.

"There are dogs."

When Larry and Stephan continue talking in Swahili as we drive along, I begin to wonder whether Franklin feels excluded. My son will claim to speak many languages, Swahili included, but this is the real thing. But he would never say anything about it, better to seem like he understands. Perhaps, in his way, he does. Once in awhile, he'll join their conversation in his own version of Swahili. This always brings a smile to Stephan's face.

On the other hand, Dr. Reiner tends to bristle at Franklin's out-of-context statements. I suppose that Larry expects a kind of "normalcy" that he'd observed in Frank's youth, prior to his breakdown. Or maybe this has to do with the doctor's age, and his experiences with previous guests on his safaris. At any rate, with Franklin he seems intent on setting the "facts" straight.

Now, Stephan says, "People are getting permits to hunt one male lion. But if you kill one, you might kill the whole pride. Because then there is no male to protect the cubs, and another male can come in and see the cubs and kill them."

"Wow, I never knew that about lions," I say. Frank says, "But I'll bet they have animal hospitals, right?"

Larry shakes his head in a disparaging no.

Stephan doesn't skip a beat. "Here? No. Just for dogs and cats. We always let nature to take place."

Frank says simply: "The enzymes."

Although in fact enzymes are active proteins found in all living cells in nature, Larry reproachfully shakes his head again, as if to say: What is he *talking* about? Larry says, "If you find a wounded animal and you try to stop and help it, it's a five hundred dollar fine."

Soon after this, Frank makes his first "delusional" remarks in some time. "My house in Boston is a restaurant. Seventeen groups cook there. Pho Vietnam. Fugakyu."

"Oh really," Larry says declaratively (and disdainfully), adding: "I've been to Fugakyu [a Japanese restaurant in Boston]."

Frank opines that the word *grassroots* refers to music. I point out that "grassroots" means something that comes from the people, indigenous.

Frank says, "Like Indians or Africans? Aboriginal."

Larry chimes in with a single condescending word: "Basic."

We are to spend our second night in Arusha, a small sleepy town when I passed through years ago, now a teeming city of almost two million people. There are no sidewalks and the crowds spilling over onto the traffic-filled streets make Franklin nervous. He stays in the car when we stop at a tourist store to look for deals on tanzanite. This is a beautiful blue gemstone that's related to diamonds, mined underground near the airport and unique to this region. Arusha's population boom is based primarily on tourism and the tanzanite trade.

After checking into the Outpost Inn on the outskirts of the city, Larry, Aileane, and I are talking about Frank by the swimming pool while he takes a brief rest. She expresses amazement at the believability of his delusions; that they are so straightforward and consistent. Then Aileane reveals what happened to her at seventeen. "I had my own issues," she says. "I have a habit of overextending myself, and I went a little too far in high school and ended up with an eating disorder. I lost twenty-five or thirty pounds over the course of about seven months.

It was hard for everybody in my family. Eventually I ended up at New England Medical Center; my kidneys were pretty much shut down and I wasn't processing anything. After that I went to a day program at McLean's Hospital for two weeks and continued doing that over the summer at the Boston Center for Psychiatric Rehabilitation. Something started to click when I went off to college."

"Franklin spent some time at McLean's and went to the BU Center for a little while," I tell her. "So you're no stranger to problems like he has." Aileane nods and says yes. I end up telling Larry the story of James Hillman instructing me to stop always correcting Frank. "I've been doing that," Larry admits. "I'll have to try to take a different approach."

At the end of the day, I have a beer with Aileane and Frank.

I say something about what a privilege it is to be traveling in Africa with Dr. Reiner, who is off resting.

"Privilege?!" Franklin scoffs. "Who's paying for this trip?"

Aileane raises her eyebrows. She considers Larry to be like her grandfather, and Franklin's retort clearly shakes her. And I'm annoyed with my son. "Well, we're paying," I say. "But it's still a privilege to be with someone who knows this country so well."

Alone later with Frank, I bring up his comment. Does he understand that the word *privilege* has a broader meaning than a financial one?

"I wanted to challenge you," Franklin says. "Dr. Reiner has a nose like this big," he continues, demonstrating the length with his hand and adding: "Nose everything."

I laugh, but only to cover up a gnawing uneasiness in my gut, as we end our first full day watching a group of Maasai dance on the hotel patio. I'm sure Frank could tell that Dr. Reiner was the least friendly toward him. While everyone else, including myself, was patient and listened to him, Larry's reactions were often negative. Could I expect Frank to respond differently based on those interactions? At least—knock wood—Larry seems to realize that a different approach is required.

Note:

1. "Major mental illness can cut across....": Paul R. Linde, *Of Spirits and Madness: An American Psychiatrist in Africa*, McGraw-Hill, 2002, pp. 56–7.

CHAPTER 11

• • •

Lost

I am here but I am scattered. Seeking stability. Safety is a concept that wears thin sometimes. I try to be kind to all but among some this idea is not respected. Reason for life is more positive than possibility of death. The world is a haven of so many things. Types of actions create conflicting results. Readiness to face each day is not always in our midst. Danger seems to lurk in every corner.

—Franklin's Journal, almost ten years
before embarking on this trip

I'VE EMAILED ETTA, WHO RESPONDS that she and Kamal had watched a National Geographic special about Africa "that went on for hours. One of the first shows concentrated on a young woman who lives in Arusha. It was so cool to get your email about being there. . . . Franklin sounds good. Probably a little overwhelmed. Big change from spending most of his time alone in his room. Please tell him how happy I am that he's getting to do this, and how proud I am of him. I'm looking forward to hearing of your next adventures."

I long for us to reach the Tarangire National Park, where the game is said to be prolific. In Swahili "taran" means river and "gire" means warthog, Stephan tells us. The next morning, for more than seventy-five miles, we travel the paved Dodoma Road southwest toward the "warthog river."

Along the roadside, Maasai tribesmen herd cattle and goats toward their enclosed circular domiciles. Many are tall, slender, handsome lads with blood-red *shuka* cloths draped around them. Walking with long elegant strides, they carry staffs to prod their animals along, some barefoot and others wearing sandals. There is also something haughty, even regal about the Maasai bearing.

As we pause near a busy marketplace, a woman picks up a rock and makes a gesture to throw it when I raise my camera. "You have to pay them a dollar first to take their picture," Stephan instructs. Soon we pass close to where Stephan grew up. "My family's *boma* is just up on that hill, Manduli hill, about six miles from here, and this is a place we used to come shopping."

When we reach the edge of the park shortly before noon, a few other all-terrain vehicles with camera-laden tourists are lined up to pay their entry fees. Once inside the gate, we see our first elephants, as well as some impalas, a warthog, and a waterbuck. The Tarangire Safari Lodge where we'll be staying for several nights is owned by longtime friends of Larry, the Simonson family, who also run Serengeti Select Safaris. Stephan's father had worked for the Simonsons and, after starting off as a mechanic, his early schooling had been paid for by them. Eventually, he'd been hired as one of their ten game drivers.

Like Larry's family, the Simonsons had originally come here as missionaries in the mid-1950s. "There were actually two missionary families, the Simonsons and the Mortensons, in a sort of competition around Kilimanjaro to Christianize the souls of the locals," Larry relates as we approach the lodge. Later the Mortensons moved on to Afghanistan, where Greg Mortenson grew up to become the best-selling author of *Three Cups of Tea*. But Dave Simonson had done post-graduate studies on the Maasai, and quickly became so beloved by the tribal elders that they granted his family a magnificent spread of their land high above Arusha.

The story Stephan heard of how the tribe came to venerate him was that Simonson became "the first American to kill a lion by using his hands in the Maasai land." That, Larry points out, was an exaggeration—but the American minister had indeed shot a rogue lion that was terrorizing a Maasai village. This inspires another recollection from Larry of a trip he'd made with his father when he was about twelve.

"Sometimes in the rainy season, it would take us two days to go all of three miles on the muddy roads. On our safaris we generally slept on cots inside an old Army issue tent, big enough for two twin beds and a kind of washroom in back, with an outer tent covering the whole thing and a double roof to keep things cool. There was also a front porch where we ate our meals and an opening that could be left open on hot nights. Inside, we slept under mosquito nets. Dad always kept a rifle in the tent, usually in a corner near the entrance. On this particular night, I woke up to a horrible stench. I raised my head and heard my father's voice whispering: 'Larry, lie very, very still. There's a lioness in the tent with us. If you don't move, it probably won't realize you're awake and will leave you alone.' I opened my eyes and peered into the gloom. There on the other side of my mosquito net—six inches from my face—was an adult lioness breathing heavily on me. Her rancid breath from the carcass she'd been eating was what woke me up. You can bet I stayed *very* still, praying she wasn't still hungry. After sniffing everything in the tent, the lioness finally walked out where she'd broken through the lining. She was in the tent for less than a minute, but it seemed like an eternity. Then my father got out of bed, went across the tent to where he'd stored his gun, and moved it under the mosquito net. From that night on, Dad kept the rifle right there in bed with him, not across the room."

Stephan pulls into the parking lot of the Tarangire Safari Lodge. Annette Simonson, the wife of one of the patriarch's three sons, emerges and greets Larry warmly. We enter past a swimming pool, boutique shop, and the high thatched roof of an open-sided lounge and dining area. Two men in green uniforms carry our bags down a long walkway to spacious twin-cotted adjacent tents. Each of the lodge's twenty-nine tents has a concrete floor and sturdy canvas walls beneath a thatched roof, screened windows with large curtains, electric lights and solar-heated showers.

The location is stunningly beautiful. The tents face a hillside where dense bush cascades into an endless valley below. We are told it's impor- tant to keep the tent zipped shut at all times. No one should walk the path to or from the lodge after dark without an escort and a flashlight. Nor should we leave any food inside the tent, lest baboons or some other uninvited guest pay a visit. "I remember monkeys took someone's pills," Stephan says. "Snakes can get inside, too, and lie on your bed."

Over lunch, a waitress looks at my son's bushy, curly head and tells him, "I like your hair." Franklin smiles and replies, "I'll cut it off and send it to you."

There is something archetypal about my son's changing of hairstyles—from putting it in cornrows to shaving his head completely—as he reaches turning points in his life. Besides the well-known biblical example of Samson, hair plays a role in the *Epic of Gilgamesh*, "pulling out his hair and throwing it away" while mourning the loss of a friend, and among the Native American Navajo, who believe that new thoughts are close to the scalp and old thoughts at the end of the longest strands of hair.

I wonder what Franklin might be manifesting this time.

• • •

Seated at a table overlooking the panoramic valley, we watch elephants crossing a riverbank many miles away. We talk about animals and how they impact you, what a powerful and ancient feeling it is being among them. Larry proceeds to tell a story about Jonathan Simonson, who has managed Tarangire with his wife since his father died two years ago. "He's a man of few words. He used to sit on the kitchen steps of his house, just outside the lodge proper, and talk to the elephants grazing in front of him. They definitely had a special sort of interspecies communication. One day he heard a flapping sound at his door, went outside, and found one of his favorite elephants with a spear through its hide. The elephant died right there on his porch. Well, Jonathan disappeared for a week after that. Nobody knows where he went or what he did. But the elephant poaching rate around Tarangire soon dropped enormously."

Late that afternoon, we make our initial game drive here. This national park is large, some 1,600 square miles, Stephan informs us. While animals live here year-round, it's easier to spot them during the dry season in September, when they gather in proximity of the Serengeti River. Unfortunately for us, we're visiting in the rainy season when the grass is tall and the animals are more spread out. But in the absence of grass during the dry season, sometimes you can see for hundreds of miles. Along with large herds of male impalas with their harems, we pass a vervet monkey nursing a baby and see a pair of bull elephants play-fighting with their tusks. Franklin comments on their huge penises. He asks Stephan what his favorite animals are. Impala and elephant, our guide says, and crocodiles in the Serengeti.

Birds, which to my surprise Franklin much enjoys observing, are splendidly abundant. Larry's favorite is the lilac-breasted roller. We spot weavers that use acacia thorns to protect eggs in the nest from scavengers . . . helmeted guinea fowl in trees that enjoy racing up and down the trunks together. . . . Fisher's lovebirds and white-browed cuckoos and marabou storks. "They are the only stork," says Stephan, "that can fly very, very high because they carry something like an air sack."

Franklin brings out his video camera and starts panning across the landscape. After a few minutes of this, I interrupt him: "Frank, you really should think about conserving your battery. We're going to be seeing a lot more wildlife, and you can't always charge up your camera at the lodge. Only at certain times of day." My son keeps right on filming.

Dr. Reiner chimes in from the front seat: "Well, don't say we didn't warn you."

Franklin glares at the doctor. He says nothing, but is clearly irritated by our interference. As we start back toward the lodge, I suggest he put his camera on the seat where it won't bounce around so much. He doesn't.

"Sorry if I'm being overly parental," I say, but half-heartedly.

"Sometimes mothering, sometimes fathering," Franklin replies.

"My own family had a little of both," says Larry. My son falls silent.

Aileane spots our first lion, asleep on the ground. Shortly thereafter arrives a family of four—a lioness and three cubs—traversing the road in front of us. It's toward the close of the afternoon and I can barely contain myself. Lions have always been my favorite animal, all the way back to my childhood and later when I traveled through East Africa. All I want in this moment is for Franklin to share my feeling of excitement. "Wow! Look at that! Frank, do you see the mother? They must be hunting!"

But Frank betrays not the slightest emotion and even averts his eyes. This hurts and angers me. Stephan tries to lighten the mood. Turning to Frank, he describes how lions can mate every fifteen minutes for as long as a week. Larry adds: "The female seems to know when the time is right. And when it's all done, she chases the male away." This amuses Aileane. But Frank doesn't crack a smile.

The lioness heads into an acacia thicket, where she's stashed a kill. It's a large ostrich. According to Stephan, the ostrich wouldn't be their food of choice. "Maybe the ostrich was sick, because ostriches are *very* fast, hard for a lion to catch. Maybe she just found a dead animal."

As rain clouds loom on the horizon, some tsetse flies invade our vehicle. Stephan says that twenty tsetses would need to bite you at the same time to run the risk of your getting sleeping sickness. "You don't need to kill tsetse flies, this is their home," he adds. But I'm nervous about them nonetheless, finding blood on my khakis in two places from squeezing the tsetses as they climb my inner pants leg. I see one alight on Franklin's shirt. "Frank, swat that thing!" I exhort him loudly. He looks disdainfully at me. "I don't want to kill it," he says emphatically, and stares off into the distance.

Larry tries changing the mood by telling another story. "My father worked for awhile doing sleeping sickness control. That program has been in place for a long, long time. Today the tsetse fly population is a fraction of what it used to be. But a lot of local tribal people had to be moved so the British government could clear the land. I sometimes accompanied my dad on his 'persuasion' visits to the villages."

Usually, the chief would invite the Reiners for a meal of *ugali*, a dumpling-like dough made from millet and dipped into a meat stew. "One memorable night, I remarked to Dad that the meat tasted unlike anything I'd ever had—sort of like pork, but somewhat different. He froze in mid-swallow, spat out what he was chewing, and said: 'Larry, put that down and don't touch another bite! Don't ask any questions, just come with me.' Then he stood up, looked over at the head man, and said politely, in Swahili, 'Chief, we're very, very full, thank you very much.' And we walked out. My dad would never say any more about this meal—but we were in an area known in the past for cannibalism. And I'm told that human flesh has a similar flavor to pork."

I flash back to a childhood memory of watching the movie *King Solomon's Mines*. Stephan says nothing. Franklin scowls and glares into the horizon.

• • •

Another memory returns. Tanzania's Ngorongoro Crater, Summer 1971: Staying at a dollar-a-night youth hostel, I'd set out hiking along a wilderness path at dusk that I was told led to the lodge about a quarter-mile away. Encountering a group of African men who'd come to a dead stop along the route, I asked what was happening. "Buffalo," one replied. He'd seen a couple of water buffalo, dangerous animals indeed, grazing off to the right and thought there might be more down at the stream where they were going to get water.

I waited with the group for about five minutes and then asked the English-speaking fellow: "Well, are you going to stand here all night?" I was young and cocky. He gave me a long look and said, "You think it's safe?" Sure, I said. He motioned me to take the lead, if I so chose. And I did, playing the role of "great white hunter" that I recalled from the old jungle movies (much to my embarrassment in retrospect), walking in front of the others, pausing, then looking back and beckoning them to advance with a forward motion of my arm. I did this several times, with my troop coming to a full stop each time I did, though at a safe distance behind. When I reached the water's edge, I jumped across. They followed suit, then ran past me and up an embankment on the other side.

But there were no buffalo, and I arrived at the lodge quite stuffed with myself. I ended up having dinner with a local Asian gentleman who built roads in the area, whom I informed that I was planning to walk back to my quarters. The man warned me this wasn't safe, but I assured him that I'd avoid the bush path and take the longer main road. Setting off after dark, I was almost beyond the confines of the lodge when a Land Rover pulled up alongside me. "I'm sorry," my dinner companion said, "but I can't let you do this. Get in, I'll drive you."

I sighed and plopped down beside him in the front seat. As we came around a curve about two hundred yards from my destination, lying in the middle of the road, as if awaiting my arrival, was a leopard. I would have made the turn and walked right into it. My heart was pounding as the driver came to a stop. We sat there looking at the leopard, which stared back at us without budging. "Man, you're lucky," the man said quietly. "They never come down here. This is only the fourth leopard that I've seen in seven years." Inside of a very long minute, the leopard rose, turned haughtily away, and walked into the surrounding hills. No further words were exchanged as I disembarked at the youth hostel. I never saw the man again, but he had most certainly saved my life.

• • •

The High Court of Tanzania has ruled that the Tarangire Safari Lodge whose operations are inside the wildlife park were negligent in ensuring the safety of a seven-year-old French boy killed by a leopard on October 1, 2005 within the precincts of the lodge. . . . Judge Sambo said it was the responsibility of parents not to let unaccompanied young children roam about, but the general safety of the boy and the parents was in no question the responsibility of the hotel or the lodge management. . . . The late Adrien Pereira was snatched by the leopard from the premises of the tourist lodge . . . while his parents and other guests were having dinner. He was found dead in less than half an hour some 150 meters from the lodge by his father and other people who joined the search mission minutes after the attack.

—The *Arusha Times*, April 4–10, 2009

Darkness descends over the Tarangire lodge before dinner. Franklin sits off by himself, sprawled in a big hardwood armchair in the lounge. He's drinking a Tusker beer when I approach him.

"How are you?" I ask.

"Why do you keep asking me how I am?" he replies angrily. "I'm fine!"

"Okay, sorry. Don't go anywhere, all right? I'll see you in a few minutes, I'm going to send an email."

Behind the front desk is a small room with a computer available for guests when there's enough power during the evening. I write to Alice:

Our afternoon trip ended with several elephants right next to the car; then as it began to grow dark, a lioness and its cubs came to the road and marched along right in front of us, which was amazing. Franklin was in good spirits earlier, very into his new camera, but then the mood changed and his enthusiasm vanished as we met the most exciting animals. I think he's tired now and wants to go to bed . . .

Perhaps ten minutes have passed when I reenter the lounge, and Franklin is nowhere to be seen. *He must have gone back to our tent*, I wonder. *I hope he had a guide with him.* I find a worker to lead me down the path. There's almost no moon, and we use both of our flashlights to see our way to tent number sixteen.

Franklin is not there.

I return to the main lodge and check the pool area. No sign of him. Dr. Reiner and Aileane are now in the lounge, having a glass of wine. They haven't seen Frank either. Again I walk the pathway to the tents, this time with Aileane and a guide accompanying. Nothing. "Would he just have wandered off?" she asks, trying not to seem too anxious.

"That's not really like him," I say. "But—he wasn't in a good place—he was pissed off at me—I just don't know."

I struggle not to reveal how terrified I am.

At last, I locate Annette Simonson. My heart is pounding in my chest.

"My son," I say, "is missing."

I begin imagining terrible scenarios. My son has wandered off without a guide or a flashlight and has fallen off the path and down the ravine. He's hit his head and is unconscious, and a leopard . . . or a pack of hyenas . . . or baboons . . . or a rogue lion . . . is closing in.

"Lions usually hunt at night," the Tarangire National Park guidebook says. Wasn't that the initial fear Frank expressed to me that day when we first talked in the car about making the trip? And hadn't Stephan spoken this afternoon about how lions have less to eat than they used to?

How silent is a kill?

"Once the animal is dead, the lions will sometimes move it to a secluded or shady spot," the guidebook says. "Depending on how hungry the lions are, they may feed quietly or if it is a large pride, eat anything they can get hold of and begin dragging pieces away as soon as possible."

How could I have been so foolish as to bring Frank to this place?

"If you find a kill with lions eating, please do not go too close as you may disturb them."

How will I tell his mother?

Annette Simonson quietly assembles staff and sends several men in different directions. I recognize Gideon, a nice young fellow who'd helped with our luggage. I see Stephan joining in the hunt. The man assigned to accompany me asks questions in broken English.

Yes, I've been down this path already. Twice.

I hear the whooping cry of a hyena in the near distance. Or is it my imagination?

"Hyenas have the reputation of being scavengers but they frequently hunt and kill their own food, and it is not uncommon for lions to steal their kills," our guidebook says.

Lightning shimmers in the distance.

We have passed our tent and are approaching the end of the path. I feel like this is fruitless because I've been this far twice already, and we're about to turn around again. But there's a light on inside tent 21. It hadn't been earlier. I glance over. And there is my son, standing just inside, talking to someone. A wave of tremendous relief washes through me.

"Ohhhhh," I call out, in a high-pitched voice: "Are you hanging out in there?"

A woman's voice responds immediately, in an agitated British accent. "Yes, he IS! And he's NOT welcome!"

Franklin pushes open the tent flap and emerges. He's staring at the ground as he says quickly, "I was really tired and I fell asleep in there. I thought it was our tent."

Later, he would explain that he'd thought the number on the outside said "16," so had flopped down on the bed and conked out. When the British couple returned from dinner and demanded to know what he was doing there, Frank responded with a yawning "whaaat?" This was followed by a back-and-forth exchange in which he told them, "This is my tent where I'm sleeping." The woman said, "I don't think so!" That's about when I showed up.

At the time, a surge of anger rises inside me. "Didn't I tell you not to leave the lounge area without letting me know?!"

Frank says nothing. Five tents down from where I found him, we unzip ours and go inside. He's now in a rage, too. He flips onto his cot while I sit down across from him. I can see the African worker who'd been accompanying my search waiting outside, off to the left, arms folded.

Abruptly, my son is what the psychiatric jargon calls "floridly psychotic." He's talking rapid-fire, ranting about devils that he saw on the road today.

"You're always being fatherly! You're not my father!"

Are we back to that?

"You can't feel anything. You're always telling me what to do!"

Big mistake, talking to him about conserving his battery.

"My name's not Franklin. It's Simon Peter."

Only later, writing in my journal, will I realize the biblical allusion.

"Dr. Reiner's always correcting what I say. Swahili isn't the real language here, with words like 'Karibu!'"

Karibu means "welcome," and is the customary Swahili greeting.

"We could write a book. I've published many already. It will take two years. I have the rights to one called *Shumaki Akidsu Nasubigi.*"

Does Frank feel left out—or even conspired against—because I'm tape-recording Stephan's comments and some of Larry's memories?

"I have a trust fund for you." He tells me the name of a bank.

I stay silent for the most part, allowing his venting to wind down. After about a half-hour, it does. I tell my son how upset I was when I couldn't find him anywhere. "So you're having a breakdown, too," he says. Is that what he wants? I think to myself. I nod my head yes.

Back in the lounge area, Larry relates to me the story about the French boy and the leopard—which he knew about but I didn't—that had been in the back of his mind. Aileane has been having a strong talk with Larry about not paying such attention to Franklin's sometimes faulty thinking. The doctor expresses how difficult this is for him because it's almost instinctual. "To me," Larry says, "he's all over the map." But he understands the consequences and says he'll do his best to bite his tongue in the future.

I remember Larry telling me that he'd initially studied psychiatry while attending Baylor University's College of Medicine, then became disillusioned about pursuing it. He'd said: "Those were the days when they prescribed many pills and used electric shock treatment; the patient would jerk and lose bladder control. It just didn't seem to suit my temperament, which was more Freudian than behavioral." Yet Aileane, I realize, is a better psychological thinker than Larry, more simpático, perhaps because she's been through so much along similar lines in her life. And Stephan, who doesn't seem to be psychological at all, is the most simpático, because he is without judgment.

Franklin has said he doesn't want to eat, but a sweet woman serving the buffet makes him a plate anyway. When I bring it to him in our tent, he's very glad to have it. Afterward, he agrees that it's time to go to sleep. I watch him take his medication with some bottled water. I lie down on my cot, my mind racing. Painfully, I realize that I'm still fitting him into my agendas, just as I have since he was a boy. The loneliness he must have felt without a father's true presence in his life! And so his "schizophrenia" forced me to notice him. But even now, after all these years, I still seek to place him within *my* context—like about when to use his camera. Of course he would run away from that, from me. I have to let him *be*. He's so used to being alone in the same known environment. But just as he knew he needed hospitalization after agreeing to go on the trip, hopefully this is also part of his process. And mine. Ours.

But also, perhaps this incident has taken us to exactly where we need to be. In the company of "the wild," the instinctual "wild animal" in and between the two of us can—and has—come to the surface.

Then I start to laugh. I can't help it. The voice of that English lady, all in a huff, resounds in my head, exclaiming: "And he's NOT welcome!" The thought of the woman and her husband walking back to their tent, ready for a good night's rest, only to find the flap unzipped and this big bushy-haired guy sprawled across their bed! Karibu!

It's like something out of Monty Python. Franklin might have been just what they needed. Oh lord, will we run into the old dear again in the morning?

•　•　•

You can count on me turning it out tonight. You see I'm not here to fight. I'm here to unite, black and white.

I question, aren't we one tribe, or am I disillusioned, do I have the wrong vibe?

Just listen to my song that is African in nature—the cradle of creation. It could be a wonderful sensation . . .

—Franklin's Journal, late '90s

CHAPTER 12

• • •

Among the Maasai

Africa, being as old as it is, makes all people except the professional invaders and spoilers into children. No one says to anyone in Africa, "Why don't you grow up?" . . . Men know that they are children in relation to the country. . . . But to have the heart of a child is not a disgrace. It is an honor.
— Ernest Hemingway, *True at First Light: A Fictional Memoir*

THE MORNING AFTER FRANKLIN'S TEMPORARY disappearance, I send an email to Etta. She quickly responds: "That is terrifying. Really sorry. Thank god he didn't really wander far." Franklin now seems just fine. "Wow, last night I ended up in that lady's room," he says, self-reproachfully. He thinks he might have left his house keys in their tent by mistake, but later finds them in his own. At any rate, I'm relieved to avoid another encounter with the British couple again.

On our ensuing game drive, while sleeping a bit off and on, Frank engages in asking questions: "Is the river customarily going to have water?" Yes, in season. "Are there emus here?" No, Larry replies, but not condescendingly this time; rather informing him that they're only located in Australia. Frank accepts this. Still, there remains some strain between my son and the doctor. This becomes obvious when, after Larry says something to Stephan in Swahili, I hear Frank mutter under his breath: "Nuremberg."

Today Frank names a yellow-crested bird as his favorite animal. Aileane likes giraffes, for Larry it's cheetahs, and of course I say lions. The morning's highlight is coming across a large troop of baboons;

moms and babies screeching away and tussling in a fig tree. On our way in to lunch, two waterbucks lock horns over a female resting nearby. A mother elephant dozes with her tusks against a tree, her baby sleeping in the grass below.

The game drivers from various companies stop to compare notes on where the animals are. One of these is an eighty-two-year-old gentleman named Eric Balson. Later at the lodge, Larry runs into him and learns that Balson happened to have attended the same Prince of Wales School that the doctor had a few years later. In the 1960s, Balson had been in charge of the Tarangire Game Reserve and was later called upon by the Tanzanian government to "help stamp out a big poaching racket." This had included the ruling Kenyatta family in Kenya, with the president's wife and daughter being "the biggest illegal dealers in ivory and rhino horn." Today, poaching and illicit sales—especially to China—have made the vaunted black rhinos of East Africa an almost-vanished species. "I know," Larry interjects. "When I was young, it was routine to see six to ten in a day every time we drove up to Bereko; now there are about thirty left in the entire region."

Balson and Dr. Reiner end up in tears reminiscing, out of a personal nostalgia that has much to do with all the changes in East Africa. Changes that seem intolerable but, at the same time, sadly inevitable. The onetime game warden shakes his head and continues: "It breaks my heart. And they already want to make a tarred road right through the middle of the Serengeti. If they do that, then bye bye Serengeti." Animals like the wildebeest would be forced away from the corridor due to the increased traffic, at a time when their habitats are already under siege.

Over lunch, Larry grows pensive and Franklin is quietly observing him. What Balson describes, the doctor says, "brings back so much." Then he tells this story: "Before I went off to school, I was out playing with some of my local friends when a man came by trying to sell lion cubs. I had no idea, but he'd stolen them from the mother somehow. But he didn't want to keep them because he knew he was gonna get in trouble. So he gave them to us boys to play with. And we used them like soccer balls. It still brings tears to my eyes. I went home and proudly told my parents what I'd been doing. I never got lashed so. My father beat me till he couldn't raise his arm anymore and then my mother took over."

A pregnant silence is followed by my son's question. What did the boys do with the cubs when they were done playing with them? "They were dead," Larry says, choking up. Frank doesn't respond, but seems impressed with his honesty and moved by the feeling.

Momentarily, Larry gathers himself and continues: "A second transformative moment I had involved another lion. I was grown by then. I went to visit a gold mine in a town called Geita, in north-western Tanzania, where some Canadian miners decided to take me hunting. When we came across a resting lion, one of them said to me, 'You're gonna take it.' I was carrying this fancy rifle with a telescopic sight. I aimed and fired and the animal dropped. And two little cubs came trotting out from under her. From that moment since, I've never been able to aim anything straight."

Perhaps these experiences, I think to myself, contributed to his becoming a pediatrician devoted to young "creatures." I wonder if Franklin might be considering the same thing about him. At the least, this confessional moment is the doctor's owning of his shadow side, but also an opening of himself to us in a new and important way.

Aileane looks at Larry. "You should tell the dik-dik story," she says. We've been seeing a fair number of these adorable small antelope with their reddish-brown coats, white-ringed eyes, long snouts, and rubbery-bottomed hooves. Stephan has said they have a scent gland under their eyes, so they can rub against a tree and remember their homes.

"I had a pet dik-dik for awhile," Larry responds hastily. "He was the cutest little guy, about a foot high at the shoulder and maybe two feet long, weighing no more than twelve pounds. Dik-diks are named for the alarm calls of the females, because as you can imagine, they would be easy prey for big cats and even monitor lizards. I could never housebreak mine, so we eventually let him go."

"No, Larry," Aileane insists. "I mean *the* dik-dik story."

Larry raises his eyebrows and shakes his head. "I hesitate to talk about this," he says.

"It certainly goes against all of my scientific training." Franklin's ears perk up. "But okay. I know this happened. I remember it like yesterday. I used to go out with a little .22 rifle and shoot small antelope. One afternoon I came across a dik-dik. This was before I had one as a pet. Well, I shot it in the flank and it disappeared into the bush.

"And out the other side, to my amazement, came a little African kid bleeding from a gunshot wound in his leg. The boy ran away. I walked over and looked. He'd emerged at exactly the exact same angle where the dik-dik would have."

Larry takes a deep breath before continuing: "This was a tribal area where the people were reputed to transmogrify, turning themselves into snakes or antelopes or other animals. You can see why I don't like to tell this story."

As a man of Western medicine, Dr. Reiner is apologetic, perhaps fearing that such a tale will make him sound crazy. Yet he is also *drawn* to the irrational—from having grown up in Africa, to inviting me to bring Franklin on this trip. What *is* normal? Africa surely is not. And Frank can suddenly relate to Larry in a way that hadn't seemed possible before. "That's a *great* story," he tells the doctor.

Might he see something of himself in the wounded boy?

We must take into account the mystical solidarity between man and animal, which is a dominant characteristic of the religion of the paleo-hunters. By virtue of this, certain human beings are able to change into animals, or to understand their language, or to share in their prescience and occult powers....he in a manner re-establishes the situation that existed in illo tempore, in mythical times, when the divorce between man and the animal world had not yet occurred.
    —Mircea Eliade, *Shamanism: Archaic Techniques of Ecstasy*[1]

• • •

Franklin takes a nap after lunch. He tells me later that he left the zipper open on his tent, and two monkeys got halfway in trying to visit him. He's beginning to notice more on our afternoon game drive: "there's a warthog" and "interesting bird" and "I smell something dead."

Around the time he mentions the smell, we come upon a dead elephant in a dry riverbed. It has no tusks. Someone seems to have cut them off. Tears well up in my eyes. I see tears in Larry and Aileane's eyes, too. Frank lowers his head. We sit in silent homage together for several minutes.

Franklin has been paying close attention to his hygiene on the trip, showering regularly and asking to use my deodorant—given the close quarters we are all sharing, a welcome development. We set off on our final day for Silalei, a large swamp and the source of the Tarangire River. It's a trek from the lodge, but the area is pretty dead when we arrive mid-morning. "It's almost eerie," Larry says, "I'm really surprised there are no birds."

Looking upon the primordial swamp, Frank recalls two boyhood moments that occurred on Martha's Vineyard—a whale that washed up on the beach and a prehistoric shark's tooth that he'd found in the sand. I, too, am in a childhood reverie—memories of going to the circus with my father, and about the first magazine that captured my fancy, *Natural History*, of which I collected every issue.

In between doing some sketches on his drawing pad, Frank makes up names of all the places he's been in Africa before and says he expects it will take two years to write his book. "How many languages do you speak?" Stephan asks him. "Thousands—a lot of languages," Frank replies, and Stephan simply nods in agreement. Larry is no longer offering any "corrections."

Joining us for a picnic lunch at a small roadside table is a superb starling, with its glossy blue back and neck. "That's like a painting," my son says, "it's so vivid!" After maybe ten minutes, he looks over and asks me: "Are you finished? I'm ready to see some more beasts!" He helps Stephan rewrap what remains of the box lunches, and we're off again.

Frank says he used to surf over in Australia, where the emus come from. "So you have been many places," Stephan says. "Yeah," Frank says. "That's good," Stephan says. Frank talks of swinging from a bungee cord after climbing a mountain in Hawaii (news to me) and of also scaling Mount Monadnock in New Hampshire (which he did as a teenager). "Would you like to try Kilimanjaro?" Stephan asks. "Yeah," Frank says. "That is 20,000 feet," Stephan says. Well, Frank continues fantasizing; he *had* spent some time in the Amazon rainforest, chiseling his way through with a hatchet, carrying his own tent and food. Sometimes, Franklin goes on, he might sleep in that same tent on Commonwealth Avenue in Boston.

Might these be metaphors indicating the reality of his inner, as well as something of his outer, life? The forging ahead on his own and the sense he must sometimes have of "homelessness." A first episode of schizophrenia, as noted earlier, tends to strand the sufferer for a long, long time—if not forever—at that late adolescent-developmental stage. Here, Frank in a sense returns to that period, pleasantly boasting with Stephan of physical prowess and feats. And Stephan responds to Frank, as always, with normalcy, this time, a "competitive" man-to-man response. He says that he himself was a good soccer player, and he also has run more than fifteen miles a day.

Stephan says he hadn't expected many elephants to be here now, but they are becoming commonplace for us, apparently still waiting for the heavy rains before moving on. Larry riffs some elephant statistics: a life span as long as seventy years, how they must stay close to water and drink more than 50 gallons a day, along with consuming four to six percent of their body weight—"but they only have one stomach, so that means bad digestion." Stephan smiles and says, "But if you take elephant poop to the Maasai, they use it to treat coughing." Larry's heard that, too, and Frank loves the idea. Maybe they should call it Robi-Turd. Ah, the natural remedies of the bush!

Stephan pulls off into a small clearing, where stands a lone baobab tree, whose vast root mass points skyward as though somehow it's been turned upside down. The trunk is hollowed out and large enough for us to walk right through. Elephants have stripped the bark during the dry season, ironically creating a "habitat" for poachers to lie in wait inside the tree. Frank and I stand gazing up into what seems an endless darkness. My son rubs his hands against the baobab's inner sanctum.

Franklin picks up his camera for the first time in awhile as we pass by a male ostrich, exclaiming "Got ya!" as he clicks the shutter. "Stephan, can I take your picture?" Soon he stands up in the Land Rover to shoot some video of a bull elephant through the open roof. When Aileane's camera battery goes dead, Frank asks her, "Want to use mine?" And to Stephan: "Your cell phone takes pictures—want me to take one for you?" Stephan passes him the phone.

The last leg of the day is, for me, a meditation. About the unquestioning nature of Stephan that Franklin relates to. It's so hard for me to relax, to let Franklin be Franklin, but Stephan's reassuring calm offers a hopeful response not unlike the land itself with its incredible variety and richness. I must represent to my son the father who's "done everything," so of course he would invent a world where he's surpassed me. In my notebook I jot down, "There must be a thin line between resentment and gratitude." Yet, through these initial days in Africa, a restructuring of our relationship feels like it's in process.

Back at the lodge, there is an email from Etta:

I hope the rest of the day went okay. I'm sure that this is, as you said, a process that he has to go through. It is a dose of reality that he could never in a million years have made up. . . . It is just so incredibly miraculous that he is there, to see, smell, and taste the African culture and people. There must be so much going through his mind right now. When I was with him last week, he at first wanted to go downtown to the Chinese dim sum place. Then he said, "No—they might not treat you so well since you are African American." So the great ambiguity that is such a source of problem in him must be right at the forefront when he sees so many African people. Who is he??? He always wanted to learn Swahili. . . . Reiner's speaking it right in front of him. No place to hide except in his illness. . . . I pray that he will get through this rocky period——and even find a way to talk or draw about it.

Now, sitting together in the lounge at dusk, Franklin says to me, "CBS News asked, 'Is Dick Russell your papa? He was a reporter who did work for *Sports Illustrated* and *TV Guide*, why didn't he stay with those two instead of being a freelance writer?'" I can't remember Frank ever before assessing my past—*Sports Illustrated* being the magazine I quit before making my initial trip to Africa, *TV Guide* being my job at the time he was born before I resigned when Frank was about nine months old.

"Hey, where's your drawing pad?" I ask him.

"Drawing," he replies, is "a feat of the imagination—and a feat of the eyes. Because sometimes you draw so hard, your eyes go sore."

While I go to write Alice, he hangs out with one of the colorfully-clad workers who tend to the pool. When I return, Frank tells me: "He says there used to be slave labor in Africa, and he does not want that to happen again." He sees the waitress who serves the evening drinks and greets her with a "Karibu!" She grins and replies, "Mr. Salsa, you're welcome." Sure enough, he wants a major bowl of chips-and-salsa. Frank always compliments the staff for the good coffee and other service, and the waitress tells me: "Your son is very polite." All of the people who work here seem to know his name. To another of the staff, he says, "If you ever have hors d'oeuvres of cornflakes with African cream, they're the best, man." The fellow loves the image. Frank informs a pretty new waitress that he's 20 percent African and 70 percent Chinese. Next he greets a European couple who are heading for the verandah, and stop to make some friendly chitchat. After listing off names for the various elephants we'd seen, Frank adds: "We saw three lions today. And if you clip their ears, there's a market run by a Pygmy where you can buy them." They nod politely and bid a hasty farewell.

Alone together again before dinner, my son goes into a long riff, during which he posits a strangely poignant moment. He claims to have heard me say, upon boarding the airplane: "I'm forever going to chase you in writing. And forever going to make you the lion that I love." (Lions are not only my favorite animal, but are also the symbol associated with my Zodiacal birth sign, Leo.)

Once in awhile, Frank invents both sides of imagined conversations that took place in the past, including a foreign accent for my voice. "You said, 'My name is Dick Russell, I come to drink with you.' And I said, 'You should be in the movies, kid.' You said, 'I'm gonna be your father in the future, because you called me a kid.' And that's the way it went." He goes on about a dictator requesting, "Call Dick Russell to Africa please." Some type of an enzyme, he continues, was taken from me and Etta: "In 1977 I decided it." (Choosing his parents? an old Jewish idea that James Hillman also suggested in *The Soul's Code*. Frank was born on January 31, 1979.)

In the next breath, Frank recalls a candy store where I once accompanied him along New York's Lower East Side, a moment which I had long forgotten.

He speaks, too, in stark declarative sentences about having lived in ancient Egypt, and mentions the boy king Tutankhamen. "I was buried in a tomb. . . . They took all my blood out. I lived anyway. They unearthed me three hundred or four hundred years later. I remember it perfectly. I remember being there with the gold." This is not necessarily delusional; Carl Jung, too, I recall, thought of himself as having lived in past periods of history.

Frank says he's getting along fine with Larry and Aileane, who soon come to join us. At which point, Frank cuts to the subject of one of his floor mates at the group home back in Massachusetts: "Has a thick white beard. . . . Female dressed as a man."

Larry joins in with a slight adjustment to the image: "*She* has a beard."

Frank: "All around. He has a spot on his neck."

"*Her* neck," Larry corrects him. Aileane is struggling to keep from laughing. I am, too. It's the first time I've seen the doctor engage in this kind of Abbott-and-Costello-like banter with Frank.

"*Her* neck, I'm sorry," says Frank. "He's on medication but never takes it. She—I call her he sometimes."

Larry: "Her he, her he." He sounds a little like a laughing hyena. "I'm really enjoying listening to this conversation!" Aileane exclaims.

I think the ice between Franklin and Dr. Reiner has definitely been broken.

• • •

We all danced to the ceremonial songs together, anyone who felt like it could.
                    —Tepilit Ole Saitoti, *The Worlds of a Maasai Warrior*

Leaving Tarangire the next morning, Stephan turns to Franklin and says: "Maasai are good jumpers. If you jump and sing a lot, women will be attracted to you."

We pass a mountain called Lepurkao, named after a Maasai tribesman who lived into his nineties with more than thirty-five wives and over one hundred children. "You think he likes all his wives?" Franklin asks, and Stephan shrugs. Larry and I need to mark territory, so he pulls off to the side. As we emerge, standing perhaps twenty feet away, observing us shyly but alertly, is a Maasai youth in his teens. He wears a black cloth, holds a spear, and his face is painted white with some checkered cross patterns that look not unlike the symbolic "hieroglyphics" that Franklin sometimes draws. I'm initially startled by the similarity. Under a nearby tree, three more Maasai adolescents sit, also with painted faces.

Back in the car, Stephan says that the boys have just gone through initiation to become *murrans* (warriors). No anesthetic is used during a painful circumcision ceremony that takes place before sunrise. The healing process can take several months. Franklin takes this in quietly, but is clearly thinking about it. *Might this trip be a kind of initiation for him?* I wonder.

Late that morning, at the base of a hill, Stephan pulls off near a large circular fence—an *enkang*—fashioned from thorny acacia branches, with an enclosed compound in the center. This Maasai village is one of two *bomas* in the area that welcomes tourists. A Maasai in his early twenties approaches our car, identifying himself in English as the son of the local chief. The requested entry fee is the equivalent in Tanzanian shillings of fifteen dollars apiece. Larry, Aileane, and I get out. Franklin shakes his head. "I'll just wait in the car," he says.

The sound of many blended female voices, accompanied by drummers, comes from behind the gate of the compound. "You have arrived for a wedding ceremony," the chief's son informs. Although it's most likely being performed for our benefit, the music is compelling. As the procession comes closer, swaying and chanting, the women are seen to be wearing multicolored garments with beaded ornaments in their long-stretched earlobes. They lean forward to breathe out, and tilt their heads back while breathing in, doing a kind of call-and-response: a lead singer for the melody and a chorus of vocalists blending in harmony.

Franklin decides to join the party. While Stephan stays with our vehicle, we follow the group as it sings and dances its way back toward the entryway. More Maasai, male and female, wait inside the enclosure. Some of the men join the dancing women, "the jumpers" that Stephan earlier spoke of. The chief's son, who is shepherding us along, says that we are welcome to participate. I'm tempted, being reminded of the moment just over forty years before in Ghana, with the medicine man standing in the center of a circle and a young fellow imploring, "The drum is calling you." I glance at Frank, but he shakes his head no. The feeling is that he has too much respect for the Maasai traditions to intrude. I realize this when I suggest he take some video footage, as I'm doing, and he asks our local guide whether it's proper to take pictures. Even though he's told it's okay, Frank won't do it. So I abstain from the dancing. But Aileane isn't given a choice. A crown is placed on her head and the Irish lass is led into the midst of the dancers. Larry is delighted.

Our host introduces Franklin and me to two other young men, who invite us to follow them inside one of the domiciles "to learn about Maasai culture." One of them says in halting but decent English, "Our houses are very small." Indeed, the circular *enkaj* is about nine feet wide and fifteen feet long. We need to duck way low to enter and then are instructed to squat on the ground. The two Maasai hunker down across from us. "Nice house, man," Franklin says. "Expensive stuff you make the house from, you know." He's dead serious, and they laugh.

It's very dark in here, despite the last embers of a fire, which Frank notices is still hot. He's curious what material they use for the walls. "This is like mud and plaster?" One of the Maasai replies: "Mud. Water. Sticks." They go on to explain that the house, built by the village women, was designed to be impermanent because of the tribe's nomadic nature. Timber poles form the structural framework, driven into the ground and interwoven with a lattice of smaller branches, before being plastered with the mud, water, and sticks—as well as some ash, human urine, and cow dung to waterproof the roof. "Urine?!" Frank exclaims, and the two Maasai react by laughing with him. Frank gestures toward the sleeping quarters behind us, says "new cot, eh?" and they nod in agreement.

Their lesson in Maasai ways continues. It's hard to believe, but an entire family apparently cooks, eats, sleeps, and socializes in here, as well as storing food, fuel, and other possessions of the household. Altogether, some 115 people live in this village. Some are Christians, while others believe in nature. The cows, goats, and sheep are put to pasture nearby, but are placed in the enclosure by night. A man's wealth is measured in terms of cattle and children, the latter being from any number of wives. Like the males, the adolescent females must go through *emorata*, female circumcision, in an elaborate initiation ritual. Any who haven't suffered the practice are generally considered not marriageable or else unworthy of a high bride price (still paid in livestock to the woman's father).

"Each wife has their own house," we're told, which the men visit regularly. Frank's ears perk up hearing that. "Would you like me to do an Internet site for you?" he asks them. Their ears perk up, too.

After about twenty minutes, we emerge to relocate Larry and Aileane, who are finishing their own *boma* tour. Outside the enclosure, a market is in progress, including booths full of beads made from numerous materials: white ones from clay and shells; black and blue ones from iron and charcoal; red ones from gourds, wood, and bone. One piece for sale, we're told, is from the bone of a lion. "You like it? Maybe for your daughter? And this?" we are asked.

A number of other Maasai collectibles are displayed at the last booth, with what seem to be high prices. They finally ask an outrageous one hundred fifty dollars for the lot. Bargaining, we're told, is expected. "No, no, no, can't afford that," I say, "I'll buy everything for twenty-five dollars." The man selling the wares suggests, "I write down a number, then you bargain by putting down another number." At which point Franklin jumps into the mix. Quickly examining each piece—this bone, that stone, that jewel—he describes their worth. "Okay, this one's worth three dollars, that one eight, this goes for eleven." Then he rapidly adds up the figures in his head. "So, altogether thirty-three dollars," Frank announces.

"Well, that's as high as I'm gonna go," I say. We walk away empty-handed. But my son has proven his mettle in the realm of the Maasai, and there's no way I'm going to trump that.

After a last stop inside a one-room schoolhouse where the children sing for us, and beautifully, Frank and I stand near the compound's entryway with the chief's son and the two companions who've been squiring us around. Frank suddenly announces to them that he plays basketball. In fact as part of the Lakers, with Kobe Bryant. (In Swahili, I'll find out later, Kobe is the word for "tortoise," although it's pronounced Ko-bay.) They look nonplussed, so I try to bridge the gap. "You know, Kobe Bryant? Famous basketball player in America?"

The face of one of the young Maasai men lights up. Backpedaling, then cutting left and moving right, he imitates first the dribbling and then taking a one-hand shot at the imagined hoop. "You mean this?" he asks Franklin, breaking into a broad smile. "Yes!" my son exclaims, and offers an outstretched hand for a high-five.

We're now speaking a universal language. As we head back to the car, the Maasai warriors take turns slapping my son on the shoulder like long-lost friends.

• • •

I'd be thinking about this morning for a long time, starting with the graceful tact and courtesy that Franklin displayed in refusing to enter the dance. He's not here to experience an exotic culture, he's here to recover and re-plant himself. Yet with the young Maasai man's simulation of Kobe Bryant and the Lakers, perhaps he is returning the compliment of some of our party (Aileane, in particular) taking part in the dance. Isn't this a way of imagining basketball, as an Americanized

Maasai dance? Reciprocity, community, and communion. That's what seemed to be happening for Franklin among the Maasai.

But also, what every young man needs: a bit of pride. Franklin could brag, tell tall tales, joke, offer something, bargain, and initiate a Maasai into the African American dance of basketball. He's a young man among young men, which is the very thing that schizophrenia prevents. (And what does the Western medical model do? It further isolates.) On the deepest, most profound level, this experience is providing an emotional, soulful, spiritual corrective. I dare to believe, a beginning to come of age for Franklin, a rite of passage—not by "going home again," but by bringing something, making an offering, rising above pride by *having* pride, and courtesy, and honor.

"*No one says to anyone in Africa, 'Why don't you grow up?'*" The honor of childhood: That is what Franklin may be recovering and this voyage is perhaps making possible, in this way hopefully making right the deficits of his own childhood.

Note:

1.   Eliade on animals: cited in Steven Kotler, *A Small Furry Prayer: Dog Rescue and the Meaning of Life*, Bloomsbury, 2010, p. 229.

CHAPTER 13

• • •

Into the Serengeti

Wilderness gave us knowledge. Wilderness made us human. We came from here. Perhaps that is why so many of us feel a strong bond to this land called Serengeti; it is the land of our youth.
　　　　　　　　　　—Boyd Norton, *Serengeti: The Eternal Beginning*

A
S WE DRIVE SOUTH ON the rutted tarmac after departing the Maasai village, Frank says admiringly to Aileane: "They gave you the crown, the Maasai warriors." She nods and Frank adds: "Then we went into a hut. Had to lower down like a goat!"

I ask Stephan if this village is similar to how he grew up. He replies: "Our *boma* was just like those, but I left when I was sixteen. I still go back because my family is there." Then he begins to reflect: "*Moru* in Maasai means someone who is old. One I knew lived to be 130 years old. My grandfather died when he was 110. His name was Sateriu. They know exactly how old he was, because of a Lutheran church built by Germans. Long ago he used to help those guys with building materials, and so from that he could mark his age. He used to walk a lot when he was that old, he was still strong, he did not carry a stick.

"Then one day going to visit his neighbor, my grandfather fell down and hit his head and he did not make it. My grandfather used to say, 'When I die, I do not want to stay in the cemetery. I want to take my bones and put them at a strangler fig tree by my house.' This tree is where they would pray for rain. Maasai believe God is inside this tree and, if you harm a strangler fig, these trees can kill you. The strangler fig always grows on top of another tree. It has very long roots and once the roots reach the ground, they start killing the other tree. My grandfather followed belief in trees, that's the church for him. So first they put him in a plastic bag in the ground for three years. But then when they dig in the cemetery, they find him just the way they buried him. My grandfather's body does not decay. And so they leave him in the cemetery another three years. Then my family pay someone to put his bones under the strangler fig tree. He still sleeps under that tree."

Strangely, about this time, a jeep going the other way has a coffin sticking out the back. When he was a boy, Stephan continues, if you saw something like that, you couldn't travel in the same direction for a month. Nor should you ever point toward a cemetery: "You point, you go there."

Stephan points out a lone tribesman some distance from the road. We can't make out what the man is wearing, but our guide says that this particular tribe lives in the bush, goes naked, and "they eat everything except hyena and vulture." This inspires a boyhood story from Larry, about the "little people" of the Hadzu tribe who lived in beehive huts and with whom he'd spend time on school vacations. "They stood about four feet tops. They were great trackers, used blow darts." Illiterate bushmen left behind when the Bantu migration headed south, Larry had witnessed their wedding and burial rituals and their hallucinogenic mandrake plants, "the basis of their witchcraft. My father," Larry adds, "didn't convert a single one!"

Out of the corner of my eye, I've been observing Franklin as these tales unfold. He stares out the window, feigning disinterest, but somehow I feel he's absorbing the stories and being strongly affected by them. As if they tap a deep ancestral chord, one that we all share.

Our next stop is the Oldupai Gorge, the "cradle of mankind," where Louis and Mary Leakey first discovered early hominids in the 1930s. I've always seen it spelled Olduvai but, as Dr. Reiner relates, the Maasai gentleman whom the Leakeys first encountered and asked for the name of the place had had a tooth knocked out. He'd tried to say Oldupai (also the name of a local sisal plant) but the Leakeys heard Olduvai, and that's what stuck.

We turn off the main road for about three miles and bring out our cooler of box lunches at a picnic area above a steep-sided ravine.

When Frank sits down across from me, I mention that his lunch is right next to mine already. His angry reaction surprises me. "I'm not your dog," he says. I pass the box lunch across to him, watch him eat only an apple with some juice and not even open the sandwiches. "You need to keep up your strength," I tell him. "I've eaten enough today," he responds curtly. Maybe he means he's taken enough from *me*.

Frank's mood lightens as we attend a lecture overlooking the gorge, which is 30 miles long and 295 feet deep. This is indeed a treasure chest of human fossils from the Pleistocene era, occupied by *Homo habilis* and his stone tools about 1.9 million years ago, followed by *Paranthropus boisei* (nicknamed "Nutcracker Man" for his well-preserved cranium) and *Homo erectus* ("Upright Man"). The findings at Oldupai convinced the majority of paleoanthropologists that humankind first evolved in Africa.

Afterward, Franklin is animated, informing us all of our common ancestry: "Europeans came from like Neanderthal, Cro-Magnon, Peking, and African." Larry, however, appears exhausted and can't keep our itinerary straight. "Are we going now to the Ngorongoro Crater?" he wonders. "No, Larry, that's five days away from now," I inform him. He shakes his head.

Deep in the bush near Lake Ndutu, we arrive late afternoon at an advertised "exclusive camp" called Millennium, which moves its tents on a yearly basis depending on where the most animals are and where we'll stay for three nights. Our African host is multilingual. Everything here is solar-powered, and each comfortable tent contains two beds.

But since our morning in the Maasai Village, Franklin has been very quiet and, upon arrival at Millennium, he lies on his bed staring at the ceiling. He won't come to dinner and my argument that he's had little to eat all day falls on deaf ears: "Why can't you understand that I'm on a diet?" He'll take his meds, my son says, but he wants to go to bed. Later, when a waiter suggests maybe he'd eat some soup and brings a bowl to the tent, Frank says, "No, I'm good." Stephan, when I describe what's happening, simply replies, "He's a good man."

I'm also worried about Larry. He'd had trouble finding the rest of us before dinner and started to wander off the beaten path. Larry might not prove as easy to find as Franklin was that night at Tarangire. But Aileane seems aware of the need to keep a close watch on the doctor.

One of the camp staff stands outside the dinner tent to scare away any Cape buffalo that might show up. After dark, everyone is escorted to their accommodations. Frank is sound asleep. After he gets up in the night to use the toilet in back, I ask him to turn off the light. "Why do you talk to me like that?" he demands. Irritated, I fire back, "For Christ's sake, it's the middle of the night!" and we both shortly fall back to sleep. I arise at 6:30 to the sound of numerous birds and animals, and awaken Frank a half hour later, who upon getting dressed grabs his camera and heads off "to start filming this area." I worry that I'd forgotten to warn him not to stray far from the camp paths. I find him drinking coffee in the dining area a bit later. Farther from civilization than either of us have ever been, everything feels tenuous.

• • •

We cross Lake Ndutu and drive across a marsh. As a herd of wildebeest passes in the near distance, a lioness hides to watch in the tall grass. "Are we waiting for her to attack?" Frank asks. We don't. He draws some hieroglyphic-like characters in my notebook while Stephan goes off-road, bouncing through the scrub and braking fast to narrowly avoid a large termite mound.

Seeing a tour vehicle stuck in a ditch at the base of a rise, Stephan stops to attach a chain to their bumper and pull them out. "We have better traction than that other car," Frank says proudly, tapping Stephan on the shoulder to add, "Road warrior." Observing nine other Land Rovers stopped on the road ahead of us, Stephan politely circles so as not to cut off their view of three cheetahs sunning themselves in the grass. Frank helps Larry climb into the backseat so he can take some pictures, then afterward lifts up his shoe and helps push him back to the front seat. Larry, pleasantly surprised, thanks him. The cheetahs—three brothers, according to Stephan—start to roll around as we move to a better viewing angle while Frank keeps filming. But something else is invisibly accompanying us. "Looks like something has been killed over there," Stephan says. We talk in whispers as he pulls over. Just inside a thorn bush, a male lion has a large wildebeest on the ground, holding on by the throat. "He's drinking the blood, or . . ." my son says questioningly. "He's suffocating it," Stephan says. It must be a bachelor male, because no females are around to help him hunt. "We are lucky to see this," Stephan whispers. "Only on TV," Frank says, wide-eyed. He hands his camera to Stephan to film with. We watch in silence as the lion moves deeper into the bush with his kill, until totally out of sight. Frank inscribes more hieroglyphics in my notebook, captioning them "Become a Lion Hunter." As we drive on, he says to Stephan, "It'd be easy to cut wildebeest with a long knife. You could smoke them, make jerky beef." Stephan nods and replies, "That's right."

That afternoon, as zebras and wildebeest leap across the dirt path in front of us, Frank requests Stephan to "stop for a minute, I want to draw this." He proceeds to fill two pages of my notebook, starting with an outline and then filling in the sketches. "Do you want to see it?" he asks Larry when finished. "I don't know," Larry says, but turns to examine Frank's work—a cartoon-like collage containing various animals and people—and exclaims: "Oh, yes I do! Wow!" They smile warmly at one another. Frank and the doctor seem to be connecting more and more.

Back at Millennium Camp before dinner, as a bug dive-bombs my red wine, Frank says: "I like these moths, or whatever they are." He once made the prescription drug Naparcin out of gnats, he adds. Two women arrive, one a lawyer and the other a physician, fresh from spending several months with the mountain gorillas in Rwanda. Frank greets them warmly and tells the doctor he worked in her hospital two years ago, in security. The women think Dr. Reiner introduced himself as "Dr. Rhino." When he starts speaking Swahili to the waiters, they stare at him bug-eyed.

The next day, as I ride along with Larry to check my email at a lodge about a half mile away, he admits: "I'm having a rough go," and adds as we start back: "I'm in a dither." Returning to the tent, he tells Aileane: "I think this is my last trip out here." Perhaps picking up on how the doctor is feeling, Franklin tells Larry how impressed he is at his having "been all over Africa."

Frank is starting to recognize and name various animals, including the difference between Thompson's and the larger Grant's gazelles. Larry doesn't think the wildebeests look very pregnant but Frank corrects him: "Those are males." Late afternoon, driving along Lake Masek, in a macabre still life, for a good ways the beach is littered with the bones of wildebeest. "When they come to drink water, the crocodiles drag them in and kill them," Stephan says.

Franklin is enthralled. Then his imagination shifts to something that happened to him once while swimming off our family's beach in Baja. "I was like an old swine in the water. I almost kicked it. These manta rays came by and said: 'I want you down underneath the water, Franklin. Water-logged.'"

Back at our camp at dusk, Frank and I sit alone having some wine. Would he like to come back to Africa sometime? Yes, he would. Then he begins to speak very personally about himself. "It's hard when people reprimand you."

"I didn't think I was doing that," I say.

"No, not you, not now, but I feel bad and get angry—very angry—because people don't understand what I am saying."

It's the first time in a long while that I can recall him opening up like this about what he goes through. It's as though being away from the restrictions and judgments he faces in American society, here among the animals, the Maasai, and Stephan—and Larry and Aileane, too, in such intimate circumstance—something is cracking open inside my son. Long-suppressed, or at least rarely expressed, anxieties are sur-facing . . . allowing other aspects of his personality—like his humor—to be illuminated as well. I feel like a witness to an unveiling.

Something Franklin says that day will reverberate in my mind: "So much that I deal with is unseen, having Pluto in 19 [degrees] Libra. But you deal with that all the time." He's right, as that is precisely where the planet Pluto was aligned on the day he was born. But how long has it been, I wonder, since he looked at his birth chart? As has been the case since he was a teenager and became interested in astrol-ogy, his memory for such details is astonishing. In terms of what I "deal with," does he mean the "unseen" as a focus of what I choose to write about? Or is he referring to what I must "deal with" concerning him?

An ancient symbol for this same degree of the zodiac is, "A gang of robbers in hiding," the keyword being divergence: "When positive, the degree is alertness to every threat against a true individuality, and when negative, abnormal mistrust of everything worthwhile." Franklin is, I believe, coming to grips with something about this.

Be beautiful and shine in your own way. Be, exist, grow, love, experience, assimi-late, build, think, consider, dream, theorize, be logical, be practical, work hard. I would like to have the initiative of Aries, productiveness of Taurus and practical-ity of Capricorn, the sensitivity of Cancer, the dreams of Pisces, the originality of Aquarius, the work ethic of Virgo, the command of Leo, the playfulness and flexibility of Gemini, the passion of Scorpio, and the flight and imagination of Sagittarius and the balance of Libra.

—Franklin's Journal, 2002

• • •

As we prepare to break camp, Stephan is in a wistful mood over breakfast: "I live in town now, but maybe later I will go back to Maasai land. I still have land there and huts. But after my kids finish school, first I would like to stay in the Serengeti; find a wife and stay there." His little girl of six attends a day school; his son is eleven and goes to a boarding school of largely Maasai. "It's expensive, a thousand dollars a year, not including books and uniform. But I don't want my son to lose his culture."

Frank has already told me that he'd like to come back to Tanzania sometime and reside with Stephan. Now, out of the blue, Stephan tells Frank that he can stay in his house and teach English. It's a confirmation of what happened in the Maasai village—Franklin beginning to take his part and place among other young men his age.

A few days ago, when Frank asked Stephan where we were going next and he said to the Serengeti, my son had responded: "Oh, we are going to the awesome place of earth." The Serengeti, Stephan explains, covers close to 9,000 square miles, "like a small country." The word *Serengeti* means "endless plain" and that is soon what we are traversing, without a tree in sight, the result of a long-ago volcanic eruption that left only raised lava in its wake.

Most leopards like a spot where they can see water, but we've yet to encounter one. "Maybe the leopards got suspended from school and are back with their parents," Frank considers. "On vacation like you?" Stephan asks. "I don't call it vacation, I call it escape," Frank says. It's mid-morning when Stephan finally locates a leopard resting between two limbs of an acacia and passes around the binoculars. Of the "Big Five," as they're known, we've now seen four—elephant, lion, cheetah, and leopard—everything except a rhino. "You can stay ten days or even a month and not see a leopard," according to Stephan.

We turn left at a sign for "Hippo Pool" and reach the Retima Picnic Site. Standing behind a wooden barrier gazing down upon probably a hundred of the beasts, Frank marvels, "they're beautiful animals."

He asks for my notebook to sketch the scene, as the hippos squirt water and make an occasional resonant honking sound when submerged.

After filling the tank at the lone gas station in the Serengeti, the new bush camp we're seeking is Dunia, which means "world" in Swahili. But it's not on any maps, as the camp shifts location regularly, and takes awhile to find. Dunia has very large, spread out tents, its own satellite Internet, free wine and beer, and reportedly an excellent chef. The Dietz lamp lit by a worker reminds Larry of his boyhood. "Look at the wick inside the base," he says. "It's a kerosene tank and the wick goes into it. You push your finger down and the whole glass section lights up, and you've got something windproof. I knew this long before I discovered you could pull a switch on the wall and get electricity."

Following a brief rain that clears the air, a Maasai man shows up in the common area carrying some of his tribe's purple cloaks. Asking Larry and me to put them on, he takes our picture. I walk wearing mine back to the tent where Frank is resting to ask him to join us. He glares at me. "What's that robe?" he says. "Do I look silly?" I ask. He says no but, when he's also offered a cloak, says, "I don't want to put that on." He then balks about coming to the campfire and wants no alcohol either. Instead, he sits in the lounge hanging out with the African staff.

I sit alone by the fire for awhile, reflecting on something that surfaced in Frank's thoughts again shortly before dinner. "I came out of a German detention camp in the 1930s," he'd said, "where they teach you trades." Sure, it's a delusion. But maybe it also reflects his feeling of being controlled, which has existed for a long time—a pattern that I see more clearly than I ever have.

• • •

A literal wake-up call—"Halloooo!"—beckons from outside our tent at 7 a.m., as I'd requested. The shrill sounds of a yellow-necked spur and the more constant call of African mourning doves have already opened my eyes. A bucket shower awaits. Out back of the tent, a worker has finished heating up about five gallons from a cistern, the bucket being attached to a pole with a pulley and rope, then hoisted up and over to where I stand waiting under a shower-head inside. "You wet your body, turn off, do soap, turn on," I'm told.

Last time I'd been left with shampoo in my hair when the water ran out. This time, success!

Before heading off again in the Land Rover, I leave some laundry outside the tent as instructed, only to worry for the rest of the day about baboons carting off our underwear. Frank is sleeping crossing an empty section of landscape, opening his eyes briefly when Stephan mentions some Crested Francolins flying by. For the first time since Tarangire, we encounter elephants and see three more leopards, which Larry thinks is a record for him in a single day. But Frank, leaning against the seat in front of him, keeps his head in his hands much of the time, tired and uninterested. I try not to let this bother me.

"Are you doing okay?" Stephan asks him at one point. "Yeah, doing okay, thanks," Frank says. Stephan asks, "Are you hungry?" "Not really, but I'm gonna eat." "We head for the central Serengeti now, where you can have your lunch," Stephan says. "Okay," Frank answers.

At the Serengeti Visitors Center, a young African named Destere greets our vehicle to offer a tour and Frank comes alive. When our guide plucks a leaf from a sandpaper tree and says it's used for washing clothes, Frank rubs the roughness on his cheek and then forehead, to the young man's dismay. "You will get injured!" he cries out. Frank proceeds to examine various bones while Destere is delighted to unexpectedly be talking in Swahili with a white-haired foreigner, Larry. As we move along, twice Frank pounds happily on my back. Back in the car, he says appreciatively of our tour guide, "He showed us everything that we've seen."

Frank recognizes a sausage tree with a vulture perched on top, and wonders what the tree tastes like. "Some think the trees are poisonous but they are not," says Stephan. "Actually the sausage tree has a potion that people use for washing." The two of them engage in further conversation, Frank wondering whether Stephan ever went to art school, and Stephan wondering "what is your future plan, to be a doctor, an engineer?" Frank says, "I do all that now." Stephan reveals to him that he'd awakened at midnight, hearing something on top of his tent, "a little bit scary," not finding out until morning that it was a tree branch. It's comforting that even Stephan gets frightened sometimes.

A torrential rain pours down that evening for about a half hour. More guests have arrived, and Dunia Camp is almost full. Across from Frank at dinner is an Australian woman in her mid-eighties, from

Perth, alongside her daughter who is a safari guide in Tanzania. Next to them is a female doctor, discussing with our African host whether malaria or sleeping sickness is more prevalent. "I got malaria," Frank tells the Australians, "in Panama, when I was building the Canal." They don't bat an eye, so he goes on that he once surfed in Perth. The older woman appreciates the alliteration.

Jackal sounds in the night . . . lion tracks near the breakfast tent in the morning. "The night belongs to the animals, as the old saying goes," says Larry.

"Some people live in the dark," Frank says in response.

We check out of Dunia. "Will driving be more difficult today because of the rain?" Aileane asks in the car. To which Franklin leaps to Stephan's defense: "He's an excellent driver!"

Now, as we cross into the Ngorongoro Conservation Area, there they are—thousands of wildebeest covering the vast plain, as far as the eye can see. The whole herd totals some one and a half million, and several hundred thousand march before us today, the single largest wildlife migration on the planet. Milk production of the pregnant females depends upon these calcium- and magnesium-rich short grasses. The wildebeest have some distance to travel yet, almost 800 miles to their primary calving grounds. Between late January and the middle of March, 80 percent of them will give birth. A newborn must be able to stand and walk within about ten minutes, or else the mother will abandon it, due to the ever-present threat of predators. "This is as good as I've seen it," Larry says, as we take turns peering through the binoculars for close-ups and attempting to take photographs, although it's impossible to capture the scale of it all.

While Stephan obtained our permit to enter this area, Larry had waited outside the ranger station on a ledge. "I'm starting to get that kind of morose feeling when it's almost over," he said. "But the best is yet to come." He was talking about the Ngorongoro Crater. At mid-afternoon, we pull over at a viewing area to look down upon the spectacle of all 3,200 square miles of it. Tomorrow we will descend into the caldera, as I had done on a bus tour a little more than forty years ago. This is the "wonder of the world" that, above all, I've been waiting to share with Franklin. But while the other four of us excitedly exit the Land Rover to pose for pictures alongside one another, he doesn't get out. I walk around to his side and offer to open the car door. He shakes his head.

"Don't bother me right now," he says.

"What are you thinking about?" I ask, puzzled.

"I'm thinking about the past. But it's private," Franklin says.

Private is probably a good thing, I rationalize, because so much of what he thinks gets voiced, no matter what it might be. But nonetheless, I feel my stomach turn over with foreboding.

> Confusion, twisted karmas intermeshed. . . . Cold nights, rats bite in the sewers of the slums. Sharing is suicide. Safety is for suckers. So where are you and I?
>
> —Franklin's Journal, ten years earlier

CHAPTER 14

• • •

Breakthrough

Madness need not be all breakdown. It may also be breakthrough.
                                        —Psychologist R. D. Laing.[1]

MARCH 1971: PERHAPS A BOND of friendship was forever sealed on this long-ago night in Africa. Perhaps, too, it was a kind of preparation for what lay ahead, in another part of the continent, forty years later.

It was night when we arrived in Accra, capital city of Ghana in West Africa. My Kansas traveling companion, Steve, and I had been dropped off by our last ride in a park full of "mammy wagons," refurbished trucks with wooden benches in back to carry as many paying passengers as they could squeeze in. Each bore a nickname chosen by the owner: BECAUSE OF MONEY ... JESUS IS ALL WE NEED ... PEACE PERFECT ... GOD IS KING ... GARY COOPER. At least they would speak English here, not French as in the countries we'd been passing through. But we had no idea where to go.

Later, Steve would recount:

We ended the last leg of our trip standing in the dark, in the middle of a lorry park. This was an English speaking country, I thought, but we heard only strange African dialects. I needed rest and calm, instead the park swarmed with strange people using their arms and hands to talk as much as they used their arms. Quickly we found a cab, asking the driver to take us to a good hotel. "Certainly," he said, and proceeded to drive in circles until he left us at the hotel of his brother-in-law. The manager fumbled with the keys and was confused over price, and charged us a high rate.

Ten years earlier, after my family had moved from Chicago to Kansas City as I approached my thirteenth birthday, our house had been only a few blocks from Steve's. We were born two months apart, and I'd gone over to see him a few times while attending the same suburban junior high and high school. But we weren't close friends; not until we ended up sharing a loft together in New York in the summer of '68. We'd each landed summer jobs there after our junior years in college and explored the big city together. Returning to the University of Kansas, the rock band in which Steve played the drums needed a lead singer and I passed the tryout to become part of the Vanilla Abstract, which earned us both some extra bucks on weekends until we graduated from KU.

I returned to New York as a full-time staff reporter with *Sports Illustrated*. Steve stayed on in school for a fifth year to obtain a degree in mechanical engineering, but joined me over Christmas to journey to Canada and to compose an article together about a draft dodger from Kansas. My friend was a talented photographer and by that summer was shooting portraits full-time. So when I opted to leave the magazine behind and see where the wind took me, we made a plan to meet up in Europe in the fall of 1970 and do more freelance stories together. He was also engaged to be married, but willing to first spend some months of adventurous traveling before getting hitched. We were vastly different personalities. Steve was shy, sensitive, and visual. I was outgoing to the point of pushy—often oblivious to someone else's feelings—and intellectual.

Hitchhiking across the Sahara Desert, we decided, could be an experience worthy of a piece for *National Geographic*. So we'd set off from Algiers, completely unprepared for what lay ahead. Early on, we waited thirty hours for a ride amid blowing sand and temperatures that fluctuated from a hundred-plus degrees by day to forty degrees at night. Our down-covered sleeping bags were no match for the elements. Later, we hooked up with a young Dutch revolutionary and his girlfriend in a VW bus, going in tandem with two Brits in a low-slung Ford Cortina. Crossing the border into Niger on a barely visible track of sand, we hadn't seen a vehicle going either direction for two days when their car got mired so badly that our bones would probably still be there had a Niger military convoy not come along to pull us out. We were then living on our last rations of stale bread and sardines, and about to run out of water.

We survived. But even for two guys in their early twenties, it had been an arduous six weeks to get to Accra, more than 4,000 miles south of Algiers. By then, Steve had grown increasingly worried that his film would be ruined by the heat and that his fiancée would give up on him and find someone else. I didn't realize how plagued he was by such thoughts, when we ended up in a hot, mosquito-infested hotel room that first exhausted night in Accra.

Later, Steve would write:

> I craved rest, but didn't know how to attain it. I had slept on the ground for so long I felt uncomfortable sleeping inside a building in a bed. The air was so thick with moisture I had to struggle to breathe. The desert had been my enemy, but at night that schizophrenic beast would calm down and take me back to rest in its sands for the next day. As the crossing had progressed, subconsciously I became more and more afraid I would never leave the desert. Had I been aware of this fear I would have tried talking it out, but it hid in the back of my head and grew stronger as my body and brain were beaten down time and again. At last, I woke to find that all my fears had jumped from my head and covered my body like locusts.

Across the room from him, I'd fallen promptly asleep. After about an hour, I heard Steve talking. He said something about being sick, but I didn't move immediately. Then he was up, pacing around the room, holding his head in his hands. "My mind," he said, "something's snapped in my mind. Dick, help me!" I jumped up, pulled on my pants, and followed him outside, barefooted and shirtless.

> This spirit of terror and fear suddenly grabbed the back of my head and let out a shriek that came from my mouth. The control of my tongue was no longer mine. The voice came again. "Help me, my mind's gone!" This scream both panicked and soothed me. I was not in control, but I'd needed to wail for weeks and finally it was emerging. I clutched my friend, sobbing with the fear that my mind was gone forever. I begged for forgiveness for the way I had acted during the crossing, as if I was pleading for my life with an executioner.

We headed toward the nearby street. Steve kept repeating that his mind had snapped. My heart pounded in my chest, I don't know when I'd ever been so scared. This was a complete unknown. We put our arms around each other and began circling around and around a fountain while a group of men stared at us. I kept trying to reassure Steve that the pressure was off, that the long difficult journey was finished and we could relax now. But he continued to moan and weep. I kept myself from choking up, trying to retain my composure. I don't know how long we walked and I talked and the fountain flowed. It was called the Liberation Circle, Steve would remember. "Dick and I walked miles that night. People may have stared, I didn't see. I didn't perceive. The only environment I felt came from within my body and brain."

When Steve seemed to calm down somewhat, we turned back toward the hotel. Passing the manager on the street, I said my friend needed to see a doctor immediately. Then out of nowhere, a young African woman appeared, holding some money in her hand. "I know you're having trouble," she said. "Do you need some money to help you get to a hospital?" I stammered, "I left my wallet in the hotel," realizing this for the first time. She thrust three Ghanian bills into my palm, hailed a taxi for us, and vanished into the night.

A simple, quiet act of kindness. A gesture that didn't have to be made. A face that passed in the dark. Things didn't seem so complex anymore. The world seemed human again.

Within ten minutes, we arrived at a hospital and were quickly ushered into a doctor's small office. The young doctor was, of course, Ghanaian. "I want to see an American," Steve said anxiously. "No Americans here," the doctor said, proceeding to take my friend's temperature, pulse, and blood pressure. All were normal. The doctor assured him that his problems weren't physical, but he knew what this was all about. He began to speak slowly and painfully, drawing parallels with his own life, letting the frightened young American know that his fears were not unique. He talked of memories he could not erase. Fleeing from South Africa on foot, walking hungry, sometimes until dawn, sore, wishing he was dead. With the aid of a hundred nameless faces, he'd arrived finally in West Africa. Alive.

No one could have put someone in Steve's condition more at ease. He gave my friend some kind of tranquilizer with instructions for its use. By the time we found a taxi back to the hotel, where the proprietor fixed some food for us at one o'clock in the morning, the crisis had passed.

> Sometimes a sound rest and a kind hand will soothe and heal the troubled spirit; recovery soon follows with only vague memories of the madness. My mind healed soon after. But for the two hours I spent as a madman, I felt I had stumbled over the edge of the world, floating with nothing for my mind to grasp, yet feeling invisible walls closing in on me.

"In times of crisis," Steve would say after I began relating the story to him of the night to come with Franklin, "it helps if you have had a similar experience in the past."

• • •

> *In the deeper layers of the unconscious space and time become completely relative . . . in the realm of the archetypes, our ordinary clock time is not valid.*
> —Marie-Louise von Franz, *The Cat*[2]

While Franklin sits sullenly in the car, the rest of us take a few pictures of each other overlooking the rim of the Ngorongoro Crater and the volcanic vastness below. Passing through the exit gate of the Conservation Area, a few miles farther down a now-paved road is the turn into the Ngorongoro Farm House where we are to spend the next two nights. It's a beautiful spot, the entry road lined with bougainvillea and the grounds a 500-acre coffee plantation surrounded by lush palms and blooming gardens. We check in at a thatch-roofed main building with a restaurant and viewing verandah. Our belongings are carted down paved paths adjoined by rolling lawns and enclosures of evergreen coffee fields. The farm is also home to 164 different varieties of birds, including the resident species Pied Kingfisher, Red Barbet, and Hybrid Lovebird.

Frank's and my spacious room is one of fifty, has a fireplace, and a phone to call the front desk. Which I do, immediately, after my key gets stuck in the lock. I ask if someone can please come to Chatu, the name on the door of our room. Only much later will I look up the meaning, and learn that *Chatu* is the Swahili word for "python."

A worker comes down to assist. A few minutes later my key is retrieved and I'm instructed in its proper usage. Oblivious, Franklin lies down on his large bed and stares up at the canopy, his eyes wide open, saying nothing. I leave him be. *This is the second night in a row he's done this, but he's been taking his medication,* I think to myself. Only much later, will I notice that he's recently been mixing up his morning and evening pills. This causes him to be more tired during the day and more wired by night, which had been happening since we entered the Serengeti. As the sun starts to set over the Oldean mountains to the west, I take a walk as far as the path goes and then back to the hotel's verandah. I sit alone there, sipping a Tusker beer, thinking of my son and how distant he's seemed for the past day or so. I decide to return to the room and see if he'll join me for a drink before dinner. I'll tell him that I'm lonely.

When I walk in, he's leaning against the wall behind his bed, drawing Asian characters in his notebook. He doesn't look up.

"You're lonely," Franklin flatly repeats my words. Then adds: "I don't speak your language. I don't know what you mean. And I don't like you. Anything about you."

He bounds out of bed and starts pacing around the room like a caged animal.

"Frank, tell me what I've been doing wrong."

"Why are you watching me?" he demands. "I'm just walking. Why don't you walk?"

"I already did," I say, "outside."

My son's eyelids flutter as he flops back down onto the bed.

"I think you have interesting things to say," I tell him, "which I write down. So whatever you'd like to talk about—I like taking you on this trip. Or maybe you're taking *me* on this trip."

Perhaps he'll appreciate that, I think to myself.

"I'm dead anyway," he says. "I'm sleeping." He pauses, and then goes on: "Dick is not a respectable name."

"What should it be? Richard?" I ask, with what I believe is sincerity.

"That's also an aftershave," he scoffs. I've no idea what he means, but will later find out that there is indeed a fancy men's aftershave called Richard James.

I sink into an easy chair across the room from him. As Frank begins to talk, I bring out my notebook. Something tells me that I need to set down my son's words. Yes, perhaps I am using my pen to hide behind, to detach myself from a painful situation so that I don't have to feel it? Still, I feel compelled to capture as accurately as I can whatever Franklin will say, wherever he chooses to go.

Only much later will I contemplate that he may have taken my doing this as a therapy session. Often when he's met with psychiatrists, they would just sit and write down things that he cannot see. This may have added to his ire toward me. Maybe if I'd shared my notes with him, he'd have had a better understanding of my psyche and who I am.

But at the time, I don't think he can see me writing. As he lies there motionless, a monologue begins. At first it is directed at me. The words come slowly, meticulously, in a deep emotionless voice.

> You've been making use of my information for the whole trip. For the wrong thing. You take my blood in the car and ingest it for the idea of being more powerful. That's what I think you are doing. You've probably controlled the whole trip. You sensuously agelessly look at me like I was your boy. But I know history in ways you do not. Where I go, the snake has been. Sixteen years after Park School, then I become the Snake King?

Yes, I calculate, that's how long it's been since he graduated. But the snake—what is it about the snake?

• • •

> *The entire process of creation took place within the green and azure coils of the plumed serpent. On several continents it was among the most important symbols of the initiate-priest. Sometimes it stands erect and is crowned, as in Egypt, or it may be winged as among the Mongolians, or feathered and plumed as throughout the Americas. . . . The serpent was a wisdom symbol, and when plumed it meant that wisdom had been given wings and had become spirit-wisdom, or illumination.*
> —Manly Palmer Hall, *America's Assignment with Destiny.*[3]

Later, as I set out to write this book, doing research into Franklin's past I would come upon a third-grade paper he once did about China. It was his choice of school project and focused on "Cycle of the Twelve Animals" that included the Chinese Years of the Pig and Dog, "Origins of the Lion Dance," and a drawing of a dragon. Frank had colored in only one page: on "the Year of the Snake."

Six months before Africa, in the summer of 2011, I'd had a powerful dream that I wrote down. I was watching two snakes going at each other—after which I encountered a thinner snake that I issued a warning about to a close friend standing alongside . . . until I realized that it was clearly intent on pursuing *me*. It kept leaping up as I continued to dodge its strikes and ended up rushing ahead of the snake down a set of stairs. There another good friend said: "That snake is *really* after you."

At that time I was reading a book by Gopi Krishna, for which James Hillman had written a commentary, about a phenomenon of the yogic tradition. The book was called *Kundalini,* which is a Sanskrit term for the primal energy of human consciousness, represented in the form of a serpent coiled around the spine. When awakened inadvertently or through ritual practices, the serpent was believed to "unwind" across the various *chakras*, or energy centers, of the body.

One of Hillman's close associates, religious scholar David Miller, had told me of a seminar on dreams in Santa Cruz, California, where most of those attending were psychiatrists. They were discussing a dream involving a snake and, as Hillman turned over the image, Miller recalled, "the audience was becoming more and more uncomfortable— appropriately, because they were unconscious of their snakiness. Finally one of the doctors said, 'Come on, everyone knows that's a phallus.' Hillman glared at him and exclaimed, '*You killed the snake!*'"[4]

It was biblical, of course, all the way back to Adam and Eve in the garden and to Matthew 10:16: "Be ye therefore wise as serpents, and guileless as doves." Mythological scholar Joseph Campbell wrote that, "Wherever nature is revered as self-moving, and so inherently divine, the serpent is revered as symbolic of divine life."[5] And the double helix structure of DNA, discovered in 1953, is shaped like two entwined snakes.

The snake motif had already come up a number of times on the trip to Tanzania. Upon first entering the Serengeti, Stephan had been talking about his ancestors. "My grandmother believes that when you die, you become a snake. You know we use wood and mud to build our house, so there are a lot of grass snakes. Whenever she sees a snake, she says 'maybe that is my husband who died years ago, or my mother.'"

While we drove through Ndutu, Frank had asked a second time, "Are there any snakes around here?" Stephan had said, "Yes, Puff

Adders and Spitting Cobras." Larry had hastened to add, "Also some okay snakes."

Stephen spoke, too, about how eagles follow the mongoose, because they know the mongoose can kill a snake, and then there will be food for the eagle.

· · ·

On this particular night in the room called *Chatu*, I don't have opportunity or wherewithal to recall any of that, as my son continues to talk. "Everybody is hypnotized by Dick Russell—Dick *Rascal*. I probably just gave you all the secrets of Earth. You don't respect me or know me. If you want me to be your son, why do you oppress yourself?" He proceeds to rattle off a list of invented words, then to talk of the robots working for him and the spaceships around here, and how "the infinite times are now: billions and trillions and pentillion octillion, nine to seventy quasars...."

Who is this that speaks? There is something oracular about the almost disembodied voice, but I can't make sense of it. Is that why I'm writing it all down? To try and later decode my son's ramblings? There may be elements of truth in what he's saying, but there are too many tangents. It's so nonlinear that I can't possibly follow it in "real time." If that is where we are ...

"I try to be nice to you, and you boss me around. If you want to push me around like that fight we had when I was at Park School—I could have hurt you then, but I didn't."

The fight when he was at Park School.... Early January 1993. He was thirteen. Things had come to a head over rap music. Frank would insist on playing it in the car. I tried to relate, to hear what he seemed to hear, but I felt many of the lyrics were full of chauvinism, anger, and outright hatred. Finally I wouldn't let him turn on the radio. And then I said I didn't want him listening in his room either. Etta agreed and pushed me to lay down the law. Frank argued to no avail, and then seethed.

In a letter to a close friend who was experiencing hard times with his own children, I wrote:

I went through such an agonizing night with Franklin two nights ago. It started with the usual problem—not getting to his homework—and

Etta and I having a stern but "reasonable" talk with him. Then came the defiance, and my no longer being able to tolerate how he treats his mom and his lack of respect for me, and we ended up in a battle royal. The first of two that night, I mean real physical fights. The second one came after he'd had to move all his stuff—record player and speakers, Nintendo game, everything—out of his room.

Frank had attacked me and it was one of the worst experiences I'd ever gone through. I was still stronger, could still hold his arms down on the bed as they flailed at me while his pent-up rage poured forth: "You bastard! You son of a bitch! Let me go!" The second time, the fight took place at the edge of a second-floor window. It was all I could do to keep us from crashing through it.

In the letter, I said: "When he finally broke down, it was heart-breaking. He sat there shaking and crying, telling me how sorry he was, how he didn't know where that rage came from, he felt like it was coming from somewhere outside him or all bottled up inside him. . . . Deep inside me, I think I've known that if I pushed him too hard, this kind of rage might erupt. So I was afraid to go too far with him."

The next day, we both felt wretched and talked quietly, pain-fully for a long while. At the time, I had seen this as a new beginning between us. But as the months went by, it was as though we had made a kind of silent pact. Neither of us ever wanted to go to that agonizing place again.

• • •

Following the line of thought in an individual in this psychic state, or "space," is quite like trying to grasp the metaphorical meaning in the lines of an obscure poem. The less one tries to transliterate it into rational talk, and the more one flows along with it, the more it speaks its own meaning.

—John Weir Perry, The Far Side of Madness

Lying on his bed, Franklin continues: "I'm a very strong man. I'm tired, yeah, not much energy. I might die tomorrow, I don't know. Whoever was in Africa replaced my head. If the 'Year of the Snake' was my brother as Genghis, I don't know."

Much later, reviewing my notes, I would learn that, in 1226, a Year of the Snake in the Chinese Zodiac, Genghis Khan had gone out to wage war from his palace on what became his last journey. What was my son tapping into?

"When I was little, they used to tell me twenty was how long I would live. Why twenty? That gave me the idea about the genie. And the genie was cursed. I've been fighting wars ever since."

A chill courses down my spine. I well remember the genie that he spoke of, almost a decade earlier when he was living alone for the first time, and then subsequently . . . the genie who had offered to grant him three wishes. I try desperately to remember: were two of these granted and a third withheld? What were the wishes? Another chill races through me.

"I was Shaka Zulu. Why are you here, Confucius? You can do anything as a genie. Why are you copying it down?"

My pen seems to suspend itself in mid-air. How could he see me writing? He's never raised his eyes.

"Africa said I came here 16,000 years ago. It's subliminal and people don't believe it, but it's true. I'm just here suffering right now. I've been dunked, lowered, guinea'd into a position here in Africa."

After beginning to speak in other tongues, he stops abruptly and says: "Languages of Kenya and Somalia," then adds: "If you want to be my guide, be a snake at the end of my lifetime."

I think to myself, *making this trip has been a terrible mistake*. My son has absorbed far too much of the African unconscious. And I don't know how to bring him back. My heart is pounding so intensely, I wonder if Frank can hear it across the room.

More than a year later, a friend familiar with the shamanic realm would tell me: "The serpent takes you to the bottom. It is relentless and will take you until you go there. And if you don't go, it will take you *down*."

• • •

Perhaps it bears repeating, what Frank wrote on a typewriter sometime in 1993–94, two or three years before his initial breakdown:

Core: White triangle with golden wings—thoughts from my inner self reaching people universally. Green circle inside the white triangle and rays in four directions. I want to give my mind to the world and the earth, to save them both. Circle is the earth. The rays are pathways for these thoughts.

<u>Limits</u>: Person enclosed in the North—my ideas are trapped in my head. Sometimes I can't express them. I spend a lot of time trying to get them out. Lightning bolts are the ideas that are trying to get out of my head. Closed eye in the West—sometimes I only see the outside of a person and can't see myself clearly. Open eye in the East—it is easier for me to see far-away things, and things on the outside. Person enclosed in the South—sometimes I don't feel connected to people. They could be having fun while I'm on my own.

<u>Attributes</u>: Star in the East—the need to understand people—tree in the South—I have more growing to do. Two faces—one black and one white represent the two parts of me learning to live with each other.

He is continuing: "There are so many curses on me, it's unbelievable that I am still here today."

What if he is right? Or am I the one going mad?

Suddenly, my son starts to recall more painful moments from his childhood. Stories I never knew. One is about a time that an older boy injured his thumb and fingers on the farm in Kansas. Another time he'd been tied up in the barn.

"Why doesn't Dick sacrifice? Came to me in a dream. You're not complicated enough."

Shit, he's telling me the truth.

"Dick Russell would never admit he is your son. I am a warrior, so be it. Whoever drinks blood from me—I thought you and Etta were doing that until I found out about the snake. It's just an image really, but when I came back I was servant to Allah, which means snake. You are more of a snake than I am, Dick."

Just an image really . . .

"I could be doing good things for the earth instead of lying in my bed and collecting things about people. When I went to the hospital, I asked them to redeem me—but they wouldn't."

I experience more chills. I don't know how much more of this I can stand. I must *do* something. But I feel frozen to the spot.

"Who controls the earth? The snake? Do we give all power on earth to the snake? Eventually Darth Vader will come to an end, using the snake."

In their visions, shamans take their consciousness down to the molecular level and gain access to information related to DNA, which they call "animate essences" or "spirits." This is where they see double helixes, twisted ladders, and chromo-

some shapes. This is how shamanic cultures have known for millennia that the vital principle is the same for all living beings and is shaped like two entwined serpents (or a vine, a rope, a ladder).

—Jeremy Narby, *The Cosmic Serpent*

Franklin starts speaking again in another language and then says "it's either Mexican or the snake kingdom of Africa. There are powerful spirits in Africa. They doused my head down with soap and said I had to become African. Questionable stuff happens. My spirit is broken. . . ."

At this point I get out of my chair and walk over to his bed. I begin to speak in a language that I invent on the spot, ranting and raving, hoping desperately to snap him out of it. Not too long after his first breakdown, something similar had worked. Unable to reach him, I'd stood by his bed and received "messages" from the radio playing in the background, talking faster and faster, until Franklin finally got up, walked over, and put his arm around me comfortingly. He was scared. Shaken out of himself. Scared for *me*. He'd told me not to worry, everything would be all right.

This time, though, my feigned "madness" doesn't work. He simply glares up at me. And, when my "speaking in tongues" winds down, he says only: "Why don't you take your face mask off? It seems as though you have been undermining me for years."

Maybe he's right—right about all of it. I sink back into my chair. I'm terrified. He goes on:

I am doing my thing as Jedi. Lost my picador place. . . . In the African way, all the spirits will gather up and say goodbye to me. Assume that all spirits will be matricized and perfected. You know what? I'll take you to the Matrix. Information from the Matrix will be bought in the future, hopefully from me, when I am part of the Matrix. So I must be brought up there.

Maybe Dick Russell could help me. When you get there, say a prayer for me. Because I don't know what that snake is doing. Drop my entrails and they're scattered out by Africa for being mean to white people in the past. My savior, the Matrix Clown, used to say things to me in my dreams.

It's the curse of the tomb of Egypt that everybody must die every night. I am speaking the Egyptian time—they have a clock, it is called the Corastone. [Egyptians invented the first timepiece, the water clock].

The time for the snake has also stopped. Put that watch of yours away in a high place—because if you don't, the Africans will find it."

My watch, a winding Hilton 17-jewel, was a gift from my parents on my tenth birthday. It had been on my right wrist, with a few time-outs for repairs, ever since. It was my oldest, most cherished possession. Forty years ago, when I was hitchhiking across the Sahara, a nomad had demanded the watch in exchange for giving me some water in a bucket from a well. I'd refused to give it to him. He drew the water anyway.

"The only person who can slow this clock down is me, by talking. I came before Adam, the original king was Alpha. Maybe you could fly me to the Matrix and we'll hang out there awhile. I don't want that star destroyed. I am right there now eating. The three wishes thing . . . I'm sorry the earth came to love money so much."

It is all too jumbled, too fast, too impossible for me to find a thread to hang onto, or any response that Franklin might relate to. It's grown dark outside. I glance at my watch. It's 7:30. His monologue has gone on for almost a full hour.

"Frank, it's dinnertime up there. Would you please come up and eat?"

He doesn't move. "The genie filled me. Please respect me. There is nothing terrible about you, you made a few mistakes. . . . There is something supernatural about it. I'm really filled up."

"Well Frank, I'm feeling pretty fucked up right now. I've got to go eat something."

He says he's going to sleep. Still nailed to my chair by a closed window, suddenly I hear a cry outside. Some kind of large bird? Probably, in the rational world. But the sound is shrill and frighteningly loud and does not abate.

"Aaaaaaaaaaaaaaaaaaahhhhhhhhhhhhhhhhh . . ."

The image of a banshee comes to mind. It feels as if something unspeakably huge is being released. Yet again, chills race along my spine. Does Franklin hear it, too? But I can't bring myself to ask.

"Will you turn off the lights when you leave?" he asks. I do so, walk out into the night, and close the door. Everything seems so still. I don't turn the key in the lock. I must trust that my son will be all right, that he will indeed go to sleep.

Among the Lakota Sioux, the guardian animal spirits often speak when they appear to the vision seeker. As Lame Deer recounts, "All of a sudden I heard a big bird crying, and then quickly he hit me on the back, touched me with his spread wings. I heard the cry of an eagle, loud above the voices of many other birds. It seemed to say, "We have been waiting for you. We knew you would come. Now you are here. Your trail leads from here."

—Michael Harner, *The Way of the Shaman*[6]

• • •

I find Larry and Aileane at a table on the verandah having a drink. I briefly summarize what's been happening, and that Franklin is really "out there."

"Will he be okay in the room?" Dr. Reiner asks worriedly, surely recalling the night he disappeared at Tarangire.

"Yes, I think so. He said he was going to sleep and asked me to turn off the lights. I don't think he'll go anywhere." My voice is quavering and I can feel my body shaking. "I need a drink."

Soon we enter the dining room to join a number of other tourists at a buffet. The food is delicious and dance music is playing and people's voices feel like they're echoing around me. It all feels surreal. I tell Dr. Reiner that I don't know whether I did the right thing in just letting Franklin talk. "There's no way to know," Larry replies, shaking his head.

Stephan joins us at our table and asks where Frank is. I tell him a little of what's transpired. "He's a good man," is all Stephan says in response. He proceeds to tell us more about his own past, starting out as a guide for people coming to climb Kilimanjaro, a mountain he'd himself climbed probably fifty times. The magic mountain. . . . I'm quietly pondering. Should I bring Stephan back to the room to see Frank? Maybe he could reach him.

No, I realize finally, I can't. Whatever has to be done, I must do it myself.

I quickly finish eating, tell the hostess that my son is sick and that I need to bring him a plate of food. I help a waiter pick out some meat and vegetables at the buffet. The man accompanies me back toward Chatu, carrying a flashlight. In our room, he silently deposits the plate at the table where I'd sat before and departs.

Franklin is angry. "I told you I didn't want to eat, the genie filled me! I'm not hungry. I'm on a diet."

"Okay." I take a deep breath. "Did you take your meds?"

I don't know how he'll react to this. Or to anything. I don't know if we'll make it through the night.

"No," he says finally. "But I will."

I go into his bag and bring out the pill-strip and hand it to him along with a glass of water. He swallows his four evening pills.

"Frank, I can't force you to eat but I'm worried that you've barely had any food all day and you won't have any way to absorb your medication. And then I don't know what will happen. I don't want you to end up in a hospital over here."

He glares at me. Then he lies back down on the pillow, rigidly staring upward, and begins again to speak in an alien tongue.

Yeah, been here before. Scared, sure, but stayed in control, got him to a doctor, things turned out all right . . . but not this time. Too much's at stake, too terrified and vulnerable. He really may go completely off his head and not come back. All my defenses, all my protections, everything that worked before—all have failed. There is just me, witness to Franklin's suffering, at least partly inflicted by myself. He keeps saying that I've betrayed him, hurt him, can't possibly understand. I've often written it off in the past as crazy talk. But now, at last, there is only the realization—the admission—that I can't go there with him, cannot understand. And so. . . .

I can't take it any longer. I walk around the edge of the bed and stand there looking down at him.

"Frank, I can't handle this. It's too much for me. You've got to help me! This is driving me crazy. *I can't understand the language!*"

Momentarily he stops talking and turns his head to look at me. "You're crying," he says.

I'm not even aware that I am. I don't know the last time he saw me cry.

"Are you having a breakdown?" he asks. His voice is filled with compassion.

"Maybe I am—I don't know." I'm taken aback, unsure what realm I'm inhabiting.

"Well, maybe *you're* the one who should be hospitalized!"

The roles are reversed. I am no longer the father, he no longer the son. I've confessed my own helplessness, and suddenly *he* is the caregiver.

I continue to pour my heart out. I talk of how much this trip means to me, having such a long intimate time with one another, how important it is for us to simply *be* together here, to take in all we have seen, how wonderful it is when he points out the various animals, how badly I feel about not being there more for him when he was young, how sorry I am for things that happened in the past.

"But I'm afraid," I finally tell him, "that bringing you here was a terrible mistake. Because of how sensitive you are, how much you absorb of the African subconscious."

He interrupts me again. "I really am having a wonderful time," he says.

So am I.

He talks about the beauty of the landscapes and the animals. "Maybe I should pick up my camera again tomorrow and start taking pictures."

That would be great, Frank.

My son is "back." And I realize in one overwhelming moment that simply the fact he could feel me—and that I could feel *him*—feel the anguish and the desperation and the love—has transformed a situation that seemed at a point of no return. He needed to find an entry into me. And I had finally opened up.

Only for a moment, his delusions rise up again, as though one final test. I cut him off. "Frank, I don't understand that world," I tell him. "I really don't. I wish I could."

"You could do more inspirational books," he tells me.

"You're right," I tell him. "And I'll need your help."

There is a pause before I add: "I don't know if I can go to sleep. You've got me pretty riled up. But I guess we should try. You still don't want to eat, right?" He says he doesn't. About ten minutes later, Franklin bounds out of bed and over to the little table where his dinner plate is and sits down.

I lie there in the dark, staring at the ceiling and say nothing until he's finished eating.

"Well, I hope it was still warm."

"It was," he says, and climbs back into bed. The African night soon envelops us both.

What has happened in the room is that I have been forced to let it all be; to let Franklin be Franklin. And he goes a long way toward becoming the plumed serpent in that moment. All of us so want spiritual things to be pure, serene. Our Heroes and our Saints, our Holy Men and Women, our Mad Monks and Priestesses—above it all. They're not; they're all half-crazy Joan of Arcs. But they have a job to do, a job that may last only for a time—or a lifetime—which may destroy them or lift them up, is as likely to crucify and crush them as to redeem and save them. What we owe them—yes, our own sons and daughters—is to *honor* them in their calling, serve them, love them, *and* admit that we are made of different stuff.

The crucial moment of that long night's journey into day is my thinking, if only for a moment, that maybe Franklin led me to Africa and not the other way around. Maybe he brought me there to teach me about who he really is, and what my role must be in his life.

> Without love, there is death. With death we return to our maker. We become dirt once again. Without spirit, we already are dead. The force of spirit and the connection to our hearts brings out the youth within us. When we contact this force, each day is a new beginning.
>
> —Franklin's Journal, ten years earlier

Notes:

1. Laing quoted in Solomon, *Far from the Tree*, p. 314.
2. "In the deeper layers of the unconscious....": Marie-Louise von Franz, *Cats*, p. 97.
3. "The entire process of creation....": Manly Palmer Hall, *America's Assignment with Destiny*, Philosophical Research Society 1973, originally published 1951.
4. Hillman and the snake: Dick Russell, *The Life and Ideas of James Hillman*, p. xxi.
5. Campbell quoted in Jeremy Narby, *The Cosmic Serpent: DNA and the Origins of Knowledge,* Jeremy P. Taracher/Putnam paperback, 1999, p. 65.
6. "Among the Lakota Sioux....": Michael Harner, *The Way of the Shaman*, HarperOne paperback, 1990, p. 75.

CHAPTER 15

• • •

In Search of the Leopard Tortoise

Life is about now and the future and the past. It is about patience. It is about learning and about teaching. It is about failure and fighting for what we believe in. It is about forethought.

—Franklin's Journal, ten years earlier

WHEN I EMAIL ETTA A synopsis of what happened between Franklin and me, she replies: "Only something as extreme as your current experiences could have triggered such a healing. Almost like an exorcism of so many buried memories. Thank god you could go the distance. But isn't that what we must do as parents?"

Later, she writes again: "Another thought. All the kind and gentle probing questions from therapy sessions really don't work with him. Or most people. Only brute reality brings about change, awakening and maybe catharsis. Of course what could have been more perfect. His world has been totally shaken up. So that the demons of the unexpressed unconscious are shown in the light. Really terrifying. . . . But this is a process he must go through to continue to heal. And us too."

The day has dawned crystal clear. Franklin asks if he could select my box lunch for me before we set off for the Ngorongoro Crater. "I got you a lot of food," Frank informs me.

"He did a great job on your box lunch, you'll enjoy that," Stephan says.

As we leave the lodge and make a turn onto the main road, a striped hyena is lying in our path, dead. We all take a deep breath. This is a very rare species, Stephan says, typically only emerging in total darkness before returning to its lair before dawn. "People on this road go very fast at night," Stephan says sadly. "In Africa, Frank, *poli poli*; that means 'go slow.'"

Maybe it's just a dead dog in the middle of the highway. And maybe not. The morning after is never really a "fresh start." It's a carrying on after something has broken; something also born, renewed, refreshed, a spirit released. An old life or form or pattern feels like it died on that long night. The snake shed its skin; the jackal gave up the ghost.

I would later read that, in the folklore of the Near and Middle East, striped hyenas are considered to be physical incarnations of jinns (Arabic for "genie"), which inhabit an unseen world in dimensions beyond what's visible to humans but can also interact physically with us. One ancient Arabic text described them as vampiric creatures who attacked by night—only brave people, it was said—and sucked the blood from their necks. However, in India, Afghanistan, and Palestine, while they were feared, striped hyenas also symbolized love and fertility, their body parts often worn as talismans. In much of Africa, including Tanzania, the striped "werehyena" is associated with the supernatural; in Nigeria, they are known as *bultungin*, which means "I change myself into a hyena."

Stephan winds our way 3,000 feet down a switchback dirt road into the ancient volcanic crater. In the car, Frank holds my notebook so that I can write more easily as we bounce along. He engages with each of our traveling companions, asking how they're doing and taking more pictures and video than at any other time during the trip. He stands to film some white storks out the open roof. In the distance we can just make out a trio of black rhinos lying in the grass behind more storks. "Little gray blurs," Aileane says, but Stephan uses Frank's camera to get a shot of the rare creatures taken right through the binocular lens. Frank shows me the picture and tells Stephan, "You got a good one. I'll send it to you." As we join several other Land Rovers observing a pair of lionesses, Frank says: "That lion looks docile, like a huge cat. Let me get a picture."

Frank makes a nice sketch of a herd of water buffalo and passes it to Stephan. "Frank, you are very good at drawing. Do you draw a lot of things?" My son says he'll send him some from his studio. And wonders if Stephan has ever thought of writing a book about the Serengeti. Frank has brought along the book, *What Color Is Your Brain?* that he picked up at the Boston airport. Now, as he shows it to Aileane, she asks what color his brain happens to be. "Orange," says Frank, "and green." Larry turns to face him. "Those were the colors of my college," he says. "Bowling Green?" Frank asks. "Wheaton College," Larry says. They both smile.

Everyone eats in their cars at the picnic area to avoid problems with circling black Kites—birds that dive for your food and don't mind if they take a bite out of your arm. Continuing on our way under a shadowy canopy of strangler fig trees, Stephan announces, "Bump!" Frank responds, "Expert lunger!"

It's hard to believe our voyage together is coming toward a close. "We have done marvelously well," Larry says. Back at the Farmhouse Lodge by early afternoon, Frank entertains a woman at the front desk by doing a sketch for her of the human body's various pressure points. Maybe he saw that they offer massages here. "Look at these beautiful gardens, all the flowers," he says outside. He is more *present* than at any time on the entire trip.

In our room, he mentions something about Dick Russell. "Last night you called me Dick Rascal," I say.

"I did?" my son replies mischievously. "Do you want me to do another talk?"

"No!" I say emphatically.

He lies down. "Well, I'll just talk to myself then. It's the only way I can get my memory down."

Later that afternoon, Frank's playing a miniature video game on the bed and asks if I'd like to try, which I do, briefly. "Do you want protection for you, from the spirit world?" he asks me. Yes, I say. "It goes like this: Sapori Shindano."

And who is to say he's not correct? Shindano is a Swahili word, Larry will tell me later, for the needle that doctors use to give an injection. Now how did Frank come across *that*?

• • •

The other one had taken out his hands (from behind his back); and he exclaimed: "Feel (thou) that which I did also feel!" and he showed the other one of his hands; and the other one's hands were altogether inside the Leopard Tortoise's neck. And he arose, and returned home. . . .

The people exclaimed: "Where hast thou been?" And he, answering, said that the Leopard Tortoise had been the one in whose neck his hands had been; that was why he had not returned home. The people said: "Art thou a fool? Did not (thy) parents instruct thee? The Leopard Tortoise always seems as if she would die; while she is deceiving us."

—W. H. I. Bleek and L. C. Lloyd, *Specimens of Bushmen Folklore*[1]

The remaining couple of days pass too quickly. We're staying again at The Outpost in Arusha. Frank compares some notes with Larry about the *Star Wars* movies and recalls when Larry's psychiatrist son Marshall came to see him the last time he was in the hospital. With a group of Tanzanian musicians, Larry sings "Malaika," the Swahili word for "angel," and a song made famous by Harry Belafonte and later Miriam Makeba. On our last day here, he and Stephan sing it together in the car.

Larry had attended boarding school in Arusha during his primary years, almost seventy years ago. It then had about sixty kids in the five grades, all white children of colonials. It's mid-morning when we show up at the school. As Larry is a venerable alumni, we're given a full tour. Today, the headmistress informs us, it's a government school and the largest in the area. There are now 840 students, including 60 in the nursery school. They are all black. And the numbers are increasing, because so many people continue to move into the city. Besides English, the children are taught both Swahili and French.

Franklin writes his name and address in the guestbook, putting his signature in Asian-style characters. When we enter one of the classrooms, the kids are on tea break. Frank is quickly surrounded by them, showing the eight-year-olds how to use his camera and even letting them take some pictures. It's a heartwarming sight. In the library, where photographs from Larry's day are framed on the walls and he recognizes some of his old classmates, Frank tells the teachers: "Excellent craftsmanship in Africa."

What Larry remembers most fondly is Kobe, a huge leopard tortoise that lived in the schoolyard in the mid-1940s. Every winter when Larry returned to Tanzania, he would make a pilgrimage here to make sure Kobe was still around. "I tell him my troubles," he says, "and end in tears." Nobody knew where Kobe came from before the Arusha School. Weighing at least 200 pounds—and probably the same number of years old, he originally lived under a fig tree, where the kids brought him water and fed him banana peels as a dessert to accompany the grasses he ate. "Several of us kids at a time could sit on him," Larry recalls. "I used to take slow rides on his back around the school."

Kobe is beloved by visitors from all over the world, from Sydney to Boston. The tortoise has a slightly fractured upper shell from various attempts to abduct him over the years but, other than that, seemed in fine fettle during Larry's last visit. "Every year, when I make this my last stop, I'm afraid they'll tell me that no one has seen him" Accompanied by one of the teachers and a couple of the students, we go in search of Kobe. Sure enough, he's awaiting us under an Odoranta fig tree. "Can we go and say hello?" Larry asks with the shyness of a boy. He approaches first. "My old friend," he says, touching the tortoise's head and offering a Swahili greeting used for knocking on someone's door: "Hodi." Turning back to face us, Larry says with a smile: "He gave me the look he always does—'Oh God, not you again!'" Tears are visible in the doctor's eyes. Franklin is moved to observe this. First he, then Aileane and I take turns paying our respects to Kobe, with light taps on his high-domed shell. "I wouldn't be surprised if he barked," Frank says, offering Larry a broad smile.

• • •

Separation is pain.

—Franklin's Journal

Our trip to Tanzania is drawing to a close. "Maybe someday I can visit you," Stephan says to Frank.

"Keep the relationship going," Frank says.

"And we will see you next year?" Stephan asks Larry.

"Inshallah," Larry says. God willing.

At the Serengeti Select offices, Frank is taciturn and pacing. It's easy to see how painful it is for him to say good-bye to Stephan. He will only shake hands and look away. After Larry does the same, I take Stephan aside to give him a tip. "I hope that we will see you again," I tell him.

"Take care of Frank," Stephan tells me, "he's a good man."

Our new driver shows up. It takes an hour in traffic to get to Kilimanjaro International Airport, then a very long wait to board our first flight. Frank is pacing, constantly bending his fingers. We fly first to the capital of Dar-es-Salaam to fill up with enough fuel to reach Amsterdam, but some kind of electrical problem keeps us on the ground for another two hours.

With the long delays, anger rises up in my son. When I start to say, "Franklin . . ." he fires back: "That's not my name, my name is Simon!"

"I thought we got through this the other night," I say.

"You're not a rapist, are you?" he asks demandingly.

I begin to dread the nine-hour flight ahead. But Frank takes his evening meds and has some food and we manage to each sleep for about two-thirds of the way. It's the next morning when I first notice the mix-up that's been happening between his morning and evening doses of Clozaril, which would account for the earlier changes in his behavior.

We arrive in Amsterdam and Frank falls in love with the city, especially the Van Gogh Museum, where we spend several hours looking at the paintings and Frank asks that I buy him several books.

According to the book *Shamans Among Us* by Dr. Joseph Polimeni: "Vincent van Gogh suffered through at least a dozen psychotic episodes. He experienced classic paranoid delusions, such as the irrational belief that the police were after him. He would obsessively translate the Bible in idiosyncratic ways. He tended to be moody, irritable, disheveled, odd, standoffish and solitary."

It's a Sunday morning when we prepare to board our last flight, bound again for Boston. Standing in the immigration line, I notice that the questioning of passengers is particularly intense, much more so than anything I've seen in the United States. I can't let my son go through this by himself, I realize.

As we approach a female security staff person together, Franklin is understandably nervous. He's looking around in all directions, avoiding eye contact with her. "Have you been drinking?" she asks. At first, Frank doesn't respond. After what seems to me an eternity, he shakes his head no. "Have you taken any drugs?" she asks. Again the silence, followed by the nonverbal no.

The woman walks over to the chief of security, an ominous-looking man standing in front of the carry-on screening machines. They talk for a minute or so before she returns.

"Are you all right?!" she asks my son loudly.

"I'm fine!" Frank exclaims at the same decibel level. Then abruptly adds: "I'm a car mechanic!"

Oh shit. The woman goes to speak again with her supervisor. "Frank," I say quietly, "just answer the questions, okay? Just yes or no. You don't need to volunteer information."

Now the chief of security beckons me over and asks what's going on. I take a deep breath. "My son," I tell him, "has a mental illness." The man is apologetic. "But he's taken his medication," I continue, "and he'll be fine on the plane. I'll be sitting with him. He doesn't get violent or anything."

The man says that someone may come around to check on us. "That's fine," I say. We make it onboard without further issue.

• • •

I have a lot of time to think on the last leg of the journey. I remember James Hillman having once spoken to his wife about my nature. My being able to relate quickly to and assimilate all kinds of people and places, he thought, would be disconcerting to Franklin, who must focus so hard on smaller details simply to be able to function.

The night of our breakthrough together, mundane phenomenon such as food had been met at first with strong resistance. As if my son was saying, "You do not understand that you are threatening the world I am in right now." But his reaction seems, in retrospect, not just compensatory. He could feel me, and change, because in the end I was shaken to my core. The very idea that, by capturing his words I could later "crack the code" of his delusions, had automatically made him into "the other." But the breakthrough occurred when *my* code cracked. It was not about being protected, but *allowing* myself to be cracked. My son needed entry into *me* . . . needed to know, too, that I felt *him*. The snake was the archetype, winding, finding our way to the root of one another.

Sometimes, where Franklin lives, there is no time—but instead all time, all races, all places. Could it be that delusions aren't really what we think they are, but pieces of a larger reality where an individual seeks to wrap their arms around something more than the everyday?

Surely, conventional psychiatrists would have advised against my taking Franklin on this trip. Just as surely, I believe, they would have been wrong.

Now, as the landing gear goes down approaching the Boston runway, I realize how much Frank is able to deftly handle the many mechanical things that I'm so inept at. I need his help, and he needs mine. We really did take care of each other on this trip.

Aileane's mother picks her up and we agree to stay in touch. She reserves her warmest good-bye for Franklin. Eddie meets us again at the airport. He drops off Larry first, then Frank. It's cold in Boston and close to ten o'clock at night when I help my son inside his house with his bags. Since we drove to the airport in Tanzania, one of my eyes has been bothering me. Maybe an insect bit me or I rubbed it too much, but it's visibly swollen and I've been trying not to touch it. "Take care of that eye," Frank says. We hug each other good-bye, the first time I can remember that happening in years.

It seems we all learned something in the course of our travels together. A few weeks later, Larry and I go out to dinner to talk about the coffee table–type memoir about his life that he'd like my help in putting together. He describes how he'd spent a good bit of time try-ing to correct Franklin but "once I got it into my head to just go along with it, then it was not an issue."

Then he says: "You know, it's the same thing with autism. I think that's a different step in the development of evolutionary life."

"How do you mean?" I ask the doctor.

"Well, there's very little difference found in studying the genes involved in the autism spectrum disorder and schizophrenia. It's the fact that we *Homo sapiens* are so intolerant that makes them the prob-lem. We could just as easily *be* the problem, and they're the norm."

Somehow, I have my doubts that Dr. Reiner would have said this before his latest trip to Africa. Or that I could have heard it.

CHAPTER 16

• • •

Touched with Fire

Such is always the mode in which the highest imaginative faculty seizes its materials. It never stops at crusts or ashes, or outward images of any kind; it ploughs them all aside, and plunges into the very central heart; nothing else will content its spirituality. . .

—John Ruskin, *Modern Painters*

NEARLY A DECADE EARLIER, AT the end of 2002, my son had handed me a stack of papers containing his writing for that year and asked if I would keep it for him. I did, and collected them in a manila folder labeled "Frank's Writings." Now, upon our return from Africa, I bring the folder out from a file cabinet and spend a good deal of time reading through his writings. The profundity of some of the pieces shakes me to the core.

The notes that I find myself jotting down are initially a kind of random comparison of qualities in father and son. My impulsiveness and tendency to move too fast: this is a trait in Franklin too, though much more exaggerated. If I can come to better terms with this, with my own obsessive nature, could he? Is his inability to focus and concentrate perhaps linked to how much I *can* do this, to the exclusion of all else? I can readily "tune out" what is around me and exist in my own world—so what's the difference really? Just as, lost in my own thoughts sometimes, nothing anyone is saying around me registers. Maybe Frank is stuck with the extremes as a constant reality. So if I can become more self-aware of my own unconsciousness, might he be better able to change? It is not as simple as "love conquers all," I realize.

But beyond this, I don't believe I ever truly appreciated what my son had recounted—and achieved—ten years earlier, when he was twenty-three and living for a time in his own apartment. Only now, as I look back, am I able to put more pieces together about what he was going through. Only now, too, am I astounded by his poetic use of language and his emerging philosophy of life. Contemplating the probably unanswerable question—is this genius or madness, or does the "madness" fuel the genius?—I realize that my son is a writer whose imagination not only soars, but whose muse can be transcendent. However it came to pass, he exhibits a wisdom beyond his years—at a place in his life where he seemed to be connecting to a source, a place not of mental illness but of revelation. After Africa, I realize that place is still there to be encouraged.

First there were his aphorisms, the playing with words, of which Frank wrote:

They need to invent a new name for my kind of satisfactory sarcasm and prolific use of sounds-likes and rhymes . . .

BECAUSE YOU CAN'T TELL TIME, DOESN'T MEAN THAT TIME WILL TELL.

STICKING WITH YOUR JOB HAS NOTHING TO DO WITH TREES AND BRANCHES.

A FORTUNE TELLER COULDN'T READ A PALM TREE. IT HAS NO WORDS WRITTEN ON IT.

NEWTON DIDN'T DISCOVER THE THEORY OF GRAVITY BY BEING HIT BY A SNAPPLE.

YOU CAN'T SAY A WORD BY YAWNING.

WHY DON'T WE CRY OVER DEAD PEOPLE IN THE MORNING.

GOD CAN'T GRANT YOU MONEY, HONEY.

8-24-02: Why study a whole book or a whole language? Why not study one word over and over. The meaning and value of one word is very powerful if used as a tool. A word is eternal. While not adequate to use in conversation, it is adept for meditation and musing.

On His Life

I like the guitar. I can play about five chords. I cannot play comfortably. . . . I love it but it is incapable of loving me or hating me. It just exists. I cannot say the same for myself. I am far more complicated. I am out there like one of the planets of the solar system, Saturn or Uranus. Go ahead you name it. I never knew my Aura to grow but it will someday when I know enough. When I play the Guitar, I react like the moon and glow internally. The sun is always there and the moon keeps changing like my emotions . . .

I am wilting because I am fighting for something which is my dignity which is the rectification of a warped distorted and altogether incomplete mind . . .

Alone, waiting at the bus. Everyone is going different directions. Thoughts scattered. Seeking positivity. Angriness. Feel as though I could explode. Don't know what to say, this happens every day, but I will succeed if I focus . . .

Believe me, it isn't easy to have emotions. To be afraid of one's self. To be afraid you have no friends. To feel like you are the only one in the world that loves and are still susceptible to all the hate of the world. I am getting a job. Maybe I will gain some consistency in life . . .

Hey beautiful! Is it just the animal in me that makes me attracted to you? Is it that beast that brings me seeking to hold you in my arms? Or is it love? OOH, what a subject. All that glossy music that we listen to and I bring up love. Isn't love only in the movies. Isn't it what they fought over in the old West. So I'm at the club thinking about you. I stare into the flashing lights and lose myself. I am getting over that Vodka and Tonic and just got some Strawberries and stuff to eat. As I look down directly in front of me, I see the shape of an hour glass. But this hour glass is colored blue pink and yellow. It is clothed with a dress. My perception is mixed between peace and absent kisses on my mind. Suddenly I have to leave the club to get some fresh air and abandon my sexual fantasies. I feel like I had been hit with a million of cupid's arrows and I can't communicate a thing. Speechless, I wait for the crosswalk light to change. I need guidance. The words "what

if?" come fragmentally into my mind. Then another sentence comes as I look at the man on the car that just turned into a sleek black cat. "Jump to see if you'll get hit." Then what happens is I become a bird, a falcon, and I become the all seeing. I become afraid and I back off as the walk sign is revealed. I think, "I just saved myself from such pain"—I could have been a paraplegic. Thank god, he was looking out for me . . .

The Downtown area is full of lights this Autumn and the numbness I acquired at the club is wearing off finally. Maybe I should do some yoga in the park. Then it occurs to me that I may have lost the girl inside the club. Maybe I should get her number. I could even bring her to my studio where we could have tea, milk, and sugar while I sketch her. I think I love her.

Satisfying each other with each embrace. Eternity has taken place in brief moments of bliss we share together.

A peaceful day is as follows. The sun is shining. The girls gather around me and I start to make a dice game. My mind is free and my work is to dedicate my time to these beautiful women. Then I preach a sermon to all around about love and kindness. Everyone begins to laugh at my jokes and everyone is alive. I feel happy.

One day I am walking through the park. It is dusk and the air is the opposite of damp. The sun is setting and the sky is full of brilliant pinks, oranges and purples. As I walk past the dusty baseball diamond I see a shadow by the fence. As I look closer, I see a small cat, looking scared. That cat was a baby and it was left alone by its mother. I had seen it before. So I think to inspect it, while I walk towards it. It begins to shy away as I chase it and I realize it has nothing to identify it by. As I run to catch it, I hear a noise ahead of me. I couldn't believe it. The cat had been hit by a car. When I was little, I would see the cat in my yard, creeping around. He had a twin too. His twin would constantly fight with him, making high pitched noises. You could tell them apart because one had no tail. Otherwise, they were identical. It seemed that they both loved the back alleys of the city. The light would expose their calico fur. In the winter time they would have thicker coats. You could see them at the park playing games and hunting squirrels.

I have no one but yet I still care. I am not comfortable but I survive. Love is hard to come by. I feel alone like the sun on a cold winter day. I am not very good at changing. My mind jumps from subject to subject. I am not satisfied. The wandering goes on. Sometimes I have no direction. So I write. I am calling out from the darkness. Shouting somebody hear me. Sometimes I barely know my name....

I am a man but my heart is heavy. I feel the weight of all. I have moments when I feel good and those in which I feel down. No day is ever perfect. Some days I feel persecuted and hated. I wish I was free. Feeling down like this, I lose perspective. I know very little about people, women, or even about myself. On days when I'm depressed I know not of form. I only know of feeling. I forget who I am. I want to move but want to stay. I am pursuing a career in Engineering, a hobby of art. I don't know where to start.

Why did the world part with Jimi Hendrix? He was great and creative while on drugs. I am straight without the drugs so far but phyciatrists [sic] make me sick in my bowels with their razmatazical matter of factualness. I'd rather be a crazy scientist because I have no order. I fit beautifully into a world of make believe and my convictions are as strong as me you see.

On His Philosophy

Blindness is a characteristic of being human. In whatever stage of life there is always blindness and always clarity. Let me explain. Blindness is our inability to see exactly who we are. We may get hints. We may see our picture in a mirror. But every day we are faced with the question, who really am I . . .

These days we live in a world of wonderful opportunities. We could work and stand together. We could take a part in making it better for all. At the same time the pressure that our careers demand leave us no ability to think deeply about our lives. At best life is fun, interesting, organized, satisfying, and challenging. Life in these times is taxing, boring, demanding, selfish, sad, destructive . . .

Simplicity should be revealed by thought in every situation.

2/27/02: Worthiness comes from practice, practice from patience. Passiveness is potential for destruction. Direction of mind, body and soul is achieved through actions based on love from the heart.

Your empty core was not the problem. Everyone suffers such human ailments. Your fruitless trail of actual events is what you'll need to repent.

If you don't know, why don't you ask. If you don't love, why don't you try. If you are satisfied with your life then you must be dead. If you put everything on others, you are of the devil, creating evil and pain for those of us that love and are good. Talk ill of your brother without cause and you are a hypocrite.

If I thought that the world revolved around me, would I be wrong? It really revolves around us all. We need to worship the center, god, in some way or fashion. . . . At the same time there is much chaos and unkindness.

Love is from the heart. Thoughts are from the brain. Thoughts mean nothing unless motivated by the heart, by the emotions. You can forget a thought and you can forget a feeling. To forget a thought is fine. You can always learn it again. To forget and not deal with a feeling on the other hand, is dangerous and potentially painful.

People need music to bring them to a point of balance, happiness and to ease the pain of living. Music is meant to be melodic not bland and boring. The vibration of music brings us all together. Music connects us with a sense of love.

Religion creates a structure to induce love from moments in time that endure, creating a life of meaning.

God is an armor to hold our ship when scary waters make it dangerous. He is the light that wakes us up each morning. He holds the inspiration of our ideas. When we have pain we must ask him to pardon and empower us. . . . We either learn to understand the god within us or we will live a fragmented life, shifting from one unformulated idea to the next.

Life goes by quickly but when you stop and quarrel mentally with it, it takes forever. All I got is time. Am I going to make it a prison or a paradise. Will I live friendly with the devil or will I sacrifice for the sake of god.

On Race

Carefully the cops and the whites try to confuse us. . . . They target us and try to tame us. They talk and their dogs bark. Why, because we are dark. The white lady expresses her fucked up desires to screw the black fugitive. Famous blacks bust watermelon rinds. Subdued they suck away the sweetness. Succumb to stitches on black and yellow man's eyes. Two seconds between the white lady's thighs.

There's this fucked up kid that I love because I was fucked [up] once about where I came from. I am mixed black and white but I am really back with wit. I am what I am and what my folks had in mind. I don't give a shit if you call me purple and yellow like the Lakers. My name is still Frank and I still speak Frankly and that's where it's at.

My roommates are watching a bootleg movie. Do they call it bootleg because it makes your girlfriend put her boot on her leg. Oh hell I could write till I become an old man with an oily nose, teaching my grandchildren phonics.

By then they will have 10,000 satellites lighting up the sky and they will have people with robotic implants that tell them the news. People will ride in hover cars with rainbow colors that they buy for the price that a skateboard costs today. Apartments will hover in the air and could only be accessed by invisible escalators that transport a person. How about those white supremacists that were responsible for killing black people. They better have guns like the dutch if they were to go against Shaka Zulu...

Is that OK with you? Or are you one of those bigots who benefits off utilizing colored people for slave labor. I bet you'd like them to fashion your Nikes for you or mop the floor from the hallway to your gold adorned room. And if they were to give an inkling of attitude you'd have them out on their asses in the street begging for money when we really need change . . .

On the Times We Live In:

Calling each other people use cell phones. Distorted waves cause static confusion.

Today we need integration, not alienation. Inspiration and not desperation . . .

Self efforts, self missions, self superiority is a disease common in America. I don't know about anywhere else. It leaves you all alone. It makes you suffer until it is all over, it destroys families. There has to be another way . . .

Sometimes I feel as though fame and name dominate our people. They begin to live for self and destroy our groups. Lives of vanity are the outcome. Comfort for the good man is sometimes hard to find. Our futures seem to be uncertain. Our fears appear as more powerful. Let us release our destruction and unleash our trust and illumination to our god. Goodness and fortitude will prevail . . .

5/12/02: These days direction in life is not evident. Each one of us is struggling for identity. Ignorance and isolation appear to be winning against clarity. Confusion is becoming a major concern in today's world. The current trends focus on mixing, blending, communicating.

The purpose though is not clear. We are capable as people to produce incredible things. Yet many lack insight. Thus, many are controlled by outer things and not inner things. The major difference is that the heart and mind are being equated to superficial values.

It is dangerous to follow a thing that is without. Likewise, do not let yourself leave or ignore the voice of your conscience or heart.

Your life is valuable. Life is work, action, love, hate, illusion, pain, suffering. These are just some basic parts of life.

Ask yourself, when my life is over what will it amount to?

The world will soon be destroyed. All of your illusions. All of your secret desires. All of your doubts are soon to be revealed. Soon everything you believed in and worked for in this material world will be reduced to ashes and dust. You will be left alone to live or die. You think everything is straightforward. Why?

Because you are blind and struggling to survive. You think not of the powerless and weak. You see them not as the same as you. If you look within, you will see that you too are powerless and weak. You can gain the whole world for the price of your soul, my friend....

The human race storms into a cataclysmic frenzy.

So why is it my poor people and my rich people, that when we have the world to work with and so many enlightened people and ideas and books and philosophies, that we cannot live together, listen to each other. Do we have to die together? Let us live!

THE GUY ON THE CORNER TALKS TO HIMSELF ABOUT HOW HE IS A GENERAL AND IS RIGHTFUL OWNER OF THE UNITED STATES. HE TAKES ANOTHER SIP OF THE BOTTLE. EVERYTHING SEEMS ALRIGHT. THEN IT GETS CLOUDY. IT BEGINS TO SPRINKLE. THE CITY STREETS BECOME EMPTY AND THE ONLY THING YOU NOTICE ARE THE BEES AND THE FLIES.

SATURDAY IS GARBAGE DAY SO EVERYONE TAKES IT OUT ON FRIDAY. YOU GOT EVERYTHING THERE. YOU CAN FIND BIKES AND TVS AND YOU CAN FIND BEER CANS AND SNAILS. ON GARBAGE DAY THE OLD CHINESE LADY COMES BY AND SORTS THROUGH THE CANS. HER COUNTERPART, THE PEACEFUL BLACK GUY, COMES WEARING A VEST FROM THE 60'S THAT HAS PINS ON IT. HIS TATTERED CLOTHES REVEAL AN OLD TATOO. IT IS HIS OLD LADY'S NAME.

. . . WHERE THE FUCK WAS GOD THAT DAY THAT IT WAS RAINING AND POURING AND I WAS BORED AND THOUGHTLESS? . . . I DON'T SMOKE OR DRINK SO MY FRIENDS LEFT ME ALONE, A SOLDIER IN THE DARK. A DISMAL FOGGY DAY PRESENTED A FEW PEOPLE HUDDLED UNDER STORE STOOPS LIKE PIGEONS. YOU NEVER WOULD HAVE GUESSED THEY HAD SEX DRIVE ON THOSE

TYPE OF DAYS. YOU NEVER WOULD HAVE GUESSED THAT THEY HAD SPIRITS. EVEN OLD LADIES GLASSES WERE FOGGY THAT DAY. THEY COULDN'T SEE A THING. THAT DAY REVEALED THE OUTER DYSFUNCTION OF THE MASSES. MOST PEOPLE LOOK SO DARNED TOGETHER IN PUBLIC.

PEACE I SAY. BUT WHO AM I ACCORDING TO A NEUTRAL PHSICIATRIST [sic] OR COMMUNITY WORKER. I AM GETTING OLDER AND WISER AND NO ONE SEEMS TO CARE. . . . I AM GROWN AND POWERFUL BUT ONLY TO MYSELF. WHY, BECAUSE I DON'T SAY MUCH. I ONLY COMMUNICATE WHEN I NEED TO. NO, THATS A LIE I TALK ALL THE FUCKING TIME. I COULD COMPETE WITH A JACK IN THE BOX. I COULD BEAT THE LOUDEST DOG IN A BARKING MATCH. I SPEAK FROM MY SPIRIT AND I GOT MORE HOTWATER IN THERE THAN A HOT COMPRESS THAT THEY PUT ON A BRUISED HOCKEY PLAYER. WHEN I WAS LITTLE I WASN'T A PAIN IN THE ASS BUT ONE IN THE HEAD. I WASN'T TRADITIONAL . . . SO NOW I'M ALL GROWN AND I PORTRAY A PEACEFUL FRAME OF MIND. I MITIGATE SITUATIONS. I CAN'T EVEN PROPERLY TELL MY PHSICIATRIST THAT I DON'T WANT TO BOTHER WITH MEDS. I ARGUE BUT DON'T WIN. IF I DID WIN THE OTHER GUY WOULD PROBABLY HAVE TO BE DEAD. I TRY TO MAINTAIN A SMILE. THE SIMPLE PEOPLE MIGHT BELIEVE THAT I BELONG TO THEIR CLICK [sic] BECAUSE I AM JUST LIKE THEM. I HAVE A HARD TIME PUTTING IN SIMPLE ENGLISH THAT I WILL NEVER BE LIKE THEM. THE ONLY GROWTH THEY WILL ACHIEVE IS ONE FROM CANCER OF WHAT-

EVER PART OF THE BODY THAT WILL SIMPLY KILL THEM.

THERE WAS A MAN THAT LIVED IN A BOX. THE BOX WAS HIS HEART. SO HE WOULD EXPLAIN TO THE WORLD THAT HIS HEART WAS SQUARE AND EMPTY. THE WORLD WOULD SAY THEY ALREADY KNEW. HE WOULD ASK WHY AND THEY WOULD SAY THAT THEIRS WAS TOO. AND THAT HE WAS STUPID TO ASK SUCH A QUESTION. NOW WHEN THE MAN REALIZED THAT HIS HEART WAS AN EMPTY BOX, HE CRIED AND WAS AWARE OF HIS EMPTINESS. SO HE HAD A PLAN. HE WOULD FILL THE BOX WITH BEAU- TIFUL PRESENTS AND GIVE IT TO SOME- ONE. THE PRESENTS WERE SHINY AND BRILLIANT. SOME WERE SOFT AND MUSHY. SO HE ASKED THE WORLD WHO HE COULD GIVE THE FULL BOX TO. AND NO ONE COULD TELL HIM. HE WAITED YEARS. EVERYDAY HE SAID GOODBYE TO YESTERDAY. THE OTH- ERS WITH THE EMPTY BOX HEARTS WERE JEALOUS AND BEWILDERED. THEN ONE DAY HE MET A WISE MAN. THE WISE MAN ASKED WHY HE FILLED HIS HEART WITH THINGS. HE TOLD THE WISE MAN, THAT HIS HEART HAD BEEN EMPTY. THE WISE MAN REPLIED THAT THOSE WERE THINGS OF THE WORLD AND THAT THEY WOULD DISAPPEAR IN TIME. THEN THE MAN REALIZED THIS AND CRIED AGAIN. HE ASKED THE WORLD WHAT HE WOULD DO. THEY DID NOT ANSWER FOR THEY DID NOT KNOW. SO HE DECIDED TO BURN THE BOX THAT WAS HIS HEART AND HE BEGAN TO LIVE ALONE, HIS HEART ON FIRE.

While Living Alone in Somerville:

9-16-02   Concern is care is confusion. Why do you look at me the way you do? You are sharing skepticism and sarcasm. Why won't you believe we could have a connection. You refuse to ignite the spark between us that could justify friendship . . .

I am achieving, moving, thriving. Being active, working, discovering. I know how to love, to hate, to feel. I feel strong, act healthy. I have no fear, resentment. I am OK, real happy and helpful. My body is dark is strong is African. I am of Egypt, Morocco, Mexico, Puerto Rico, all lands. Being as me I am made to be free . . .

Living alone is not easy. Trying to maintain when everything seems strange. I want to be left to complete things to be passionate. Unpredictability surfaces in the world. I feel alienated and stressed. I think everyone hates me and especially women. Conspiring around me people know my name and everything about me. I am hated. Creepy people wander around. Devilish dead ugly rude people point fingers at everyone. . . . I cannot love every woman. I only need one. But why can't I love the world? Because the world is insane. Mouths filled with trash, speaking of sickness and hatred. Ugly sinful people justify madness and play with a lover's heart. The whole world joins them to an empty cause. Together they pillage an honest man's haven. Direct the kids or they won't just destroy themselves but you too.

Since when did I become a slave to the computer? Hurry up and print faster. Don't make any noise. It isn't as though you are having sex is it. So loud people are talking in the next room. They are enlisting themselves guiltily into nonsensical and dramatic conversations. If they were my kids I'd whip them into shape. Well really I'd just give them the evil eye . . .

Maybe there will be a dinosaur that will scare the shit out of me and eat the shit. Shit would be the only money I would pay him to run away and get back in his Jurassic cage. You know what, fuck the dinosaurs. They died off millions of years ago. Get that through your bony cranium!

I don't belong to you succer, and sucker has a c and not a k because it gives me no kick and allows you to see. Did I studder? Well I probably tripped because it's dark in my mind. About as dark as a butt naked African and prematurely

birthed and deformed hoot owl. You'll never recover from this abstract sermon especially if you ARE religious. To me it's as good as honey from a bee hive. Careful, don't get stung! . . .

Wasn't it the flying monkeys that got killed in oz. Poor ugly degenerate creatures. And that wicked witch just melted like a candle stick into this green shit that woulda made you sick if you saw it . . .

I used to know this old lady that smoked brown cigarettes. Maybe she liked brown dick and liked it thick. In the process her dog would hump her leg like a deprived sexual thief. I wonder what they did at night? I think she taught her dog to speak and he would call "One Nine Hundred, Hot Clit" on the telephone. And maybe her dog wasn't partial to her. I think he dreamed to be an army sergeant so he could make love to young army Virgins. Anyway he was a horny little thing. When she died he would make love to her tennis balls.

You know those horny toads? I think they go both ways. Bisexually content. They spit semen and their dicks get as hard as cement. Maybe they solidified the AIDS Virus. Could be they have a passion for death and wanted people to disappear so they could take over the earth. Really though they are the softest harmless little buggers. And their skin looks kind of brittle—especially when they are toasted by some homeless dude with a lighter.

On the Nature of Being

Forces control us that we know not the source. One day everything is satisfactory. The next is terrible.

I am that water, that steam, that influence. That power, that product, that entrance. I am the feeling, the light and influence. I represent that medium, and structure of the new age. Flowing is the spring that brings us to that feeling. Liberation of spirit away from luxury. Lecture upon lecture about the ills of society. We keep going, time goes on.

Rejuvenate us. We are quiet and we are loud. Lost and found. Foul and clean. Savory and mean...

You sold out and couldn't take it. Life crumpled you up like paper and threw you in the trash. Now you reek of destruction. Death and dismay. Wondering how did I get this way. It's pretty simple—you lost your faith. Fortunate for you, you now have joined the crew of losers. Listening to their tower of babble, you enjoy yourself. Self pro-claimed leader of a tribe without direction. When did you begin to live like a bullet, where will your trail of emptiness end. A bullet stops eventually.

He disappeared, not here anymore, gone. Traveling through the portal was a long, laborious process. It was all light, different colored light. For a moment he was transfixed between heaven and hell. His soul could be lost. At the same time there was always the danger that his soul could be captured in the light and sold for a high price to someone who had lost their soul.

Note:

1. *Specimens of Bushmen Folklore*: Full text at www.sacred-texts.com

PART 3

Call of the Shaman

If your psyche is disordered or deficient or overcharged, blocks are created in you that prevent comprehension and remembering. To open up the channels in you so that whatever energy you need can flow freely is not the task of the teacher; it is the task of the shaman.

—Malidoma Patrice Somé, *The Healing Wisdom of Africa.*[1]

• • •

CHAPTER 17

Double-Edged Homecoming

After all this work, don't let us go berserk. Prepare us, protect us.
—Franklin's Journal, 2002.

F OR HIS THIRTY-THIRD BIRTHDAY NOT long after our return from Africa, my friend Eddie, his wife Candy, and I take Frank to lunch at Legal Seafoods. He talks a little about our trip and the animals he'd seen, but is largely silent. My son apologizes for being "so out of it." He says he hadn't been this way earlier at his house, but had watched something on TV "and maybe someone put a curse on me." We drop him off at home soon afterward.

At least Frank has been able to articulate what he's going through, which is a change in itself. Another friend recalls how difficult anyone's return can be from an exotic place, as if a piece of their soul is still over there; she herself had experienced this acutely coming back from the Amazon, with visions of indigenous Yanomani pursuing her in dreams. And Frank, who has difficulty processing anyway, would doubtless have a hard time coming back to American "reality."

When I share some of the story of our African experience with my literary agent over the phone, she says: "Franklin found a father, but you found a son. Anything you do now will be reconnecting on that level."

I come to a decision. I can't go back to LA and continue to see my son only every few months as I was doing. I can't leave him alone again after such a profound time together. Alice and I discuss her coming to join me soon in Boston, which she does. I call Frank the day after his birthday. He's now all right and, when I ask if he knows what the problem was, he says: "Drugs in the wind or something." Then I tell him that I'm going to stay on the East Coast and Alice will be coming. "That's great, Dick!" he exclaims, suggesting that he knows of some yoga exercises that could enable us to have a baby.

He's still somewhat disoriented when we go to a mall to pick up more shelves for his room. But we assemble them together. Then, while we clean his whole room, I realize he needs a wastebasket and laundry bag and a hook on his door for a bathrobe. From his storage area in the basement we bring up a DVD player and four small speakers, and I'm impressed with how focused Frank is in setting up all the wiring. Any delusions seem to have all but disappeared.

And, most heartening of all, he wants to go back to school. "Whatever I have to do," he says. It's been a decade since he attended the Franklin Institute. Now he's intrigued by Lincoln Technical Institute, which has a location in Somerville not too far from his house. I make an appointment for us to meet with the assistant admissions director. The school has about 300 adult students, who take courses in computer repair, massage therapy, or to become a medical assistant. Concerning the last, the administrator wonders, would he be squeamish about blood draws? "Oh no," Frank replies, "I've had a lot of experience with those. Of course, it's not like tracks from heroin or something." She raises her eyebrows and leans across the desk. *Has he ever had a problem with that?* she asks. "Oh no," Frank says again.

Another question is whether he's ever been arrested on a felony charge. I jump in to say that he hasn't. But after a brief pause, my son interjects: "Well, I did get arrested once. I took off all my clothes by the river and was naked, and the police saw me." *Oh shit*, I think to myself, he never told me about *that*. Once again, the administrator's eyebrows come up, but so does a smile. "But you didn't go to jail for that, did you?" she asks matter-of-factly. "No, no," Frank says. A bit later, when he asks if they wear uniforms at the school, she says that's a good question. Yes, they have T-shirts with the school name. "Can you wear blue jeans?" Frank asks. No, only khakis or dockers, she replies, and adds: "But just remember: you have to keep your pants on." They smile at one another with mutual understanding.

Frank opts for the curriculum offered in computer repair. Next step is a twelve-minute aptitude test on a computer. After taking it, he whispers to me that he's done poorly. How does he feel about the test? the administrator asks. "Oh, I felt okay but I don't think *you* will!" Frank exclaims, saying he'd only answered 30 of the 50 questions. "I didn't tell you," she says, "but nobody finishes it."

He's charmed his way into acceptance and I'm just along for the ride. Frank pats me fondly on the head. We tour the spacious classrooms, informed that they help you find a job upon being certified. It looks like he'll receive a Pell grant and have most of his tuition covered through student loans. Others at the school come up to congratulate him.

Orientation is coming right up, and Frank already wants to get his books. Classes will be from 8 a.m. to 2 p.m., four days a week, all the way from mid-February to November. My son is excited and determined. Privately I explain to the administrator about Frank's history and situation. She understands and says she'll watch closely for any agitation.

Frank has an excellent first week, up at 6 a.m., and catching the bus to school, while going to a gym in the same building after class. He's wondering if it's possible to eventually be off the medication. I tell him about some research suggesting that many people's condition improves as they grow older and that it's certainly not something to rule out, or at least be able to cut back on.

"When you can make it seem like you know something, that's half the battle in life," he says one day, and the wisdom in that statement makes me laugh. He comes over to Fort Hill to study with one of the men who used to help him when he was homeschooled. The computer courses are clearly not easy, like learning a new language, but I've not seen him this devoted to making something work in many years. Etta finds the change in our son quite miraculous and knows it couldn't have happened without Africa and the relationship that he and I have repaired.

Suddenly, his house gets word from Social Security that Frank's monthly benefits have been cut off because he has more than the allowable limit of $2,000 in his bank account. Frank is a mess. He gets on the phone with me and begins ranting about his many accounts and the Mafia and dealing drugs and white people and how he needs a sleeping bag if he's going to be out on the street. I drive over to his house right away. As we cruise around, gradually he comes back to himself. "It's hard to be safe in today's world," he says, adding: "You know how to do that and at the same time have an agenda. I can't do that, and it's frustrating." He also says how hard it is for him to express his emotions. "Well, it's hard for me too, Frank," I tell him. The next morning, the money problem will turn out to have been a clerical error.

Shortly thereafter I'm called to a meeting with his teacher and the school's education director. Frank did pass the first module, but is having a hard time taking the tests and with focusing in general, although he's been on time every day. They're concerned about whether he's getting enough sleep. They apparently really like him and want him to succeed, but it feels very tentative. *Is the pressure simply too much for my son?* I wonder.

It's not been an easy period for me. Besides my ongoing concern about Frank, difficult and painful issues have arisen both with my writing work and domestic life. As I'm taking Frank to his psychiatrist, he notices tears in my eyes. "Are you all right?" he asks, alarmed and adds, "Do you want me to change the station on the radio?" It's playing older folk songs, which he knows I used to love. "Do you want me to rub your back?" I'm deeply touched at his concern, as Frank rubs both sides behind my neck while I drive. He says he knows some medication that might be good for stress.

"I'm having a hard time," I explain to him. "My life seems to be in upheaval. I'm running into brick walls at every turn."

I feel my son take a deep breath. "Oh, that's why you felt like that," he says. I thank him, for noticing and for asking.

The difference in him is tactile. But by springtime, frustration is building in him. Twice he speaks of how everyone else in his class has been using computers all their lives. He falls into a mind-set that hasn't happened since our breakthrough night in Tanzania—back to the Matrix, talking about Hitler and the far right. Sitting in the car in a mall about a mile from his house, I take a chance: "We can be honest with each other, can't we, Frank?"

"No, you're not an honest person," he says.

"Frank, I'm worried about you," I persist.

He bolts from the car and announces that he'll walk home. I try following him through the mall, first by car and then on foot, but he wants nothing to do with me. So I leave him be. *Has anything really changed between us after all we went through in Africa?* I wonder. *Can it?*

I call his house forty-five minutes later and he's come in. I tell them of my fear that he can't handle all that's being demanded of him in school. But when I phone again the next morning, Frank has arisen early and gone on his way to the bus. That night when I call, he begins by apologizing for his behavior.

I fly out to LA for a few days to retrieve some files that I need to finish my biography of James Hillman. Upon returning, Frank asks how long I'm actually going to stick around Boston. Hearing that I've no plans to go anywhere, he reports that sometimes he has to be a Titan to keep from going underwater like the *Titanic*.

Patriots Day in mid-April is a holiday in Boston for public schools and Frank is "very worried" about whether he might have classes anyway. I get hold of the admissions director on her cell and it turns out he does. She's proud of him for being so concerned. That weekend he comes over to my house to do some interviews for his class. It turns out to be a Jungian personality test on "the types"—which I read about during the course of my Hillman research—and Frank asks questions of me, Alice, and another friend. On the way home, he brings up again whether I'm really remaining in town. When I respond in the affirmative, he turns to me and says, touchingly, "You're one of the purest hearted people I know." He calls later to inform that he got an "A" on the paper based on his psychological interviewing: "I just wanted to let you know." I shout into the phone, "That's awesome!"

• • •

My love is like an eagle's bones set to dry in the sun. Once flying high trying to reach the sky something happened and the eagle died. The flesh disappeared revealing the magnificent skeleton. Large and standing still, the vultures assumed positions staking claims on the flesh. The spirit left the bones. Now it flies high and free amongst the transient clouds that mark the emotions.
—Franklin's Journal, ten years earlier

Memorial Day. Frank is waiting for me outside his house, wearing oversized sunglasses, very nervous upon getting in the car and staring rigidly ahead. He's grown a mustache and a small goatee. En route, when I say he seems very distracted, he replies, "I'm programming my mind—and my body, too." After a quiet lunch, I speak to the staff at his house. One says that Frank had seemed "off" for a couple of days and, when she asked to see his pill strip containing each day's medications, he said curtly, "Not now."

Not too long ago, I knew that Frank had to leave school early because of dizziness. He'd asked me to hold his arm and steady him when we were out. It's now mid-June, and Alice and I are boarding a bus en route to the Martha's Vineyard ferry when Etta calls. She's come to visit Frank, but he's experiencing terrible vertigo. She will end up taking him to Cambridge Hospital for a CT scan, which thankfully shows nothing unusual, though his blood pressure and heart rate are both elevated. In the emergency room, pacing back and forth, he wonders aloud to his mother why he can never cry. Before taking a pill that quiets the dizziness, he briefly talks about suicide. Etta doesn't bring him home until after midnight. She cancels her return flight to Baltimore and checks into a motel. We talk on the phone about whether the dizziness could be a side effect of the Abilify medication that's been added by his therapist to help provide more energy, or whether it could be psychosomatic due to the stresses of school. We both well remember how hard he'd been working at Commonwealth, but unable to concentrate, just before his first breakdown.

Frank shows me his midterm exam with an excellent grade of 93, but says the teacher for this module nonetheless wants to fail him for lack of class participation. He loves going to Lincoln, he says, but had missed another day—"I was comatose, having heat stroke." None of this bodes well. Next time I pull up at his house, on a hot summer day, my son is standing outside holding his wallet and his keys in a woolen winter skull-cap. Becoming paranoid while we're having lunch nearby, he leaps up from the table before finishing and says he'll walk to pick up his laundry—which he does, even though it's more than a half mile away. His mother and I concur that he needs to see his doctor soon, that something is awry with Frank's medication.

> June 27, morning: He hasn't gone to school for two days and has decided to quit. Too much studying. This is the wrong decision, I tell him, and we'll be out a lot of money in student loans. Wrong thing to say. He'll pay me back, he says. No further discussion allowed. He hangs up. Etta says that what counts is that he *finishes* something, "but he's shutting down." The defeat in her voice is tragic. We had dared to hope again.

Jim, one of the staff at his house, can't understand it, pointing out that Frank had an overall GPA of 89. But Frank claims that a teacher told him "I don't like you, you're a nigger," although he hadn't reported this. And says he's planning to file human rights complaints against Jim for pushing him to stick with school and against me for persisting in telephoning him. I insist to staff that they need to administer his medication again, rather than let Frank do it himself, but they say they can't without his doctor's checking off that box on the official form. Once again, the bureaucracy at its worst; I dread what's likely coming.

Etta talks to our son for about a half hour, who says he simply can't continue at Lincoln Tech and asks her to please explain this to me. I go to see him, and he's relieved at my saying that his decision is all right with me. I fill out paperwork at the school for Frank to take a medical leave of absence, resuming as much as six months later if he wishes. For the first time I learn about Section 504, federal legislation, which accommodates students with mental difficulties if the particular disability meets certain criteria for modified assignments, untimed testing, frequent breaks, and smaller groups to work in. But why didn't they ever tell me about this before? Even though the education director confides that his own father suffered from schizophrenia, hence he'd grown up in that environment and understood! I don't get it. Is it all about simply running students like sheep through a money mill?

Dr. K., Frank's medication therapist, calls after their monthly get-together. My son is refusing to continue taking Clozaril. It's the required blood draw again. He's likely been skipping doses already. The danger is, after two days, you increase the risk of affecting the white blood cell count and so must start over at the lowest possible dose. Frank is willing to take a different medication and, to the doctor's surprise, has requested Haldol. As far as side effects, that's one of the worst antipsychotics, so Dr. K. will try having him take something else. He goes on to say that he's witnessed this many times over the years, someone beginning to make progress after receiving a lot of help, then ending up "regressing and decompensating." *God, I hate their therapeutic language,* I think to myself. It's a heartbreaking phenomenon, the doctor adds; just as people start to get better, then they do worse. I hear him sigh as he concludes, "This is another chapter in a long story."

At his house Frank refuses to take the newly prescribed Seroquel alternative and, within a day or so, is back in the hospital. Maybe this is something he needs to do, his mother feels, to make choices beyond what his parents have done for him. We're told he's "disorganized, but cordial and polite." There are no available beds at Cambridge Hospital, which I'd requested, so he's taken by ambulance to the Walden Behavioral Care Unit out in suburban Waltham. Frank says I'm not his father or his guardian and I abused him and he wants no further contact with me. He's malodorous and refusing to shower, a fuck-you to the whole human condition. They call all this an occurrence of "very rapid decompensation." I gather some clothes for him in a bag and drive these to the hospital. Waiting at the locked entry, staring at the sign—"Please ensure that unit doors are secure"—thinking, *how many times have I seen those words?* In the hallway I visit with his doctor, a kind African American man named Dr. Love. He seems to have an effect on my son. Within a couple of days, Frank showers and does agree to a blood draw for resuming Clozaril, but will need to restart the dosage while continuing on Seroquel.

I've been working on a book proposal, with the idea of a "happy ending" in Africa. My literary agent writes me: "You can find the heart [to continue] if you don't deny what's happening now. This doesn't have to be a completely wrapped-up story. There is the poignancy of not knowing, if you can be honest about it."

My close friend, Melinda, who takes medication for bipolar disorder as does her daughter, writes to me as well. She and I haven't had a chance to talk since the trip to Africa but, as though tuning in to what happened between us there, she says:

> Franklin needs time to himself to re-sort some things. Your book is NOT about just the trip to Africa, but Franklin's struggle to find a soul. His soul. . . . He's too wise not to have one, somewhere. But he keeps losing it, can't keep track of it, this is where his mind messes him up, it's insidious.
>
> Why don't you try going where you CAN'T go, where the journey is too impossible and then frightening. And when you seem to be there talk from THERE. Maybe you'll speak the same language, if just for a minute. Then at least he could tell you what's WRONG, even if he does it by telling what's wrong with YOU! Sometimes these substitutions are necessary. Just dig his world. Dig what life is for him . . . pretty flimsy

and dangerous. Unreliable…let Frank choose the language. Let him direct the play for awhile. Not you. Drama!!!

Is it possible that Franklin has a legitimate concern about the drug and needs to try something which approaches his lack of clarity in a different way?

On the medications, he's still isolating and refusing to socialize. He tells the nursing staff he wants to remain in the hospital and not return to his house. According to the weekend notes, he's said: "I'm back to being half Egyptian." Melinda, hearing of this, writes me again: "He's talking real stuff, it's just symbolic, images. If you can see the half-Egyptian, like get him in focus: he can tell you more, just because you know him in that moment, and are willing to accept his symbols." Sage advice, I feel.

As the level of Clozaril gradually is increased, Frank initiates conversation with staff—does someone want to play cards?—and works his fingers using a stress ball. In early August, I go to the hospital to discuss discharge plans, the first time I've seen or spoken to my son in a month. He wonders if we might make another trip together next year. He's filled out some job questionnaires in his own private language. He writes down an "Einstein formula" in my notebook. He asks, "Were you made to look like Lee by the CIA?" He's referring to my book on the Kennedy assassination, and to Lee Harvey Oswald. Oddly enough, in my twenties I was once told by someone who'd known Oswald well that I bore a physical resemblance to him.

On the next visit, we talk about returning to his house. "But what if Henry calls me a nigger?" Frank says of one of his floor mates. My response is immediate: "Then tell him to fuck off!" Later, I advise trying to ignore him instead, but the emotional reaction seems to have gone over better.

He's almost ready for discharge. Frank fills out a list of needs when told that the staff at his house are planning to do some grocery shopping for him. I arrive for a mid-afternoon visit. Alone together in the visitor's area, our conversation begins with a role reversal. "I'd like to see you healthy," Frank says, "not drinking a lot of wine and things." I point out that the long-time cyst on my neck has been removed, and he's pleased to hear that. I tell him that I love and care about him; he says he does too and adds: "You say 'I care about you,' but really it's traditional."

He then continues: "I was an asshole for hurting you in 1993, I'm sorry about that." He's again remembering the fight we had when he was thirteen, which had come up on the breakthrough night in Africa. "You didn't really hurt me," I say. "But I grabbed you by the neck!" he responds. There's nothing more to say. Perhaps this ends it forever.

The woman in charge of his house is going to talk to Henry, I tell him. Frank replies: "It's those military tactics he uses. 'Are you fiercer than me?' Henry says. I didn't know all he wanted was Chinese food. But it's expensive, you know." Later Frank says, "It makes me sad being there, all those guys out on the porch smoking." I ask if he'd consider returning to Earth House for a few months. "I'm not ready for Earth House," he says.

He talks about all the jobs that he'd like to apply for: puppet master, librarian, archaeologist. *The symbology is so him*, I think to myself. He goes on: "Or a linguist, I forgot about that. Or a salesman, merchandise creatively, almost like Clarence and Olive." My father had been an advertising executive who created marvelous jingles, my mother a composer of piano music for children. Frank must know these things, but it's been years.

At the bottom of an application to work at a Subway, Frank has signed off with Asian-style characters. I suggest that he not use these, because prospective employers won't understand the language. "I don't know if you'll remember this," I say.

"I remember everything you say," he responds.

"You've gotta realize," he says, "one hour for you can be like seven weeks for me. . . . I took a seven-year vow of silence back at Commonwealth School and it turned out to be eighteen years, or 165 months." Has he actually calculated, in an instant, the amount of time that passed since that painful period?

"I don't like to look like Barack Obama." Why not? I ask. "He looks kind of Chinese, but he needs to look black for some reason."

"We've gotta get into the unconscious, so we know what the hell's going on," he says.

As I prepare to depart, I stand up and walk over to him. We do a long fist-handshake kind of dance and I find myself exclaiming, "Ah so!" which cracks him up.

Frank is excited that the staff from his house are coming to pick him up. I've bought an air conditioner for the window of his room, which he says makes it "just about perfect." Talking about jobs again, he says, "I might surprise you."

"You always do," I say.

On the drive home, I contemplate that as Melinda suggested, we've been communicating within *his* boundaries, which are limitless. A place where, curiously too, all of his life memories are. And how vivid they remain, detailed to the year!

While his thoughts can still be all over the map, despite this latest setback I feel like it's different than before: That Frank is able to bounce back quicker and to a more solid place. I have faith that our intense time together in Tanzania did rearrange something, inside both of us, that didn't and can't simply disappear. We didn't end up back on square one, at least not for long.

I feel, too, that he's ready for something new . . . that it may be right around the corner . . . that perhaps I can help him find it.

CHAPTER 18

• • •

A Quest for Alternatives

Shamanism is a great mental and emotional adventure, one in which the patient as well as the shaman-healer are involved. Through his heroic journey and efforts, the shaman helps his patients transcend their normal, ordinary definition of reality, including the definition of themselves as ill. The shaman shows his patients that they are not emotionally and spiritually alone in their struggles against illness and death.

—Michael Harner, *The Way of the Shaman*[1]

WITH ATTENDING SCHOOL NO LONGER in the picture for Franklin— at least right now—what else might spark his interest and get him out of the house? Part of Etta's recent work has involved studying and teaching music therapy, and there turns out to be a possibility of this, not far from where Frank once lived at Aberdeen House. His mother and I visit the Expressive Arts Therapy Center in Watertown, which offers free sessions in both art and music. The director spent the first eighteen years of her life in Cameroon. Patrick, himself a musician (as well as a trained therapist) who is close to Frank's age, could see him for 50-minute-long weekly sessions; piano, guitar, drums, and African instruments are all available. We sign him up.

Frank is quickly engaged. When I go to pick him up after his first music session, he greets me enthusiastically and asks that I come in to check out a large African drum. He's got considerable energy—riding his bicycle around the neighborhood, doing push-ups and sit-ups outside his house. He suggests we might do a hip-hop adult education dancing class together.

Next time, arriving at his house, I see him emerge suddenly from below the deck out back, wearing a maroon corduroy shirt and carrying his guitar. It's a stunning image, thrilling actually. "Been playing some tunes?" I ask, and he nods happily. In the car, he asks: "Which do you like better, the written word or the psychic word?" That's a tough question, I say. He goes on to describe how six normal senses exist, but many more psychic ones, and also several Haiku, along with a fair number of "wolf senses."

We're looking for a new restaurant he knows called "Red Bones," but he can't quite remember where it is. In Davis Square, Frank points to a girl passing by on the street and says I should ask her. "She won't know," I say under my breath. But I ask anyway, and the girl points us in the right direction. Following a hearty meal of ribs, Frank marches ahead back to the car, saying "Come on, Dick."

Heading back home again, Frank suddenly tells me, "My planet is not still the Dog Star." I know that Sirius, colloquially known as the "Dog Star," is the brightest star in the night sky. Frank does not elaborate. Then he mentions Eddie (whom he used to sometimes refer to as his father) and the fact that he has a 10 Degree Sagittarius Mid-Heaven in his astrological birth chart, which Frank says can be the cause of some trouble. Could he really be remembering this obscure detail? When I get home, I look up Eddie's chart. And Frank is right on the money. He must have memorized this years ago.

When I reach Etta to tell her about our "psychic day," she reveals that she'd spent a long day discussing alcohol and kids at her school—followed by Frank calling to say he'd like to come to Baltimore and have a drink with her.

At music therapy, he plays what I find to be quite a remarkable short improvised piece on the piano while Patrick accompanies on the drums. Frank has started going to the two-hour weekly art therapy classes, too. "You're a wonderful guy, Dick," he says after one of these.

En route another time, Frank asks if I ever dreamt about deep-sea diving or playing soccer. Never soccer that I can remember, but quite a few dreams about being in deep water. I ask about his own dreams—I can't remember ever talking about this with him before—and he says he recently had one about a dragon visiting him and wondering whether he could also fly. "And before that, I had a dream about day lilies."

Something seems to be shifting in Franklin's psyche, or perhaps simply coming more to the surface in a concrete way. But it's a good thing that I accompany him to see his therapist, Dr. K. The last hospital had never sent over any records to the doctor, so whether Frank needed a new prescription was unclear. Later, house staff will tell me they'd called Dr. K's office several times to discuss this. The ongoing ineptness of the system! I call the hospital and they finally fax over the discharge papers to the doctor, and the pharmacy straightens it out on their end. Meanwhile, Dr. K. has suggested to Frank that, by Christmas, he's going to try upping the Abilify and lowering the Clozaril to see how that goes. "Couldn't we have Christmas a little early?" Frank asks.

Sometimes he seems on the verge of cracking up with laughter, as if playing some kind of game with the doctor. I recall that, as a child, he went through a whole thing about needing glasses when he knew his eyes were perfectly fine—to mess with the adults, he later confessed to me. But at the same time, I notice that Frank is developing a disconcerting way of moving his lips slightly, as if talking to someone. Might this be a side effect of his medication?

The medication dime is about to drop for me . . . and hard.

• • •

The time has now come to call an end to the psychopharmacological revolution . . . [it] now has to meld into a quiet world where drug therapy . . . will be joined by other approaches as equal partners, preferably working together in harness rather than in conflict.
        —Peter Tyrer, Editor of the *British Journal of Psychiatry*, August 2012[2]

While browsing in a local bookstore, I'm drawn to a paperback by Robert Whitaker called *Anatomy of an Epidemic: Magic Bullets, Psychiatric Drugs, and the Astonishing Rise of Mental Illness in America.* The author is not an advocate, but a former *Boston Globe* reporter whose series on the pharmaceutical industry led him to write the book *Mad in America*, and this is his follow-up. And what I read is not only appalling but terrifying, if not entirely unexpected.

The figures are staggering: Since 1987, a fifty-fold increase in sales of psychiatric drugs, from $800 million to more than $40 billion. This has coincided with a vast increase in people receiving government-funded psychiatric disability payments (with all medication costs covered by insurance), from 1.2 million adults twenty years earlier to four million adults in 2007. And now the reach has extended to children—from 16,000 diagnosed with mental illnesses necessitating psychotropic medication in 1987, to more than 600,000 today.[3]

Perhaps the biggest revelation is that while antipsychotic drugs may prove effective for short periods, their long-term use often causes deterioration of brain function. Schizophrenic-diagnosed patients who've been on medication for years, and then stop taking it, generally relapse in worse condition than before. Yet studies by the World Health Organization comparing schizophrenia outcomes in developed countries like the United States versus nations like Nigeria where the drugs weren't generally available found a much higher rate of recovery *without them* within two years in the poorer countries.[4]

Since Robert Whitaker lives in the Boston area, I arrange a get-together where I impart some of my story about Franklin. During out meeting, I learn a great deal from this impassioned man who started the Foundation for Excellence in Mental Health Care. Even someone at Eli Lilly, the pharmaceutical company I'd sued on Frank's behalf, has recently admitted that the drug paradigm has not worked. The new president of the National Alliance on Mental Illness is an African American woman—long-diagnosed schizophrenic—who at fifty was able to slowly leave medication behind. However, Whitaker tells me that the Clozaril my son takes is the most effective, but also especially difficult in terms of withdrawal once you've been on it for a long time. Also, epigenetic changes that it can cause in the brain may prove irreversible.

There are no easy answers; it's a real Catch-22. But support is crucial, Whitaker adds encouragingly. He agrees that Franklin probably didn't have enough support from the school where he'd enrolled after our Africa trip. Also, treating someone so afflicted in a "regular" way, as Stephan did so beautifully with Frank in Africa, is critical. Whitaker recalls a Quaker group in the early 1800s, which used to have "mad people" look into a mirror until they could see a normal face.

Whitaker is to give the opening speech at a two-day conference in Maine toward the end of September, called "Innovative Solutions to Building Recovery with Alternatives to Psychotropic Medications."

I make the two-hour drive up from Boston. The most striking part of Whitaker's PowerPoint presentation is that medical experts have doubted the long-term effectiveness of antipsychotic medications for a very long time. Since hyperactivity of the brain's dopamine system had been theorized as the root cause of schizophrenia, most of the newer drugs (interestingly, not Clozaril) were aimed at blocking dopamine receptors by as much as 70 percent. However, the brain tries to compensate by becoming "supersensitive" to dopamine, with the drugs triggering an increase in the density of dopamine receptors. Which, over the long haul, makes patients more biologically prone to psychosis and worse relapses upon withdrawal of the drugs.

But since the early 1980s, studies had generally been geared toward finding favorable outcomes; indeed, the drug companies themselves often wrote the articles for medical journals. It's as though the drug companies have *designed* their products to ensure a lifetime of dependency.

And virtually no long-term research existed into the results of tapering slowly off of these medications.

In 2003, a fourteen-year-long study of more than 500 schizophrenia patients, overseen by Nancy Andreasen (editor in chief of the *American Journal of Psychiatry*) reported that MRI imaging tests showed a decline in brain volumes related to the antipsychotic drugs, including decreases in both white and gray matter. "The prefrontal cortex doesn't get the input it needs" and gradually atrophies, Andreasen said in 2008, because the medications "block basal ganglia activity."[5]

Yet the drug model has become so ingrained in our culture that I couldn't recall a whit of doubt ever being raised by Franklin's doctors about whether he should stay on his medication. No one talked about alternatives. No one mentioned that Loren Mosher, in charge of schizophrenia studies at the National Institute of Mental Health in the 1970s, had conducted an experiment comparing conventional treatment in a hospital setting to the Soteria Project that he'd initiated. This was a group home environment with minimal use of antipsychotics. At the end of two years, the Soteria patients had "lower psychopathology scores, fewer [hospital] readmissions, and better global adjustment" than those treated with antipsychotics. And only 31 percent who remained *off* these neuroleptics after leaving the program ever relapsed.[6]

Hearing all this—hearing an older woman ask, "Were we human beings before we became a diagnosis?"—on Franklin's behalf I feel cheated, even conspired against. "We are surrounded by sudden genetic epidemics," says Dr. Miles Simmons, "and Big Pharma is laughing all the way to the bank." He and other speakers discuss the value of nutritional supplements, such as the orthomolecular approach that had proven so beneficial for Franklin at Earth House. But would he be willing to do this again, having abandoned the vitamin regimen (with no argument from his Boston therapist) soon after leaving their program? David Oaks, founder of MindFreedom International, talks of the need for a nonviolent revolution in the mental health system. As appealing as this might be, I know it's not Franklin's style.

Then, during one of the audience participation periods, I hear a woman's voice in the back of the room raise something about . . . shamanism. The speaker onstage offers no response. But my curiosity is piqued. I'm in the middle of reading *The Horse Boy*, which my publisher recommended as a good model for what I'm planning to write. It's a father-son story recounting how author Rupert Issacson's little boy, a victim of severe autism, begins to improve after learning to ride a neighbor's horse. As a travel writer, Isaacson is then struck by a wild idea: to take his son to Mongolia, the one place on the planet where horses and shamanic healing intersect. My reading the book not only connects to my trip with Frank to Africa, but brings to mind several times when he has made reference to Mongolia and horses over the years.

Now, taking a break from the proceedings, I find myself in the outer hallway standing near a young woman. Although I hadn't been able to see the face of the questioner, I have a curious feeling that she's the one who tried to bring up shamanism. I guess right. Carin Seadler is a psychiatric registered nurse in Maine who does some shamanic work part-time. After talking for a few minutes, we decide to have lunch together. As I speak very personally about my son, Carin says there is a woman who has mentored her, and who I really should try to see. She writes down the contact information for Kaye Lawrence, who doesn't live that far from Boston.

• • •

Franklin is quite intrigued by what I find out at the conference. When I mention Carin saying of him, "You never know, he might even *be* a shaman," my son's face lights up. "Oh, that was very nice of her!" he exclaims.

He's excited, too, about my embarking on a book proposal about us and our trip, but adds: "Don't you think you ought to learn a little Swahili for that?" He writes down some subject lines in my notebook, largely having to do with where we'd stayed and about the food. "Do you see how much you need me?" he says with a big smile. This is a pattern that continues over our next visits, him jotting down more ideas for me. Once he writes Asian-style words above some graphics and proceeds to "translate" these into English: "I'm Chinese style . . . I love Tanzania . . . I speak Swahili . . . I am justified . . . Figure it out . . . I answer."

I have a dream where Franklin is saying that Africa had helped him to "operate," and in the dream I'm wondering whether he also means "cooperate."

In "real life," he writes down my name in Swahili. He says it means "deference."

Interestingly, Etta has recently come across a scholarly article from the *Journal of Music Therapy* (1985), comparing its "guided imagery" technique with shamanism. "Both processes involve the use of music in attaining an altered state of consciousness for the purposes of healing," wrote a therapist with Salt Lake County Mental Health in Utah. "The techniques suggest maps of consciousness that are strikingly similar."

Before trying to contact the woman whose contact information Carin gave me at the conference, I see what I can find about Kaye Lawrence online. There isn't much. She is definitely not tooting any shamanic horn; the word isn't even mentioned. She is a registered Play Therapist for children and holds certification as a school counselor, with an undergraduate degree in music and theater. She uses a "non-judgmental, empathic and strengths-based approach in work with people of all ages . . . and [their] mental health struggles."

I send Kaye an email, including some background about myself and a synopsis of what happened during the breakthrough night with Franklin in Tanzania. "What's happening between us continues to fascinate and often amaze me. I've learned a great deal from my so-called 'crazy' son. Whatever direction I might help him find in life, I love him very much." Kaye responds that Carin had mentioned I might be getting in touch. "I can tell your heart has been opened by your life," she writes. She knows of James Hillman, "and Carl Jung has been a spirit guide of mine." We schedule a meeting. "It's not just me that you get, but a whole team of energetic beings who are in relationship with me," she writes. Although I'm not a person who goes in for New Agey solutions, her words somehow ring true.

I ask Frank, "Do you know what a shaman is?"

"Yeah, something to do with medication," he replies.

I explain that a shaman deals with the spirit world, which he knows a lot about. "Yeah, I know several shamans," Frank says.

Later that same day, he asks, "What do you know about Malcolm X?" Frank is attentive as I relate quite a few things. When I'd taken my first trip to Europe upon graduation from college, I'd devoured *The Autobiography of Malcolm X* on a ship across the Atlantic. It was then, and remains, one of my all-time favorite books. But never before have I considered that maybe Malcolm X was a kind of shaman.

> *Human salvation lies in the hands of the creatively maladjusted.*
> —Dr. Martin Luther King Jr.

• • •

Mid-October 2012: In a rental car, Alice and I make the two-and-a-half-hour drive to rural Maine. Shortly before 11 a.m., we pull up to a large yellow farmhouse with Tibetan flags marking the driveway and walkway. A barn, obviously in construction, is attached to the house and two chickens are pecking at the yard.

Strangely, I can't get the car radio to turn off; not even when I take the key out of the ignition. In frustration we give up, ring the doorbell, and hear a dog barking inside. No other response. We're back in the car, still fussing with the radio, when a woman in a long dress emerges. She has a pleasant open face and starting-to-gray auburn hair all the way to her waist.

The car radio shuts off.

Kaye Lawrence greets us each with a hug. Inside the house, we're introduced to her part-collie, Conner. We walk through a mudroom into a kitchen with a braided blue rug on the floor and bright yellow cabinets. Kaye brews up some English breakfast tea in a blue enamel pot, and then leads us to her adjacent conference room carrying our two large cups on a tray. We take the couch, Kaye sitting across from us in a large high-backed oak mission chair, a wood-burning stove in a corner.

She has a kind of wispy, ephemeral presence, like someone out of a fairy tale. She does "sand play" with children suffering from autism and Asperger's disease. Kaye was originally from Asheville, North Carolina, but moved with her lawyer husband to this forty-seven-acre farm with its own water source and has been here since '93. Later, she would elaborate that she has a law degree and briefly practiced in New York as a litigator. Indeed, as a legal intern with the Southern District of New York, she'd been part of the environmental protection unit and worked briefly with Robert Kennedy Jr. on a Hudson River case. "I'm very much identified now as a shaman and psychotherapist—floofy stuff by the standards of many," she says. It hadn't been an easy transition. She'd been a Buddhist for ten years, while people kept asking weird questions about whether she'd seen a particular shaman and sent her links to various websites. She wanted nothing to do with all that, but finally gave in. The calling was bigger than her personal desires.

"Do shamans, as a friend of mine suggested, live mostly in the world of the unconscious?" I ask. "I'd say we live in the energetic world, with the other foot in the physical, but we visit the unconscious of those with whom we work. And we certainly have a presence in the collective unconscious as well, being very comfortable with experiencing archetypes and synchronicities. Jung certainly had a shaman's mind. I guess it would be fair to say that shamans are conscious of the unconscious! I love the 'out there' physics that says maybe there is no matter at all—it's all energy."

She walks over to a copy of Jung's *Red Book* resting on a nearby table, which is open to a painting that the psychologist once did depicting three planes of consciousness. A tree grows out the top of one side, roots reach down on the other side. I'm reminded of Hillman's "soul's code" theory about the acorn containing the future oak. Kaye uses the painting to point out the several realms where higher, middle, and lower spirits reside.

Before we arrived, she had been upstairs in her "treatment room" meditating about Franklin. I'd sent her a picture of the two of us in Africa, and her first impression upon seeing his face was of someone who'd been on a lot of medication. When she communicated with his "being" today, Kaye says, it made her cry. "Such a sweet soul," she says. I tell her more about our trip and his fantasies connecting to publishing or building, as well as his savant-like ability since his teenaged years in memorizing people's astrological charts. "He might indeed have shamanic abilities," Kaye says, and has the idea to send me her birth chart and show it to Frank, and see what he might say.

After about an hour of talking, she asks if we'd like to see the treatment room. At the top of some very narrow stairs, Alice stands stock-still in the doorway. The small room, she will say later, felt so "charged" that she couldn't enter at first. Pictures of Kaye's ancestors are framed on the walls, all the way back to her great-grandfather. Again I flash back to the upstairs guest room in Hillman's house where I had often stayed, whose walls were lined with similar ancestral photographs. Next to Kaye's forebears is another framed picture of a red-tailed hawk. "This was the first animal spirit that came to me," she says. On a wall in the back of the room, alongside a hanging quilt of the upper, middle, and lower worlds, is a curio owl.

Accompanied by her dog, we go outside to walk. Kaye points downhill at a body of water on her land. Her attorney husband was able to secure legal protection to keep the beavers here from being trapped. "Also, the pond is serving as a test site for technology placed there by the Maine Department of Inland Fisheries and Wildlife," Kaye says, "and a biologist who is a beaver expert to assist landowners who want to preserve their habitat—from towns that would prefer the dams be destroyed, due to road flooding that occurs during heavy rains and snow melt. So far, so good. It's working beautifully and the beavers have enjoyed peace from the town road commissioner since the installation!"

We pass through a dark pine grove. It feels enchanted. "I work very closely with a spirit population that the Celts were aware of called Sidhe or Sith [Dwellers of the Mount, the Shining Ones, or the Peaceful ones]," she will later elaborate. "However, a large portion of my work—and joy—is in building a solid relationship with the spirits of place here, and the compassionate spirits of the three worlds who are connected with the land and beings here."

We pause by a little dock above a pond where Kaye and her friends sometimes swim, then climb a steep path to a wooden cabin that's used for drumming sessions during periodic "weather circles," a form of spiritual ecology designed to heal our relationship with weather. It has a sleeping loft and a downstairs with a small kitchen. Later, back inside the house, we see a black-and-white shorthaired cat, staring at us from a glassed-in door that leads out to the barn. "You must be very special," Kaye says, "Phil never shows himself to strangers."

She relates a story: "My cat started life with us as 'Philippe,' but quickly we knew that his true name was 'Phil.' He is very attached to me, and also very tuned in. Years ago I did a healing on him when he began having an asthma attack. He calmed down and slept all night against my stomach. Next morning, I was sweeping the porch at our summer cottage downeast, and see him running toward me with something in his mouth. Phil stopped and looked me in the eye, then dropped a beautiful crow feather at my feet. Then he went back to his cat business for the day."

Where should we go from here? she wonders as we sit down again. Alice asks frankly whether she thinks it might be better if Frank either went back to Africa to see a shaman or saw a black shaman in this country. Kaye nods in agreement, not at all put out by the question. She does know of one man in the proximity. Since she's already communicating with Frank, she can ask his permission to find out more along these lines.

On the way home that night, Alice suddenly remembers: "What about trying to contact Malidoma?"

• • •

I first heard of Malidoma Patrice Somé from James Hillman, who mentioned several times that I ought to interview him for the biography and that he might even have some unique insights into my son. Malidoma's second book, *Ritual*, contained an acknowledgment "to James Hillman for his encouragement and support. . . . It is his vision and determination that have helped me to move with greater ease within American culture. He has become for me a psychological touchstone to this rapidly changing modern world."

Hillman and Malidoma were both among the leaders at a series of men's retreats organized by poet Robert Bly and storyteller Michael Meade in the late '80s and early '90s, held in the woods of Mendocino, California; West Virginia, North Carolina, and elsewhere. This was where Malidoma had initially told the remarkable story elaborated upon in his autobiography, *Of Water and the Spirit*. He'd been born in 1956 into the Dagara tribe in a small village in Burkina Faso (at the time, the French West African colony known as Upper Volta). He was the grandson of a renowned indigenous healer, who foresaw that the boy had a curious destiny—to somehow build a bridge between his African culture and the West. The name Malidoma means, "he who makes friends with the stranger/enemy."

When he was five, Malidoma's Christianized father made an arrangement to hand him over to Jesuit priests, to be indoctrinated in their distant boarding school along with children from other African villages. There, whenever caught speaking anything other than French, a rotting cow's skull would be placed around their necks. At the age of twenty, following an attempt by a priest to abuse him, Malidoma ran away and, over the course of several arduous weeks, made his way back to his village. He'd forgotten his native language, unable to communicate even with his own parents. A council of elders considered whether to reject him as having been corrupted by the white man. A decision was made: to see if Malidoma could withstand the ordeals of a month-long initiation that customarily took place when a boy entered puberty. Some of the tests involved journeys to "other worlds."

Malidoma passed all the trials and gradually relearned the Dagara language and ways. He then went on to gain a degree at the university in Ouagadougou, capital city of his country, followed by twelve years of Western education. Malidoma would earn three MAs and two PHds—first studying at the Sorbonne in Paris, ultimately gaining a doctorate in English literature from Brandeis University near Boston. Over the past two decades, he authored several books, including *The Healing Wisdom of Africa,* endeavoring to bridge the cultural gap with the West.

For Malidoma was, at the same time, a shaman—inheritor of the esoteric techniques practiced by his grandfather. He traveled the world conducting workshops that introduced Westerners to ancient Dagara wisdom through different kinds of rituals, with emphasis on the importance of ancestors and community. He also held private, forty-five-minute-long divinations with individuals who came to him seeking insight and guidance for particular life problems.

I'd known little of this in 2008 when I arranged a telephone interview with Malidoma, concerning his relationship with Hillman and the American men's movement. At the end of my conversation with Malidoma, I had brought up the subject of my son. Franklin was then twenty-nine. Hillman had suggested it might also be useful to find out how mental illness was regarded in Malidoma's culture.

When I described Franklin to him, Malidoma responded:

> In my culture, it's contemplated as a particular being having broken into the field of a person's vision. It's like when the other world is dialing the person, the person doesn't know how to pick up the phone. But the calling, and the waiting, drives the person nuts. So my village has a way of dealing with that. It has to do with just keeping the channels broadly open. And when that happens, then the person's job is to differentiate between extremes of communication—what is *this*-worldly as opposed to being *other*-worldly. Then they know when the other world is taking over, and they can behave accordingly. Usually, people like this are extremely spiritual.

At that time, I already knew that Franklin possessed psychic ability, at least insofar as tuning in to what I was thinking. I already knew, too, that there were patterns to his sometimes delusional thought process— recurring fantasies, as it were. But to consider Franklin's behavior as somehow governed by "a particular being having broken into the field of a person's vision" or "the other world taking over"—in 2008, this was an entirely new idea to my rational Western mind.

I mentioned to Malidoma that I'd long wanted to introduce Franklin to African culture. "That would be really helpful," Malidoma said. "If you can get him to Africa, there will be something there."

He was so right.

Now, four years later, I find a website online. Malidoma's calendar says that he will be doing divinations in Ojai, a little more than an hour from LA, in mid-November. That's less than a week after I've already planned to be back on the West Coast, where Alice needs to spend time with her new grandchild.[7]

I don't fit in. . . . I need a medicine man to help me out.
—Franklin's Journal, late '90s

Notes:

1. "Shamanism is a great mental and emotional....": Harner, *Way of the Shaman*, p. xix.

2. "From the Editor's Desk," by Peter Tyrer, *British Journal of Psychiatry,* 2012, 201:168.

3. Statistics on psychiatric drugs: cited by Robert Whitaker in presentation, "Psychiatric Drugs: Problems and Solutions," September 20, 2012, at conference on "Innovative Solutions to Building Recovery with Alternatives to Psychotropic Medications." Sponsored by CCSME, Freeport, Maine. See also Whitaker's website, www.madinamerica.com.

4. World Health Organization study: Robert Whitaker, *Anatomy of an Epidemic: Magic Bullets, Psychiatric Drugs, and the Astonishing Rise of Mental Illness in America*, Broadway paperback, 2010, pp. 110–11.

5. Nancy Andreasen: quoted in Robert Whitaker, *Mad in America*, Basic Books, 2010, pp. 297–8.

6. Soteria Project: www.madinamerica.com, March 8, 2012.

7. As you read the remainder of this section, you may wish to refer to the science about shamanism and schizophrenia in the Epilogue.

CHAPTER 19

• • •

A Man Named Malidoma

In the West there is a similar saying, "I knew it in my bones," which refers to a deeper, more elemental knowing than is possible through rational thought. . . . I wonder if those in Silicon Valley who shave stones to their essence and put them in machines of memory perhaps already know somehow that stones have always managed information. . . . If the information out there echoes the information inside of us, could it be that the great turmoil of unrecognized wisdom within us is forcing us to race along the information superhighway, hoping that we will discover what we already have?
—Malidoma Patrice Somé, *The Healing Wisdom of Africa*[1]

As soon as we're seated in Fugakyu, Frank's restaurant of choice for the day, he asks: "So how long has it been since you were in LA?" I tell him not since March, but I'm going soon for a short visit. I mention Malidoma's name. Frank says he's heard of him. I run down a little about him as a shaman, but when I bring up looking for alternatives or adjuncts to the drugs he takes, he says he's not unhappy with his medication right now.

When we get back in the car, I ask Frank if he would like to take a look at someone's astrological chart that I brought along. "Whose is it?" he asks, and I say it's the woman I just saw in Maine, Kaye Lawrence. He picks it up and, over the next several minutes, describes what he sees in the symbols. This is someone "into the occult thing, like Chinese stuff," Frank says. Also someone with a good memory and imagination; a "traveler" with "creative impulses" and a "spacious astrologer." Then he places Kaye's chart back on the dashboard.

She responds by email to my "report":

> Franklin's comments about my chart made me smile. . . . I was able to check in about him earlier today. Here's what happened: When I first journeyed with some of my spirit guides to Franklin, he seemed hesitant and a little distrustful. Shortly, what I will call his "Wisdom Self" appeared and explained to me that Franklin had experienced some mistreatment in his life and tends at times toward being a bit suspicious. Then Wisdom Self explained my presence there to Franklin, and he relaxed and gave his consent for me to go forward with a check in. One of the strongest messages I received is that all interventions should be gentle and progressive, so he isn't overwhelmed. . . . Also, I was told that working initially with a man would be better for Franklin, in that the mother/ancestral work would be less jolting coming from a grounded, peaceful African man. . . . I was told that a check in after he has worked with the African healer for awhile would be appropriate for a more detailed process of going forward.

Not long after Kaye responded to my email, a woman named Yetunde from Malidoma's office calls. According to her, Malidoma has often said people diagnosed with schizophrenia are actually shamans. Later, I contemplate that perhaps the cathartic monologue by Franklin in Africa was a kind of shamanic teaching for me. Yetunde suggests that I might want to schedule back-to-back divination sessions, as this has worked well for individuals with complex situations. For ninety minutes, the cost would be five hundred dollars, which is not cheap, but I go ahead and schedule a rendezvous in Ojai.

I pick up Frank from his music therapy class, to which he's brought his guitar. At lunch I mention again that some people think he might even be a shaman. He smiles, pleased, and replies, "Well, I like astrology. And I'd like to study shamanism."

I begin reading in earnest Malidoma's first book, *Of Water and the Spirit*. I've had a copy for several years, but for some time it's been buried at the bottom of a box where it got wet when my basement flooded and remains waterlogged. Turning the crinkling pages, somehow I find this appropriate. The book is very visual and evocatively written. Revelatory are passages about the strong relationship between grandfathers and grandchildren, each being so close to the "other world." I find myself thinking a great deal about James Hillman and realize that this must be the first anniversary of his death. I also recall many moments from my youthful past—the voodoo ceremony in Paris, the medicine man with whom I danced in Ghana—as well as Stephan's stories in Tanzania about his grandfather not deteriorating after death and the banshee-like cry of release outside the window of our room as Franklin's otherworldly monologue in Tanzania wound down.

And to my surprise, Malidoma offers a new definition of something that—in terms of my son at least—I'd always believed was a sign of contempt:

> The aura of disgust that elders love to create around themselves is the result of their having to let go of certain social pretenses, and especially of their unyielding concentration upon the spirits. They don't have any spare energy to invest in being polite. Among the Dagara, the more you dwell in the other world, the more you shock those who don't.[2]

• • •

One man needs the eyes of another man to see what the shadow of the tree hides.
—Malidoma Patrice Somé, *Of Water and the Spirit*[3]

In the car I show Malidoma's book to Frank and he reads out loud from the description on the cover. I tell him that I've scheduled a meeting with him in California, and he smiles. Frank wants to take a walk around Jamaica Pond—unusual for him—and it's good to be out in nature together. He admires a flying swan, notes a nice-looking piece of bark on the ground, and says he could make pancakes for me out of a walnut tree. Heading off again, he says I should be a tour guide for the Lakota Sioux, whose reservation in South Dakota we'd visited when he was twelve. "You look like a Lakota," he says, "you feel like a Lakota; it's really complicated to become a Lakota." We stop at a mall so he can get a winter coat, hooded sweatshirt, and pants.

Vinfen, the organization that staffs Frank's group home, holds annual goal-setting meetings for its clients, and Etta flies in from Baltimore to attend his. Frank sits between the two of us at a long conference table. Marc, the clinical director, says to our son: "You're not the same person as a year ago." Well, he's thinner, because he's been working out, Frank says, and adds: "Is that what you meant?" Marc continues, "Your illness has taken awhile to subdue. I don't know if you can conquer it." Frank says he thinks he can.

For much of the next hour, he does a lot of the talking, expressing strong interest in pursuing new activities, perhaps yoga or tai chi. Not school: "College puts me too much on edge." Marc counsels that, while Frank has a lot of ideas, "I'd rather see you do one or two things well." Frank brings out a book on welding from his backpack and Marc suggests maybe he could combine welding with art. "I could learn to be more social," my son says. He makes everyone laugh when discussion comes up about his visiting a potential new group home residence, saying: "How many headaches can you get a day?" The meeting concludes with the program director saying that she'd be pleased to take Frank to an arts center in Brookline next week. "I didn't know you liked me," Frank says. Everyone laughs again. "How could anyone not like you?" I say incredulously.

Next day, after his art therapy, Frank says he thought the meeting went well. He mentions, for the first time I can recall, that he'd like to be involved in some programs where he could make friends. At his request I drop him off at a Learning Center sponsored by the providers of his group home, where he wants to take a yoga class.

A few days later I sit in an anteroom outside his music therapy, listening to Franklin drumming away and playing some xylophone and piano as well. Seeing Malidoma's book in the car afterward, he picks it up, "translating" into Swahili what's on both sides of the cover. When at lunch I read aloud a passage from where I am in the book, he exclaims: "What a wonderful story!"

On that note, I depart for Southern California.

• • •

In 1972, a few months after my return to America from traveling around Africa, I'd received a letter from the medicine man with whom I'd danced in Ghana, translated by a boy in his village.

You told me you would come here again. I prepared some things for you to collect but as you failed to come I spoiled them. Please let me know the time you may be here so that I can do something for you to take back to your country. . . . I shall pray for you to achieve success in everything you do and live longer. Please soonest reply needed. Tell me your present condition of health.

Your lovely friend,
Bosomfor Sekyere

How curious that, forty years later, I am making my way to another rendezvous with an African "medicine man." It's a cool, mid-November morning along a winding road on a quiet residential street. After missing the driveway twice, I press a button that opens an automatic wooden gate. Inside, to my surprise, the grounds are quite spacious. I park near the gate and walk past several buildings, including one covered by a geodesic dome. Except for some chickens and a rooster that decide to follow me, nobody seems to be around.

This is the Temenos Center for Wholeness, located about eighty miles northwest of where I live in West Hollywood, surrounded by hills and mountains in the small valley town of Ojai. Sometimes referred to as "The Shangri-La of Southern California," Ojai is home to a retreat center dedicated to the teachings of Krishnamurti (who once lived here) and the Krotona Institute of Theosophy, as well as Temenos, a Greek word meaning "sacred site."

My appointment with Malidoma is five minutes away and I'm uncertain where to go. Finally I notice a small, hand-lettered sign on a door toward the back of the compound: "DIVINATIONS." An arrow points to the left. Around the corner is a small white stucco house, with a few empty chairs outside a closed door, apparently the waiting area. I hear laughter inside and take a seat.

At 9:45 a.m., precisely my appointed time, two women—one black and one white—offer good-byes with "blessings" as they emerge. I leave my shoes outside and walk into a small room with two straight-backed chairs facing each other and a bed on the floor nearby. An African man of medium height stands to greet me with a warm smile. He has a round open face and is simply but elegantly dressed, much like the picture on the back of his book, wearing a checker-patterned woven hat and similar cloth shirt above gray slacks and sandals.

"Hello Dick, I am Malidoma," he says, beckoning me to sit down across from him. Our knees are almost touching. His secretary, Yetunde, has said that it's a very good idea to tape the session, since there is so much to take in that needs to be contemplated later. Besides, she says, Malidoma will not remember what he spoke about. I need to make sure that my machine makes no distracting humming sounds.

I turn on my cassette recorder, then hand across a typewritten statement that I was also instructed to bring, explaining my reason for being here. The page briefly recalls our phone interview four years earlier about James Hillman and then gets into Franklin.

> You told me that introducing him to Africa might be very helpful. It was. Last January I took my son to Tanzania to witness the wildlife migration on the Serengeti Plain. It was a life-changing experience for both of us. Toward the end of the journey, one night Franklin went through a frightening "other-worldly" experience. Lying on his bed, he spoke for an hour of being taken over by the Snake God, of a genie who had returned, of going into the Matrix. "Africa said I came here 16,000 years ago," he told me.

"Mmmm . . . mmmmm. . . ," Malidoma says as he takes in my words before exclaiming: "The Snake God!"

My statement continues:

> Knowing how psychic and sensitive he is, I feared that Franklin had opened himself too completely to the African unconscious. Only when he was able to feel my desperation, anguish, and love for him, did he return to an earthbound reality. Today, we are both living in the Boston area and are closer than we have ever been. He is enjoying music therapy and art therapy classes. Knowing that the medications he takes have severe side effects, I have been looking for alternatives or adjuncts that could enable Franklin to live a more fulfilling existence. . . . When I saw that you were to be in Southern California at the same time I am visiting, I wanted to seek your help in-person, as we already have a connection through James Hillman. It may be that something ancestral is involved in my son's struggles.

When he finishes reading, I show Malidoma two photographs of Franklin; one from a decade ago and another of the two of us together in East Africa. The shaman breaks into a broad smile. "Oh, what a face, what spirit!" he exclaims again. I tell him I've also brought along some of my son's writings, if he'd like to take a look at those later. "Yeah, eventually I'll take a look," he says, "because usually when people like this write, you can tell through the stream of consciousness about the type of imagery that they are familiar with." Malidoma's voice still bears traces of a French accent from his youth among the Jesuits; English was, after all, his third language.

Between the two of us, on a small table, is a white cloth that contains a circle at the center. Around the perimeter of the circle, and also used to divide it into quadrants, are five colored stripes of black, blue, green, red, and white. Within the circle rest a number of objects—many cowrie shells, stones both precious and plain, coins from various countries, a ring, and a key.

"Okay," Malidoma says, "with your strong hand, bring it down here and spread these shells and other objects clockwise on this surface." As I hesitantly bring my arm forward, I tell him I'm left-handed. "Yeah, that's your strong hand," he says. I begin to move the objects in a clockwise direction. "Just keep going, and I'll tell you when to stop."

After perhaps ten seconds, Malidoma does so. He leans over the table, peering intently at the pattern I've formed. While I wait anxiously, he takes some time to "read" it. "Mmmmm . . . everywhere. It's so out there. Just everywhere. Wow." Only later would I consciously notice that the majority of the materials had ended up on the left side of the circle, which Malidoma said represents the "other world." Since I'm doing this on my son's behalf, the images I've positioned on the divining table seem to belong to the reality that he often inhabits.

"All the energy being stirred up through this process," Malidoma says, "is involved with this: the essential term is art, period."

Going back through some of Frank's journal writings from the late '90s, I'd recently discovered that he'd written: "I don't have the desire to be a carpenter or a mechanic, but I do want to be an artist. This title has few limitations—musician, painter, sketcher, model, engineer, designer." In 1999, when he was hospitalized for the second time, Frank had spoken of someday being a social worker and artist who would teach kids. In 2002, my son wrote: "Really you should be an artist. But an artist is about condensing ideas into time. You don't have much patience."

Malidoma continues: "The way this pattern is laid out, there is a certain perception of the choreography of this world that is like a mirror of other-worldly scenarios. And he is in the middle of that.

Almost like two magnets, each pulling the other, which means a person like this is a clear participant in two world realities."

Malidoma goes on to describe my son as being "like a bridge"—not between cultures or traditions, but rather between dimensions. "The consciousness that he is in touch with is one that he wants to bring into this world, to make known." Ordinarily I might have dismissed such statements as "New Age jargon," but there's something about Malidoma that I instinctively trust. Something, too, that resonates in terms of subjects Franklin has often brought up over the past several years.

"Your job with him is to hold the space," Malidoma continues. (I wonder if that is what I ultimately did for him on that frightening night in Africa.) "Anyone involved in a job like his is going to need an assistant, someone who is always looking at the whole thing from this dimension—with the mind as a translator—someone with the capacity to explain this complex stuff. Because you have a mundane experience that he doesn't, and your mundane experience coupled with the natural disposition that you have, to approach him from an angle of understanding as opposed to an angle of suspicion, puts you in this unique position—to be able to convert the things that he puts out into a sequence that is understandable. In a way, you are more like his biographer."

I take a deep breath and reveal to Malidoma that I've indeed begun working on a book about Frank and all that we've been through together over the years. The shaman laughs. "Oh, that's what I am suspecting here. Because you have a way of discourse that allows you to make a very substantial contribution not only to him, but to all others like him who in this world are labeled as clinical cases. Your job is basically the humanization of the spiritual emergency, such that people can gradually step away, distancing themselves from the easy labeling of clinical psychotics, schizophrenics, which is a reflection of a profound misunderstanding. Because the structure of the world afforded by people like this has not been studied sufficiently."

Malidoma continues: "This is something that is extremely important for you. Your role as such is, you are here to change the angle of approach to energies like these that are being carried. It's not a fair approach to look at him as sick. It's an indictment that seems to say that skills of this sort, frequencies of this nature, are not allowed. This is really a major discrimination."

He points to Franklin's picture. "Look at this. This is a vibrant man with a huge spirit."

Is Malidoma simply telling me what I want to hear? No, it doesn't feel that way. Rather, a confirmation of what I've only recently begun to fathom. A metamorphosis that had emerged on our trip to Africa is, through this African man, taking further shape.

Malidoma closes his eyes and continues: "He draws all the time because he is good at delivering blueprints. And your job, down the road, will be to look at the pieces that he channels, like hieroglyphics to be deciphered."

I think of the mysterious "hieroglyphics" that Franklin draws so rapidly, resembling Asian characters and captioned often with English translations, filling entire notebooks.

"You will start to align these together by sections, out of which comes an evolving sequence that makes sense. That's the exotic part. This is a very interesting project. You see, it is not his job to make it linearly clear enough for people to understand. Therefore you are being challenged to be a very, very astute observer, to be able to convey the scenario in lay terms. Because it's almost a parallel technology that he's privy to. If you want to put it into a shamanic context, shamanism as the study of various alternative technologies."

Ultimately, Malidoma foresees, Franklin will survive the labeling and be able to work with others like himself, because he understands the extremes and can "join with their frequencies. So that these people are reconciled with their genies, becoming conduits of a paradigm that the world needs. There are more and more individuals coming into this world with the gift of bending the sensical realities we are living by and expanding dimensionality. Down the road, the teachers of these things will be people like Franklin. But for now, it will be mostly your being able to follow him and record the steps of his initiatory journey. This has been going on for years, and the end is not there yet."

Malidoma opens his eyes and looks intently into mine. "The thing about it is, he chose his father very carefully, knowing that you have what it takes, almost like sponsoring or vouching for him—with the risk of being labeled as having been infected by him. Because it is the result of intense observation, and intense alignment with these kinds of frequencies."

Chills course down my spine. Malidoma points to the apex of the circular pattern and then says: "This genie cannot be removed. It is not there with him to do damage, but to enhance qualities, to contribute to the breakthrough. That's why the genie comes from water. This is consistent with the ultimate intention of the plan, which is to contribute greater flow to human consciousness. More often than not, what stops people from breaking through into a parallel reality is something missing in the imagination, which kind of makes them go in circles."

Continuing to re-vision Franklin, Malidoma adds: "The intensity of what is going on here is completely off-scale, like only otherworldly presence can trigger this much pain. That is a whole lot bigger than the kind of local community inside which gifts can be tested and shared. This is why he needs a broad space of operation. That is to say, to be in touch with various experiences in the world that broaden your son's perception of *this* planet. That's why the intuition you had to take him into Africa was so right, and will need to be repeated again."

Suddenly Malidoma changes the subject. He asks where things stand with my biography of James Hillman. Volume one is complete, I tell him, and will be coming out soon. I add that Hillman had also offered me some great advice about my son. "That is why what you are doing is not any different," Malidoma says. "Because you know by now that James Hillman was toying with schizophrenia. Were it not because he came across *very* strong things in terms of his perception of the psychological profession, it is the kind of thing that could have toppled him over the edge. That's why he basically lived on the edge all his life."

As far as I'm aware, Malidoma doesn't know about the breakdown Hillman had experienced late in 1952, a breakdown that led him with his new bride to Zurich and the Jung Institute shortly thereafter. Before this, Hillman was intent on becoming a novelist, not a psychologist. In the biography, I quoted Malidoma on his later experience with Hillman at the men's group retreats in the early '90s:

> With a group in North Carolina, I introduced for the first time a radical ritual, in this case a water ritual. That was when I noticed James Hillman's genuine interest in ritual—and the demonstration that he actually knows something about it. In the middle of the week, he called me to his side in the bush, asked me to take a piece of leaf and put it in the water and brush his body with it. Which is something we know in my culture as a cleansing. So for me, to see that fortress of a mind become

ritualistically alert, and trusting an African guy to help him with some kind of energy that he needed to be cleansed from—oh, that really got my respect.[4]

But I haven't said anything to Malidoma about quoting him, and so am taken aback when he now begins to discuss "a number of rituals that you need to be aware of, as a grounding agent of Franklin's energy, one that is vested in humanizing his being. They are very simple, but they address themselves to the ocean." I am to bring some specific natural elements to the water's edge—organic milk, apple cider vinegar, spirits such as vodka or rum, and an ear of Indian corn—and follow carefully Malidoma's instructions to offer these to seven waves as nourishment for Frank's psyche. It's a ritual that will need to be repeated over time, and with incantations, eventually I should bring Franklin to the ocean and watch as he performs it, "with a quality completely different than yours. That's when you are going to be able to draw a comparison, as part of the layout of his biography."

Once more, Malidoma emphasizes my *holding the space for Frank*, "in order for him to find his way, without influencing anything. The eclecticness is that every piece will have multiple faces and you will have to circumnavigate these faces. Only after that will you have your own epiphany, which will finally nail down the ultimate meaning of it all. And when that happens, it's like a transmission will have happened, simply because you have been exercising a kind of meditational approach to something that was handed over to you by him. . . . You find yourself, like Joseph Campbell would say, in a forest of symbols, like some kind of—I don't know—Harry Potter character who has entered an unknown geography. In this sense, Franklin is the gatekeeper."

• • •

> . . . *we are told of the . . . Pygmae who do not exceed three spans, that is, twenty-seven inches, in height. . . . Aristotle says that the Pygmies live in caves.*
> —Pliny, *Natural History*, AD 77–79

Malidoma now begins to talk about the "little people"—the Kontomblé as they are called in the Dagara language, meaning beings from the Other Side of reality, the world of Spirit. They reside at an *actual gateway* (he emphasizes the words) in a cave outside of his village, behind what appears to be impenetrable volcanic rock. They occasionally will show themselves. Malidoma says, "Personally I'm curious about how Franklin can react to the little people. A person like this is very likely to understand the language they speak, just like that!" Malidoma snaps his fingers. "Most people I take there—of course some can't see them, others can hear but not see, and only a few people can hear and see them at the same time. But no one understands what they're talking about, because they speak a different language that looks like Aramaic or some kind of ancient . . ."

I turn the tape over and the machine stops recording.

About a half-hour will pass before I notice this, a half-hour during which Malidoma speaks further about the Kontomblé and warns also of the danger involved in encountering them, that someone who crosses into their world may be claimed and not able to return. A half-hour when I tell Malidoma about Franklin's curious drawings in Asian-style characters, which I remember the shaman referencing as "like cuneiform writing." A half-hour, too, in which I show Malidoma the pieces that Franklin had written in the immediate years before his teenaged breakdown (and described earlier in this book)—about seeing the four directions and the "white triangle with golden wings," about finding himself elevated above a pyramid and then slowly passing through a long tunnel. Malidoma addresses the images breathtakingly, eloquently. And I'm initially devastated that these moments weren't captured—but perhaps they were not meant to be. Perhaps I must come to their hidden meanings myself.

I tell Malidoma the whole story of the night toward the end of our Africa trip. The chills racing through my body when Frank spoke about the genie: "Means it's true," Malidoma says. How my son had stonewalled my effort to "speak in tongues" in trying to bring him back: "Your frequency wasn't even noticeable!" Malidoma exclaims with a chuckle. Then Frank's abrupt return to earthbound reality when he sees me crying by his bedside and begins to take care of *me*: "He shifts back and forth between parent and child, this is fascinating!" And my son's telling me that I could write more spiritual books: "What is implied is, because he can give you the material."

Malidoma envisions one final task as our divination session draws to a close: "a need for reconciling ancestors"—a subject that will soon become a keystone in both mine and Etta's lives.

For now, though, Malidoma shakes his head and offers these parting words: "I mean . . . being with a person like Frank, there can't be a dull moment." Oh no, I say, and Malidoma laughs.

He emphasizes the need to go slow, a gentle approach, mirroring what Kaye Lawrence had observed.

"I would love for you to meet Frank sometime, but we're not ready yet," I say in the doorway.

"No, it will happen when the time is right, you know? It's like our meeting today was quite—you couldn't plan it. It was meant to be."

Malidoma hugs me good-bye and beckons in his next patient, who is sitting outside on a rock.

Later, sitting down in my office to transcribe the tape of our session, I notice another mysterious thing. When I'd been almost knee-to-knee with Malidoma in those two straight-backed chairs, his voice had seemed completely normal. But on the cassette, it's strikingly different, with a rising-and-falling cadence that's reminiscent of my visit with a trance medium many years before. It's as if what Malidoma had told me came disembodied, being drawn from an invisible source . . . as if he wasn't always physically there in the room.

Later, too, after looking up some things online about Burkina Faso and the "little people," when I try to watch a YouTube video about Malidoma, it won't keep playing—and my computer temporarily shuts down.

• • •

Early in December 2012, I head for a beach to perform my assigned libation ritual. A friend knows a spot in Malibu likely to have very few visitors. I stop at a Whole Foods and a liquor store to gather my supplies, and it's raining when I reach the Pacific Coast Highway. I'm thinking on the way how Malidoma doesn't know that Franklin was born under the sign of Aquarius, the "water-bearer." Pulling into El Pescador State Beach north of Zuma after an hour's drive, the rain has stopped. A young couple in a fancy convertible arrive simultaneously and walk a dirt path down a long hill ahead of me. We're the only ones there. On the shoreline I watch them nestle in among some rocks and walk about a hundred yards to the far end of El Pescador. The surf is up and some of the waves are quite high. Wading into them in my bathing suit and a T-shirt, I invoke my son's name. I ask the spirit of the water for aid on behalf of Franklin's psyche, as I first empty a pint of organic milk into each wave crashing ashore, and indeed there are precisely seven of these as Malidoma had said there should be. Soaking wet, I repeat the ritual with the apple cider vinegar and then a small bottle of vodka—"spirit to spirit"—and then I walk back and forth, including once backward, speaking Frank's name periodically as I flick kernels of Indian corn off my thumb and cast them individually into the water. The latter is a "planting" that Malidoma had said didn't need to happen all at once, so I use only about a quarter of the ear.

Down the way, the young couple is swimming and I've gone unobserved. The day is overcast but with a gracious stillness, and I can feel a presence in the soft wind. I bow to complete the ritual and thank the spirit of the water, offering a second moment of gratitude when I again reach the top of the hill. I look down at my watch, my oldest possession. The water ritual has taken a little more than a half-hour.

> *By ritually putting what we do in the hands of the gods, we make it possible for things to be done better because more than we are involved in getting it done. Also, willingness to surrender the credit or our accomplishments to Spirit puts us in greater alignment with the Universe.*
>
> —Malidoma Patrice Somé, *Ritual*

Notes:

1. "In the West there is a similar saying….": *The Healing Wisdom of Africa*, pp. 177–8.
2. "The aura of disgust that elders have….": Malidoma Patrice Somé, *Of Water and the Spirit: Ritual, Magic, and Initiation in the Life of an African Shaman,* Arkana paperback, 1995, p. 76.
3. "One man needs the eyes of another man….": *Of Water and the Spirit*, p. 77.
4. "With a group in North Carolina….": Dick Russell, *The Life and Ideas of James Hillman*, Skyhorse Publishing, 2012, pp. 287–8.

CHAPTER 20

• • •

Holding the Space

B ACK IN BOSTON APPROACHING THE end of 2012, driving around again with Franklin, I'm telling him a little about my time with Malidoma in Ojai. "I know his family," he says. "They sell rice, pork—and ghosts." After I describe the water ritual I did at the beach, he says he also performs rituals—"like Navajo, where they sew patterns called glyphs."

Frank looks terrific, says he's been exercising and is down to 193 pounds. "You're a handsome dog," I tell him. "If I was a dog, I'd be a greyhound," he says. He wants to go to a bookstore, where he selects volumes on feng shui, knitting, origami, Japanese language made simple, and a Greek-English dictionary. The last, he says, is because Greek has similarities to other languages that he writes in.

A staff person at his house informs me that Frank recently came home carrying a big atlas. So I begin thinking about other trips he might like to take. Maybe China, or Machu Picchu, or back to East Africa with Dr. Reiner next June? Perusing some catalogs, he says matter-of-factly, "India's the place." Impulsively I make a reservation for a few months down the road with a tour company in Cambridge, told that a full refund could be available inside of a week. I call Etta, who can't quite believe it and expresses some concern about crowds.

That night I wake up at 2 a.m. thinking about the same thing, then fall back asleep to a detailed and scary dream. Along with a couple of friends, I'm sleeping in a single bed atop a cliff in a rugged area. I'm worried that I might get up in the night and fall off the edge. And that's what happens, though I dream nothing about the actual fall, only of waking up on the ground pretty badly hurt. More friends are attending to me. "At least I'm alive," I say to one, trying to move. At the end I'm on my feet and walking past some of the younger people in my family on a beach, who all realize that something has happened that I'm not talking about.

Mentioning to Franklin about the teeming population we'd encounter in India, he says he could handle it. But Alice also feels this is a bad idea, because it's hard enough for a normal person to absorb such a culture. For all the progress Frank's made, there could be a regression. Maybe later, but not now. Why not continue my libations at the Atlantic, and let the spirits instruct me?

I'd written to Kaye Lawrence seeking her advice as well. "I would think that Franklin would need some consistent grounding experience before undertaking something like this," she responds. "I haven't been to India, but know many who have, and the consistent report is that there is fairly constant sensory/nervous system overwhelm. Franklin is so sensitive to energy that without a reliable internal tether, I would be nervous as well at this point in his process."

When I give Frank what I expect will be disappointing news—fabricating a story that the tour company called and the India trip is full-up—he doesn't skip a beat. "Okay, let's go back to Africa then," he says.

Kaye also writes me that, while part of Frank's grounding can come from energetic sources, "another source could be his relationship with you as you hold the 'father' container of love and protection." I haven't told her what Malidoma said about my job being to "hold the space" for him. Definitions seem to be constantly emerging.

• • •

The connectedness between humans and the animal world is very basic in shamanism, with the shaman utilizing his knowledge and methods to participate in the power of that world . . . the power animal is a purely beneficial spirit, no matter how fierce it may appear. It is a spirit to be exercised, not exorcised.

—Michael Harner, *The Way of the Shaman*[1]

Kaye Lawrence does a remote check-in on my son and we talk about it over the phone. A week or so earlier, Frank had said: "You can tell a lot about their art by how someone holds their brush." When Kaye "visits" him he is sitting outside on a chair alongside an easel and a palette, holding a brush and painting. She tells me that she doesn't really know how much this is metaphor or how much is concrete. But it's as though she's interrupted him. However, Frank seems relaxed and pleased to see her. She asks if it's all right to speak and he says yes, then at some point turns away and continues with his painting. His "deepest Wise Self" comes forward and resumes the "conversation" with Kaye. Franklin ritualizes spirituality through his art, she learns. It's about making the invisible visible. Kaye also says: "My feeling about Franklin during the check-in was his delight about becoming truly known."

Also during the check-in—and here Kaye hesitates before I ask her to please continue—"well, this star stuff came in," she says reluctantly. What do you mean? I ask. "One of my shamanic teachers was an astrophysicist at Carnegie," she goes on, "so I did some journeying to black holes, photons. But I'm not versed in constellations. However, with Franklin's soul genetics, Ursa Major or Arcturus kept coming up. My left brain is saying: I hope they're not telling me that Franklin is some kind of star person—how would I explain *that* to Dick?"

I take an inward breath and ask her again to please continue. This had arisen, Kaye says, in context of asking Franklin's "deepest Wise Self" what lay behind his desire to travel to India or again to Africa. "It's part of a consciousness shift. I find this with the autistic community; these are the most intuitive spiritual beings, they can put their consciousness all over the place. Franklin has the experience where it's very normal for him to be part of this unified consciousness of certain beings. I don't know how else to put it. And it feels very familiar to him to be within cultures that manifest this more clearly than the United States, which is very differentiated and individualized. So there is a comforting aspect within that."

Not too long ago, I would have found this too strange for words. But it was certainly what Malidoma had tuned in to, in his own way. Then Kaye brings up something else: "What was very strong is . . . a spirit animal is with Frank. I kept getting symbology of a bear, I think a black bear. With indigenous people in the United States, the world is considered so fraught with danger that a child couldn't make it to adulthood without at least one spirit animal accompanying. And why do we freely and abundantly bestow upon our children teddy bears (and other stuffed animals) and rattles? Rattles are used in shamanism for many purposes, for example calling in the compassionate spirits, inducing shamanic trance and sealing a person's energy field to keep someone's energy in and inappropriate energy of others out."

After our conversation, I do a Google search on the two constellations Kaye had mentioned. Ursa Major has been seen as a bear by many distinct civilizations, part of oral traditions dating back more than 13,000 years. Along with Orion and the Pleiades, Ursa Major is one of the few star groups mentioned in the Bible and was pictured as a bear by the Jewish peoples. Arcturus, brightest star in the northern celestial hemisphere, was known by the ancients as the Guardian of the Bear. Additionally, Black Bears once had a long-range habitat across the North American continent, with sightings from Florida to Alaska, and were revered by Native Americans. With the Lakota Sioux, for example, a shaman called Lone Bear told an ethnologist that the ordinary word for bears was *mato*, but spirit bears were termed *hunomp*. Bears are the oldest verifiable sacred animal.

• • •

If you lose track of your identity, you have the totem animal to remind you of it.
—Malidoma Patrice Somé, *The Healing Wisdom of Africa*[2]

Behind the wheel with Frank, I ask if he ever dreams about bears. "Oh yes, I had a dream about a bear two or three nights ago." The bear had greeted him thusly: "Hello . . . good fella." Its name was Kunsa. In the dream Frank says he told the bear, "Give it a rest." I crack up laughing. He'd then said to it, in Swahili, "You're the bear that I love." He asks for my notebook and jots down "spotted bear" and "red woods," though he's not sure whether that refers to the redwood forest or to something else. Frank then proceeds to fill a page with Asian-type characters, which he labels (among those I could decipher) "spirit" and "bear." Later, when I ask if he recalls any other dreams about bears, he remembers one saying to him, "You're getting smart. I want cookies—right away!" And when I mention Ursa Major and Arcturus being constellations of the bear, Frank quickly and easily pronounces both of these back to me.

"There's a book I want to show you," I say as we continue our drive. "It's in the backseat." It's my copy of Carl Jung's *Red Book*, which the Swiss psychologist had worked on for sixteen years through a technique he called "active imagination." It consisted not only of text but remarkable color illustrations of mythic imagery, which "had burst forth from the unconscious and flooded me like an enigmatic stream and threatened to break me," Jung wrote. These had begun with visitations from two figures, an old man and a young woman (Elijah and Salome), accompanied by a large black snake.

Franklin cradles the Gutenberg Bible-sized *Red Book* in his lap, slowly turning the pages and immediately impressed. "I want this book," he says. He's especially fascinated by Jung's calligraphic script. "Is this Arabic?" he asks. It looks something like Arabic, but is actually old German, I tell him. "Old German," he repeats. Then he draws two designs in my notebook whose origin, he says, is Egyptian.

Frank wants to try a new Portuguese restaurant not far from his house, "sort of tucked away like an old napkin." He orders the pork, because "it helps you to remember." I tell him the most important thing I feel I have to do is to help him fulfill his destiny. "How so?" my son asks. I don't know, but it's important. "You have an important destiny, too," he says.

I never know what might be coming next, and Frank brings up a conference on sugar that's scheduled soon somewhere down South. "People don't like yellow molasses, so that should be fed to the animals," he says, "but two bottles of milk and corn would be better." It's a curious harkening to the water ritual assigned me by Malidoma.

On the way to Harvard Square to pick up some magazines, Frank speaks first about a gas on Jupiter that heats up and then rapidly cools down, causing cold spells that can be balanced from Saturn, then about the rings of Saturn having loose atoms, which reach the jet stream and heat up the air and land in Argentina and Peru. He buys a *Popular Science* and a magazine devoted to the life of Jesus. When we stop for a visit to Fort Hill, he stands outside the kitchen before entering, where a daughter-in-law is sitting next to her baby in a high chair. "I have to wait a minute," Frank whispers to me, "and check out the energy."

> *Mental disorders . . . have always played and continue to play a key role in evolution. Perhaps they are the secret advantage we have over intelligent machines.*
> —Susanne Antonetta, *A Mind Apart*[3]

• • •

By mid-December, I've scheduled a meeting to attend in Baltimore and bring Frank along to visit his mother and Kamal. At the airport, when Frank shows nervousness putting his computer through the inspection machine, a fellow with Homeland Security questions me about him. What is our relationship, what do I do for a living, do I go to Baltimore often, how many bags did we check?

Arriving without further incident, the next morning Etta and I accompany Frank to the Baltimore Museum of Art, which he greatly enjoys and asks me to buy him a couple of books and a Japanese Hiroshige calendar. Back at her house, I show Frank some pictures of his ancestors that my brother's wife just sent me copies of. Maybe he should write a book about them, he suggests.

While we're in Baltimore, Etta tells me she would prefer to see Kaye Lawrence before encountering Malidoma; she has a very positive feeling about her and would feel more comfortable initially with a female shaman.

In terms of Franklin, however, Alice feels strongly that I should try to bring him to meet Malidoma sooner rather than later. I write to his office assistant, Yetunde, asking about his upcoming schedule. She responds that Malidoma will be in Jamaica in mid-January, doing a workshop and then individual divinations. I call Frank and he wants to go. I book the flights. It's only a few weeks away.

On Christmas Eve, Frank emerges from his house carrying a book on "communicating with the public," from his last course at Lincoln Tech before he dropped out of school.

I rejoin Alice in LA for the remainder of the holidays. On a sunny day early in January, she accompanies me out to Malibu as I conduct my second water ritual. El Matador Beach, adjacent to the first one I visited, is a lovely spot at the base of a cliff with many seabirds perched on large rocks just offshore. It's high tide, but there's still room for me to walk along the water carrying my libations. While watching a dolphin cavort nearby, I receive a phone call from Frank's closest childhood friend. They've not seen each other since Eddie took them both bowling a few years back, but they're out to lunch somewhere and text me a picture of themselves. Another reconnecting.

I'd earlier written to tell Malidoma how moved I was by our time together in Ojai, but no response has been forthcoming. Now, following my second ocean ritual, I come home to find an email from him, the first I've received directly. "I just returned from Africa and I am barely recovering from a bad cold. It was nourishing to have an entire session on your son. I felt deeply honored and uplifted in a very unusual way. Thank you for the opportunity."

When I pass along Malidoma's message, Etta emails back: "So much happens in the realm that we cannot see."

A few days prior to departing for Jamaica with Franklin, I fly out to Boston. It's still January, but Frank is exercising outside in the cold when I get to his house. You'll need to prepare an autobiographical statement for Malidoma, I inform him. "What language shall I do it in?" my son asks. He'd like to speak with Malidoma about drumming, he says. I suggest he bring along some drawings to show him.

Frank doesn't want me to stay and help him pack, says he'll do it himself. There's some snow in the forecast for the morning, so we'll need to get to the airport early, to which he agrees. Before heading home, I say I have something to give him. It's a CD of his grandparents' music, made from 78-rpm recordings and one old cassette. "Do you have it with you? Let's pop it in," he says as we pull into his driveway. A stillness descends in the car as we listen to my father's soaring operatic tenor against my mother's piano accompaniment. Frank glances over at me—as if to observe how moved I might be—and grins. As the first cut ends, he says, "That's enough for now, I'll listen to the rest upstairs."

"It's quite beautiful, isn't it?" I ask, as I eject the CD.

"Yes, it is," my son says with sincerity.

Notes:

1. "The connectedness between humans and the animal….": Harner, *The Way of the Shaman*, p. 74.

2. "If you lose track of your identity....": *The Healing Wisdom of Africa*, p. 261.
3. "Mental disorders....": Susanne Antonetta, *A Mind Apart: Travels in a Neurodiverse World*, Jeremy P. Tarcher/Penguin, 2007 paperback edition, p. 141.

CHAPTER 21

• • •

In Jamaica

The larger the soul the greater the suffering. From suffering comes beauty. Bob Marley preached and taught it when he said "One Love, One Heart, Let's get together and feel alright!"

—Franklin's Journal, 1999

IN MID-JANUARY 2013, ALMOST A year to the day since we left for Africa, I wake up at 3 a.m. and sleep fitfully until 5:30. A couple of inches of snow are on the ground in Boston, and it's still coming down. I call ahead to make sure Frank is up. I'm pondering how much to tell him about Malidoma before we see him in Jamaica.

At his house, my son is already downstairs waiting. The fellow on duty hands me his medications, with a note of instruction. Going through airport security, they examine his carry-on, which turns out to have a set of metal computer tools inside. Why he is bringing these, I have no idea. "Are you going to work?" a woman asks him. "Yes, I'm a teacher, of Spanish," Frank replies. Soon after that, I interject, "We're going on vacation to Jamaica." The woman raises her eyebrows: "I thought he was a teacher and was going to work." Frank and I respond as one voice: "Oh, that's after." Whew, once again we make it through.

Our flight is delayed, and I'm worried about missing our connection in New York. An hour goes by and we're parked on the runway when the de-icing trucks arrive. The water pours down over the window above the wing where I'm sitting, which seems fitting as I read about water rituals in Malidoma's book, *The Healing Wisdom of Africa*.

Coming to a section about the making of large clay pots in West Africa, I reflect on how much Franklin enjoyed creating these in high school and taking a Saturday pottery class in more recent years.

And there is another description, which takes me back to when Franklin was living alone in his own apartment and gathering old motors and other metal parts off the street. Malidoma writes about a young man in his maternal family who, after his father died, "began acting quite unusually. Not only was he speaking out loud by himself most of the time, refusing human companionship, but he was also quite inexplicably collecting scraps of metal. The little room he occupied in the compound was crowded with random metal objects, from bicycle parts to old tin cans, radio antennae, and dead light bulbs taken from flashlights. From these pieces of scrap he made things that appeared to be almost functional."

Malidoma's explanation gives a new slant to Frank's obsession:

> The urge to collect is the natural response of the human psyche to an aesthetic object that speaks directly to it, stirring memories that lie deeply within. Collecting confirms the indigenous belief that the human psyche reads and understands symbols and that the attraction to beauty is a function of psychic awareness. I think museums are born out of the West's confused response to things that speak directly to the psyche.[1]

When we finally take off, Frank is persistently massaging his arms and shoulders. I'm wondering if his nervous energy is related to the Abilify that his therapist has prescribed, which helps counter the sedating effects of the Clozaril. Landing in New York, our next plane is just boarding. It's a four-hour-long flight onward to Jamaica. Frank wants to fill out his own customs-and-immigration form and then passes it to me to fill in the gaps. He's listed "Teacher" as his profession and checked off "Married." Okay, what the heck. But then, for a question as to whether you've been in any other countries over the past six weeks, he writes down "Africa" and invents a home address in Brookline that's also not on his passport. Besides "Vacation" as our reason for traveling, he writes "Conference." I envision more problems going through Customs. "Frank, I've got to fill out another one." He shrugs consent.

We make it into Montego Bay, the country's largest city after Kingston, with no problems. Frank finds it "just like Tanzania, all the drivers waiting." An older gentleman named Winston is on hand to meet us. At rush hour, our driver takes quite awhile to get through the city; then its single-lane roads along the west coast en route to Negril. We journey past some sprawling resort hotels as well as through a number of small fishing villages, where reggae music pulses through the streets and the scene is frenetic and lively.

It's dark by the time we pull into the Rockhouse Hotel, past the sandy beaches on the cliff side of Negril. This is where we'll stay for the first couple of days, before catching up with Malidoma following his workshop. "I don't know about you, but I like this place," Frank says, meaning Jamaica as well as our abode. We're helped with our luggage down lovely stone paths to a second-story room, overlooking almond and palm trees with the sea beyond. Walking in, Frank announces with excitement: "There are Lakota Sioux here!" Yet again harkening back to the first big trip we made together when he was twelve.

Frank walks out onto our front balcony and begins pacing back and forth "for exercise." Then, as we walk to the hotel dining area, he exults: "I *love* you for taking me to this place!" He is never this effusive. Lying on his bed after dinner, Franklin's lips are moving silently, mumbling to himself—or to an invisible someone. "Are you talking to your genie?" I ask, flat out. He grins and says no, but he's talking to some spirits and adds: "You know what I mean!" I smile and say I do. And maybe I'm actually starting to.

The next morning, he puts on an emblazoned T-shirt that he bought before we left. It depicts a big computer-like object saying "I am your father!" on one side, and a smaller computer saying "Nooooo!" on the reverse. At breakfast overlooking the rock ledges that taper slowly into the sea, I remark on how good-looking Jamaicans are. "Like Tanzanians," Frank replies.

I decide to then tell him about the water ritual I've been doing at Malidoma's behest. He's especially interested in my plucking off the individual kernels from an ear of Indian corn and offering these to the ocean waves. When I bring up what Malidoma saw about Frank's genie being a water spirit, he says "Poseidon," and adds "Astrology." I mention that Malidoma is interested in helping him find his purpose in life.

Outside our room a bit later, he whispers to an unseen entity in another language. He will spend almost the entire day in a chair on our balcony, contemplating and drawing and absorbing Jamaica. Around 5 p.m., I go to the pool area for a drink and read the opening chapter of a book by Michael Harner that I've brought along, titled *The Way of the Shaman*. It contains the following passage:

> We need to communicate intimately and lovingly with "all our rela-tions," as the Lakota would say, talking not just with the human people, but also with the animal people, the planet people, and all the elements of the environment, including the soil, the rocks, and the water.[2]

I read the passage aloud to Frank. "That sounds like a Mende prayer," he says. I've never heard of Mende, and figure that he has probably invented it. But when I later sit down at a computer outside the reception desk and do an online search, sure enough the Mende are one of the biggest ethnic groups in Sierra Leone and belong to a larger tribal people in West Africa. Many Mende believe that all human and scientific power is passed down through secret societies. A guy behind me who's waiting to use the Internet notices what I'm reading and asks, "Secret societies in Jamaica?" I glance back at him. "No, West Africa, my son somehow knows about them."

I think to myself, *he's mentioned Sierra Leone before, could it be pos-sible that's where his ancestors on his mother's side came from?* I show Frank-lin what Malidoma wrote in the concluding paragraph of his *Healing Wisdom of Africa*, first in his own Dagara language and then the transla-tion: "May all ancestors join forces to wake up our spirit and put good thoughts into our psyche. Then we shall see the good that awaits us and accept it." Frank reads it quickly and says, "Nice poem."

Then he asks: "What should I talk to Malidoma about?" I say that Malidoma will probably do most of the talking, but he should have some things prepared. "I'd like to talk to him about pottery and paint," Frank says.

"Yeah, he writes about clay in his book." I explain that I've brought my tape recorder so his session can be listened to later, and suggest he say something in his introductory statement about how the medical world has labeled him a paranoid schizophrenic but he is wondering how to find his true purpose and lead a healthier life. "That's fine," Frank says.

"This seems like the beginning of something important."

"I know that," Frank says.

"For me anyway, it really began in Africa."

"I'd like to do some drawings for Malidoma," Frank says.

And that's what Frank proceeds to do for the next half hour. He starts with one that he captions "Elephant Bird." Simultaneously, I turn to a page in *The Way of the Shaman* depicting four ways to depict an eagle as a "spirit animal." I turn next to a drawing of a tunnel, and recall Franklin writing when he was sixteen about passing through the tunnel. He hands me his quick sketches one at a time, sixteen altogether before he says he's finished. They include a "Still Life" with a sewing machine and what looks like either a boat or a bowl, "Anglo Saxon Template" with his glyphic-like characters, a long cross-encased penis, what appears to be a coffin, a series of three masks, a centipede-like creature beside another mask. The last was "Scene Labyrinth," the lines indicating a tunnel. "Can I have those back? I want to put inscriptions on them," Frank says, and begins to add symbols to each drawing. All this transpires while I am re-reading the transcript of my divination session with Malidoma in Ojai, where he spoke of the pattern I would begin to see eventually in my son's otherworldly drawings.

For two consecutive nights, Frank reports having animal dreams—the first time about a growling dog that turns friendly and a troop of baboons, the next about visiting a zoo with giraffes and llamas.

• • •

Winston picks us up again, heading about fifteen minutes farther up the coast to where Malidoma is staying, at a wellness center and spa called Jackie's On the Reef. It's some two and a half miles past Negril's famous lighthouse on West End Road, behind a chain-link fence and an unlocked front gate.

In the entry hallway, a print of the Mona Lisa faces a larger painting of an African tribesman holding a spear. Visitors enter a large pagoda-like common area with concrete floors, limestone-covered walls, and a soaring wood-beamed ceiling probably fifty feet high whose circumference is lined with stalks of bamboo. Along the floor below, beside a few daybeds, are massive crystal geodes, little shrines with totemic objects, and piles of self-help and spiritual books. A corrugated tin roof serves as a rainwater catchment. Stone steps lead down past the bougainvillea, hibiscus, cactus, and aloe plants, toward a covered massage area and a small saltwater pool carved out of the rocks, where

Caribbean waves wash up and gently over you. Above the beach, pieces of coral that broke off during a hurricane are fashioned into what the proprietor calls her Stonehenge. The four-and-a-half-acre property includes several across the road for raising organic fruits and vegetables.

Franklin's and my room is called The Dome, a circular thatched hut with three walls and louvered wooden shades, camping chairs, and wicker tables. Two bamboo beds face the sea. There is no radio or TV. Since the temperature is in the mid-seventies in January, the lack of A/C is not a problem. The adjoining bathroom is partly open to the air, with a solar-heated stone shower.

When we go to check in, Frank and I fill out some forms, of which he writes that what he's looking for here is "good Jamaican food and building relationships." He checks off that he'd like to learn meditation and yoga. The first order of business is a therapeutic massage, which Frank declines ("I don't want people here touching me," he says privately), but he agrees to have a facial.

At around five o'clock, Frank is sitting at a table in the common area, reading a magazine about "The Art of Tantra," when I go for a beer. Jackie Lewis joins me at the bar, an elegantly dressed African American woman who I guess to be around seventy-five. Once the owner of a highly successful boutique clothing store in New York, in 1987 she'd left it all behind to pitch a tent along this undeveloped stretch of Jamaica's west coast and spend the next seven years building her New Age retreat. When I mention to her the trip that Franklin and I took to Africa, Jackie says: "It gave him confidence." She then continues, stating "Generally, handicapped children have different"—I finish her sentence, interjecting "qualities." Jackie says, "No, it's not that, it's gifts." I feel badly that I interrupted her, and speak of my son's psychic abilities. "He lives in another dimension," she says. I'm somewhat taken aback at how quickly our hostess seems to be in tune with Franklin.

"Here comes Malidoma now," Jackie says. I turn to see him walking down some steps toward us. He looks very different than I remember from our formal time in Ojai, dressed here in a casual polo shirt and slacks with close-cropped white hair. He doesn't recognize me either at first, though he'd seen the two of us arrive and figured that must be Franklin and me. "I hope I've brought him at the right time," I say. Malidoma responds: "We'll know tomorrow." Frank has spent most of his time so far in Jamaica sitting alone, I say hesitantly, looking out on the scene or reading. Malidoma says simply: "He's processing." I then tell him the Lakota Sioux and Mende poem anecdotes. Malidoma's eyes widen as he wonders aloud, "What frequencies is he tuning into?"

> *. . . Along which secret aqueduct,*
> *Oh water, are you coming to me,*
> *water of a new life*
> *that I have never drunk?*
>
> —Antonio Machado, *Last Night as I Was Sleeping*

When we arrive at dinner that evening, it is the first time that Franklin and Malidoma will officially meet. They shake hands, greeting each other warmly, as if this is not the first time. Eight of us sit down family-style at a dining table, Jackie at one end and Malidoma at the other, with Frank and me on either side of him. At first Frank doesn't want to participate in the nonsectarian prayer but he acquiesces, even taking the hand of Malidoma and an older gentleman to his left. The other visitors are primarily from the East Coast: a woman from just outside Boston who enlisted Malidoma to come, a schoolteacher from Philadelphia, and a fellow from Albany, New York, who once attended men's retreats where Malidoma and James Hillman were among the group leaders.

Our meal of locally landed grilled shrimp has barely begun when Frank turns to Malidoma with a question: "Do you cut your hair every week?" Since Malidoma's hair is quite thin on top, I'm hoping that he doesn't take offense. Malidoma smiles and replies, "No, once a month." Frank rubs his own full head and says that he himself has a "Rwanda curl." "Rwanda, eh?" says Malidoma. "I used to have an Afro like yours back in the 1970s." The three black women at the table say that they did as well. Frank grins and again turns to Malidoma. "So you're a writer, huh?" Malidoma says yes.

At Frank's request, the waiter delivers some pepper sauce to the table. "Would you like to try some?" my son asks Malidoma, who agreeably shakes a few drops onto his food, tastes it, and winces at how incredibly spicy it is. He glances at Frank, who has proceeded to shower the sauce onto his diced tomatoes and then add still more ground pepper on top. Pouring it on a bit thick, I ponder, to see how impressed Malidoma might be with the powers of his palate?

Malidoma recalls, on an earlier visit to Jamaica, encountering the sculpted Buddha in the corner on a very dark night and asking, "How are you?" He was a bit offended that he received no reply. When he speaks of tonight's beautiful sunset, Franklin nods and says knowingly: "Sun conjunct Jupiter and Mars, or Mercury." Shortly after dinner, Malidoma leaves the table and Frank soon retires to our room. As I hand him some ice water to take his pills, I notice how he seems to be in good spirits. I'm starting to nod off when, from his adjacent bed, Frank laughs out loud and says, "You're funny sometimes, Dick." I guess we're still having a conversation.

My dreams that night are intense. In one, I enter a room to encounter an old friend. We begin talking about UFOs, when I realize that I'm being interviewed on TV. Then I see footage of some aliens doing all kinds of curious things. I wake up, eyes riveted to the thatched ceiling.

At 7 a.m., I arise to deep vibrant tones emanating from the nearby "temple" area. A woman there is sounding a series of Himalayan bowls using different gongs, surrounded by several other women seated on cushions, eyes closed and palms up and out. After the session ends, I approach Jackie. Mentioning that Frank seemed very quiet last night, she says reassuringly, "Yes, but also very observant, I saw that at dinner."

Back in our room, I decide to show Franklin the piece he wrote as a teenager that described going through the tunnel. Although it's only a little more than a typed page, he spends a long time reading it, as if reliving something, and then says, "I like this article I wrote." He asks if I'd like him to read aloud from a book on Tantra, and I say sure. He opens to a random page and, after a few minutes, looks over at me. "You from East India?" he asks, adding before I can answer: "Didn't work out too good." I crack up laughing. He reads some more, then starts "drawing Sanskrit" interspersed with "part Jamaican, as Bob Marley," and then back to the Tantra text.

Malidoma is running a half-hour late, but around mid-morning we walk over to the house where he's staying. He's alone outside in a straight-backed chair, shoeless in blue slacks, with his white cloth divination shirt on. "Are you ready for us?" I ask. "I hope so," Malidoma says. We're his third consecutive session. I plan to let Frank be with him for forty-five minutes and then return to turn over the tape, and either join or let them continue, whatever feels right for all.

Frank has already handed Malidoma some pages of his calligraphy, or hieroglyphy, or Asian characters, or whatever they are. "You write Chinese?" he asks my son. "Yeah," Frank says matter-of-factly. Malidoma turns to me and exclaims: "This is the first non-Chinese who writes Chinese that I know of—oh my God!" I pass him my son's written statement about why he's come. "You can go," Frank says. And I do.

It's a slightly overcast day. I sit for awhile in the common area, watching a fishing boat maneuver through the waves, while violin music plays in the background. I've gone back to our room to read when Frank surprises me by returning five minutes before his session is supposed to end. "Oh, you were there forty minutes," I say.

"Forty minutes? It could have been four years!" he replies, somewhat breathlessly. Then he taps me on the shoulder, points to the door, and adds, "Good luck."

I walk back to where Malidoma is still sitting. "I am overwhelmed by what I saw," he says, also seeming breathless. "There is no equivalent, no frame of reference. It is so unique that it sent me kind of spinning. It just reaches you and grabs you and throws you again, oh my God."

"He does that to me a lot, too," I say.

It will be later that day when I go off alone with the tape recording of the divination session. It begins:

> "What I want you to do, Franklin, is use your strong hand and I want you to spread these shells regularly by moving the hand, spreading them on this surface until I tell you to stop. So make sure you touch as many as possible, and when you are satisfied with it, you can leave."
>
> "My left hand? I can leave?"
>
> "No, once you are satisfied with it, you can stop doing that. . . . Position these wherever you want, however you want." The silence of the tape indicates this goes on for a little while. "Yeah, that's good, very good. I can see now you've touched pretty much all of them."
>
> Frank laughs heartily and says, "Smells good."
>
> Malidoma starts laughing, too. "It is good."
>
> "Yeah, it's a good game."
>
> "It shows a lot of the energy that is yours." Then he says with genuine puzzlement: "Why do they call you schizophrenic, you're not schizophrenic."
>
> "I had a schizophrenic—a lot of Africans never get schizophrenic, but Indians, they have a thing in Lakota Sioux called *Wasi*. A ceremony. They even use a shotgun sometimes."

"Wow."

"They just aim it up in there. If you're not careful—you better run, you know."

Was Frank making up the word *Wasi*? I Google it. It is indeed a Lakota word, used derogatorily for non-indigenous people, especially whites. *Wasi'chu*, which translates "taking the fat" or "greedy person," is still used in reference to those who covet Native American resources for their own profit. This had been referenced often in *Black Elk Speaks*, which I seemed to recall Franklin reading while in school. Maybe also in the film *Dances with Wolves*, which was set on the Lakota reservation and which I'd taken my son to see. Or did this relate to our visit to the reservation together more than twenty years ago? How did *Wasi* lodge in his memory bank, oddly related to the word *schizophrenia?*

"This is scary indeed," Malidoma is saying, but also laughing.

"I'm sorry."

"No, but that's fine, I think you've got something here to show the world."

"Yeah, I think so."

"Now I'd like to see those drawings that you have." Franklin hands some over. "Oh my goodness."

"You can have that."

"Oh, okay. This is amazing—this looks like Egyptian. . . . And how did you see these shapes, these forms? They just come to you like that?"

"Well, those ones, there's a watermark on the back so nobody can steal it. . . . One of those was written in Arabic, I think."

"So you also know Arabic?"

"Yeah, I'm not that good, but I'm good enough."

"This is fascinating."

"Yeah, you also fascinate me."

"It is exciting you know, because what it tells me is that you are in touch with a universal consciousness. And also that you live in a state of timelessness. See, the sequentiality of time and space only applies to you if you want it to. Otherwise you can find yourself here, and then go far into time, then come back so fast that nobody notices. This is why you look like a messenger of the cosmos. You process so much data that sometimes you are in multiple places at the same time. And yet, you still look like you are here in body and flesh, sitting in front of me, when in fact it's *everywhere*. There is something about that that also makes you, as you sit here, look like you are a sub-space antenna. Picking up messages from so far away."

Frank has been saying "yeah" and "uh-huh," but now he laughs. He asks Malidoma if he's from Senegal or Nigeria.

"No, from near Senegal, it's Burkina."

"Burkina Faso."

"Yeah"—Malidoma laughs again—"you see, you know it."

"I respect—lot of respect—I'm trying to learn how to be, you know, a nicer person."

"That's why—your knowledge of geography, the different places in the world, it's just outstanding."

Frank laughs and says, "Thank you, or should I say, 'Dashi.'"

"Dashi! And also the knowledge of language, universal language, it's just amazing."

I will later look up *Dashi*, too. It's of African origin, historical meaning unknown, but a name sometimes given to female babies. The Internet site I find says: "People with the name Dashi . . . fight being restricted by rules and conventions."

Pointing to the pattern that Frank has made on the divination cloth, Malidoma speaks of how "it gets you in touch with the ancient Mayan, Egyptian, and Native traditions. Here, I even see Dogon cosmology."[3]

"Oh nice. This is an ancient game. From Atlantis or. . . ?"

"Yeah. The other planet that is called—"

"Pluto. Neptune," my son interjects.

I envision Malidoma shaking his head. "That's right. All these energies . . ."

Frank points to certain rocks that he moved around to form the pattern. "I love these. These are special rocks, old, quite old."

"Very old indeed. . . . The way you know things is unbelievably calibrated. And so far beyond the normal human consciousness, I mean somebody"—

"Somebody could walk up to you and be angry at you for that, though."

"That's right, because you're so far advanced. This world is borderline, just skimming the surface."

"Yeah, I know."

Malidoma asks Franklin whether he does sculpting or some other form of art. My son says he does pottery, but needs "to do better to work with it." Malidoma says it looks from the shell pattern that there are other places in the world he needs to go. "I think so. What do you recommend?" Frank asks.

"Here it looks like a place that has ancient vibration. And when you get there, it will feel to you that you lived there before."

"Nice."

"You will start hearing sound—voices—and images that will confirm this. Because here it looks like, once upon a time, you were an engineer, and you helped to shape different form, creating sacred geometry. . . . This knowledge is still with you, right now."

Frank asks Malidoma to choose which of his drawings he wants to keep. He selects one "complex enough that I can sit with it and meditate. There was another one here, this reminds me of a space device, traveling at a tremendous velocity." Sacred geometry, he adds, is a big part of Frank's identity. "And this is why—the thing that you are sick"—

"It doesn't show?"

"It doesn't show here."

"Give 'em a call for me if you could, you know, in the hospital, tell 'em that. Write a good note for me or something," Frank says.

Malidoma tells my son that he'd "love to stay in communication, because there's something about you that is fascinating to me. And has nothing to do with someone who is ill. No, it's someone who knows so much, that this knowledge must be respected and catalogued and arranged. I know that your father does some of that. I mean, last time, when he showed up, it was all about you. Because I couldn't see him as separate from you. And the work that he is doing is really beautiful. And I wonder, how is this translating in terms of your dream and your vision?"

Frank points to a piece on the table that he says "represents me, represents the conversation." It's a very old piece, he adds. Some of the objects, Malidoma tells him, "are smaller than others, for a reason. But in the end, they are all meant to vibrate at a specific energy. And that energy is helpful in deflecting certain kind of frequencies." Frank chuckles. Malidoma asks if he can keep his drawing of a bird, "because this is also a sign that shows how your spirit can fly."

Malidoma continues to interpret what he sees in the divination design: "The light that shows here is not of this world. How could that be connected to the body that is sitting in front of me, I have no clue." Frank is still drawing. "Yes, you've been there. Through various tunnels. And it has led you to various worlds. And it looks like you've *left something of yourself in those worlds.*"

Listening to the tape, I wonder: *Could that be what happened when he was a teenager? And eventually triggered his breakdown? Or am I going too far out there?*

Malidoma goes on: "You have a very big heart, too—that is constantly open to a specific tune and frequency. In your sleep are travels, journeys where you interact with various things. Entities. Non-human entities."

A bit later, Malidoma asks Frank to choose two of the objects and place them somewhere new in the circle. Frank does so. More now seems to be revealed.

> Somewhere down the road, there is a part of the world that you will need to be at physically. This one has geometric structures that are located out in nature. It is not in a city. These are two homes that belong to you. And one of these is going to create an epiphany, some awakening in you, that is going to settle any and all of these things that make people think of you as being ill, schizophrenic, when in fact you're not. And when that time comes, a new life that is very rich, very beautiful, colorful, will come into place. This is something that is inevitable, you're not going to stay in the same modality after this. All of this is taking you to somewhere that looks like the top of a structure, it's pyramidal. You've got to go to Egypt at some point. And the other place looks like somewhere in South America.

Long ago, sometime in the late 1990s, Franklin had written in his journal:

> In Egypt, the man stands alone, perched upright and staring at the great pyramids. He lets his mind wander into the past where great civilizations rose and fell based on these pyramids and the pharoahs. The sculpted rock encasing tomb after tomb, passage after passage, intrigues him. The geometry of the big mass of rock seems perfect, shaped by a master. Some say it was music that built the pyramids. Imagine that: a man or woman with a flute, and making massive rocks to move. I'm sure that kind of music would move me. Or maybe the music was so beautiful that it moved folks into working to build the pyramids. Music is food for the soul. . . .

In this place of peace, people come on pilgrimages to see the pyramids and the great sphinx. They have been rediscovered and uncovered from the desert sands where they were built. The desert was a blanket that protected them from the outside world. These tombs held mummies that were secured in their sarcophaguses in rooms full of gold and riches for the afterlife. Sacrilegious people stole from the tombs (grave robbers). There were legends of curses that would be inflicted upon those that entered certain tombs. Scientists, archaeologists defied curses and paid the price. They were killed soon after entering. So, what does that say about the Egyptians? Did they practice magic? Did they know the supernatural world? Their mysteries are yet to be deciphered.

Now Frank asks Malidoma if he can read to him from a magazine he bought upon arrival in Jamaica, with Bob Marley on the cover. Malidoma says, of course. The article says:

> People . . . exchanging stories, ganji memories of each other like the marble games of childhood, exaggerated tributes to innocence . . . recognized by half a century of repetition and remembering into legend. From different islands in the same sea, with diverse histories, and the same grand chronicle we share. Which continues in us, in our children, in this city, far from the trees under which our naval vessels have been buried in the previous century . . . whose dense wood was so heavy it provided ballast for the slave ships in Africa.

When Frank finishes, Malidoma says, "That's fascinating. The thing about it is: there's something about that that relates to you. I was trying to see it here, but it's much more sophisticated than I think I can deal with."

"Well, can I call you? Letters?"

Malidoma says both would be good. They exchange contact information, and Frank takes his leave.

It turns out that they are both born under the sign of Aquarius, the Water Bearer, one day apart.

• • •

His father exclaimed, "Arenquiapaa! Oh my goodness!"
When, I wonder, would anyone
Not have a story to tell

After returning
To the village?

—Traditional narrative, Tununak, Alaska

After I tell Malidoma what Franklin said upon returning to our room—"Forty minutes? It could have been four years!"—he bursts into laughter.

"That's true! I felt like I was here *forever*, because he took me on a spin, and then came out, landed me, and said, 'I'm gone.' Oh my God!"

"He ended the session?"

"He ended the session, so it felt like *he* was the one doing it for *me*. But he did ask gently, can I go now? I said, of course." Malidoma then describes more of what had transpired. "Because there is no indication of an emotional or energetic condition, it's an expansion of such a magnitude that it made me dizzy. Because it goes into galaxies, planetary structures, dimensional vortexes, almost like what the Hubble telescope shows."

It's now time for my session, begun by pushing the shells and other objects in a clockwise direction. When Malidoma tells me to stop and begins to divine the pattern, a look comes over his face that seems pleasantly surprised. He points to two stones, one clear and the other orange. He explains that he'd asked Franklin, toward the end of his session, to move things around a second time. And after he'd spent some time rearranging, Frank had taken those same two stones from the center and placed them carefully on the right side—in almost precisely the same spot where I'd moved them a moment ago.

The orange stone had to do with a kind of healing related to the ancestors; the clear stone had to do with structure "or what you call the purpose that is mandated by ancestors," Malidoma says. "Now what were the chances that you were going to move them almost exactly like this? That's why I can only see how intertwined your two paths are. It simply means that the one needs the other as much; there is a kind of reciprocity that made both of you a team. Where all of that is going, will reveal itself in time. The journey is an ongoing one. And there won't be a dull moment!"

He points again at the clear stone. "This is the area of focus, ancient wisdom, ancient choreographies and processes connected to structure. That's what also comes out in his drawing. These are the items of some kind of awakening that he is slowly moving closer and closer to. And you are the monitor of that. Certain initiatives that you've got to take on your own, on his behalf, will help accelerate something that looks here like a homecoming. It will have a cathartic component to it, a time when perhaps the medical establishment will say: no, he's not schizophrenic anymore, or something like that."

There was unfinished work with ancestors. I would find myself stretched "beyond what might be called limits," taken to a "cutting edge," in order to discriminate what is needed to "house a complexity such as Franklin." Malidoma references what the French-African writer Aimé Césaire called "the voice of those who have no voice," meaning that "it doesn't just limit itself to Franklin, but your role and your mission in this life has always been that."

I would contemplate this later in terms of the subjects I chose to write books about—the likelihood of conspiracy in the Kennedy assassination, the genius of African Americans, endangered fish and whales, a biography of an under-the-radar psychological thinker. And now, it seemed, my own son.

I speak of how Franklin is always the unexpected, he'll go silent and not want to do anything, until suddenly—"There is this burst," Malidoma interjects, thrusting his hands forward, "revelation that's completely in contrast with the previous calmness and inactivity when nothing is going on, it's flatlined. Then, boom, there it goes."

Malidoma continues, "The amount of patience that is needed is unbelievable. Eventually there are codes to decipher." (The codes again!) "Symbols and emblems to bring together, in order to create a kind of whole that explains a mystery, you know what I mean?" It's important to observe what comes in intuition and dreams, he adds.

But the key, as Malidoma had seen before, is that the time will come when my otherworldly son needs an escort into 3-D reality. "It is *this* world that needs to factor into this knowledge he already has. But he's going to need to hang on to your arm, because he doesn't want to fall off. You see, there is no introvert or hermit of an isolated life associated with the process that is developing. It is meant to become extroverted someday—and you play a fundamental role in this. I mean, without you, forget all of this, just plain forget it—it's gonna be medical establishment contributing to deeper and deeper mess until oblivion sets in." Malidoma points again at the pattern. "The devotion is even outside of the circle. It comes from a different sphere, somewhere else."

After listening then to the tape of Franklin's time with Malidoma, I run into him again later in the afternoon. I tell Malidoma I could sense how happy Franklin was to be recognized by him. "He was just like a colleague!" Malidoma replies, and laughs. "It's a wave-length. Particularly when he asked if he could write or call me, I realized he is *that* relaxed. Also that he would sit there and write all those things. There's so much hope. He *will* make a breakthrough."

Returning to our room, I find Frank sitting on the edge of the bed with his head down, facing the door. "What's up?" I ask as I enter.

"I don't want to talk right now," he replies gruffly. I sit down in a chair looking out to sea. In a bit I ask if he wants to be alone. He says he does. I leave and walk down to the water. Years ago I would observe such behavior and immediately worry, go into "doctor mode." I would start trying to detect what was wrong, what I could do, how I could interject. Now when I realize that he'd probably like to be left alone, I ask him, he tells me, and I depart without resentment or judgment. This is how the bond between us has grown. Frank knows that, no matter where he is mentally, I'm there to help when and *how* he'd like me to, rather than my pulling the "I'm your father and I demand you tell me what's wrong."

It's getting dark. Despite these realizations, I can't help wonder: *Is it something I've done that angered him?* There is no way to know. Nor will Frank come to dinner that night. He simply lies on his bed star-ing at the thatched roof. I want to bring him along to a club where everyone else, including Malidoma, is going to listen to some Jamaican drummers. But Frank simply shakes his head. I stay behind, too. Alone at Jackie's On the Reef, we read awhile and go to bed early.

When I arise a little before seven, Frank is still sleeping. Going for coffee, I run into Jackie and speak openly of his night of silence and my fears. She says: "He resonated with Malidoma, because he so lives in that other world, too. And he *wouldn't* want to talk about it. You want to serve him, but really all you can do is hold the space for him and be patient. You're the one who needs to learn from him. He's a savant. He's in his own little world and you must honor that."

However, Jackie goes on, "He's a master game player, because he doesn't want to get too close." She recalls being with Frank the day before, and his talking to her about what he was reading when he abruptly stepped back—"he read me," as she puts it—and then resumed their conversation. But his silence was okay, "so long as he's not in a dark place." She doesn't think he is.

Franklin is indeed in good spirits when he gets up. I suggest he change his clothes (he's been sleeping in the same ones since we got to Jackie's) and he does, putting on his swim trunks and a T-shirt for the first time, saying that he needed to clean up. I bring him a cappuccino. He's very talkative as we sit in chairs across from each other, looking out to sea. Eventually, I tell him, I hoped that through this process he'd be able to cut back on his medication. "Maybe so," he says, looking at me intently. He mentions being a deal maker or game maker— tuning in to Jackie's metaphor—"like the game we played yesterday, with Malidoma."

Momentarily he adds: "I guess the way I am built is for privacy. I think if I can open to people more, I would be a happier person."

I go for more coffee and this time encounter Malidoma, and tell him what Franklin just said. "He's back!" Malidoma exclaims, a broad smile crossing his face. "That's perfect." Like Jackie, he felt it was normal for Franklin to have gone mute the night before. "I thought of going to see him and saying, 'let's go have some fun.' But then I thought, 'No, let him be. He's not lost somewhere.'"

Later that morning, my son and I walk together to say good-bye to Malidoma, who is outside talking to Jackie. He gives Frank a bear hug and says he'll text him, and my son turns to ask me, "Does he have my phone number?" I assure him that he does.

• • •

When the ceremony was over, everybody felt a great deal better, for it had been a day of fun. They were better able now to see the greenness of the world, the wideness of the sacred day, the colors of the earth, and to set these in their minds.
—John G. Neihardt, *Black Elk Speaks*[4]

At the breakfast table, Frank and I are joined by Jackie and two of the women from the group, and he is very at ease with everyone. Sometimes he takes things too personally and gets emotional, he says. Jackie concurs and says he needs to be aware of assuming things.

"You sound just like that Tantra book!" Frank says, making every-one laugh. "But I'm not gonna bullshit about it."

"You can, we wouldn't know," Jackie says teasingly. Frank talks then of his travels, some of them with me. "Dick's a good guide, a Leo." He himself likes to go by being a Capricorn, "but my birth certificate says 1-31-79 [sign of Aquarius]." The table gets into talking about yoga and Frank decides to demonstrate several positions with his arms. He ends by pretending to wring his own neck. Everyone howls. He's in rare form.

A little later, when I pass by my son leafing through a book in the common area, he glances over and says, "I'm learning." Patting him on the shoulder, I say, "I know."

Jackie tells me, "He's comfortable with us now. He's opening up—like a flower. And he'll be better by the time he leaves here."

Even though Malidoma has departed, I've scheduled us to stay for a couple of extra days. While Franklin does the Reikian non-touch therapy, I decide to try the Himalayan bowl treatment. Tanya, a New Yorker who studied with a "master bowl teacher," uses bowls made from twelve different kinds of metals (including meteorite), mostly from the seventeenth or eighteenth century. The bowls are fired and hammered, which deepens the sound. Her cymbals are known as tin-shaws. "I am calling in the ancestors here," she says.

I lie down on my back with my feet propped on pillows. Tanya begins by sprinkling sage with a feather "to cleanse your aura." The gongs of different vibrations resound in my ears and at the back of my head, as well as to a bowl placed for awhile on my solar plexus, and continue on for a timeless half hour. I see many colors, ranging from yellow to purple and then turning completely dark and all white, depending upon which tone I hear. While no visions other than the colors appear, it feels as if I am on a long journey and perhaps trav-eling far into space. Once or twice appears the image of a tunnel. I think of Franklin and our traveling together. Afterward, when I open my eyes to the tinkling of a chime, I'm surprised to find tears rolling down my cheeks. *Was I crying in some other dimension?* Tanya advises me to take some deep breaths as I did in the beginning, slowly return to consciousness, and turn over on my side before trying to sit up. When I do so, I seem to see every single leaf on a nearby tree, as if I'm high on a psychedelic substance. She plays a few more notes from a short distance away and says, "You've been vibrated. Be sure to drink some water, because the water in your body has been shifted." I'm warned that sometimes people feel dizzy when they get up, and I do indeed feel a bit disoriented.

When I arrive back in our room, I find Frank in a good mood. The Reiki lady had rubbed some things on his arms, he says. Did she do energy work above you? I ask. "Yes, she did." Then he returns to the common area, reading a book called *Sacred Women*. I can't remember when I've seen Frank so relaxed.

Late that afternoon, we head for downtown Negril with two of the other guests and Jackie at the wheel. Having some food on the beach, Frank looks up from his jerked chicken to ask her, "That apartment back at the hotel, is it yours?" After a bit of back and forth, he adds: "Guess I should get to the point, I want to live there!" At another point, Frank brings up Malidoma. "After that game we played, Malidoma told me so many things. About my destiny." He names off a couple of these, and then exclaims: "And King of Nigeria!" The ladies howl again. Jackie offers a refrain: "Just tell 'em Malidoma sent me!"

We drive on to a big resort, where on satellite TV the New England Patriots playoff game is about to happen. I'm a huge fan, but Frank isn't, and the drunken tourists and general chaos are too much for him. He has a piña colada and soon goes off by himself, sitting well above another section of the crowd watching some Jamaican drummers. I find him later looking at some brochures in the lobby. With the Patriots hopelessly losing to the Baltimore Ravens, we leave early in a cab back to Jackie's. There Frank sits on the edge of the bed for awhile, saying that he's thinking. Twice in the night, I awaken to the echo of the Himalayan bowls inside my head.

When I wake up, Frank says good morning to me in some other language. While shaving I hear loud and clear my father's voice singing a beautiful piece that my mother wrote for him, "How Sweet the Moonlight Sleeps." Frank tells me, "I'm so glad you took me to this place."

A little before eleven, Winston arrives and we hop into his minivan to make a two-hour drive to the Roaring River Park in Petersfield. Its limestone caves, according to Jackie, possess healing mineral waters.

Beyond a meadow full of water lilies and hyacinths and an ancient cottonwood tree, past a stone aqueduct where the waters run turquoise jade, we enter a subterranean passage lit by electric lanterns. Inside Roaring River Cave are underground springs, pools, and thousands of limestone formations that our ganja-smoking young cave guide observes resemble various types of animals as well as humans.

"It's beautiful," my son again says reverently.

Frank doesn't want to, but I put on my bathing suit and make my way carefully through some jagged rocks to sit under a cool mineral waterfall. "Dunk your head under," our guide suggests, and it feels fantastic. I stay in for about ten minutes before we resume our tour. Around a bend, several young Jamaicans stand tucked back into an elevated cavern: "the music compartment," our guide says. They strike pieces of bamboo with a stick and play a set of stalactites like a xylophone. Frank claps his hands happily beside me until the percussionists end with "When the Saints Go Marching In" and a shout of "Ras Tafari!" We continue on, ducking under large stalagmites to enter a "sanctuary," where people come to meditate. "The stillness in here is unbelievable," Frank says reverently.

Back outside, we're shown a spot where Bob Marley supposedly used to wash his dreadlocks. Given that one of Marley's band members did live near Roaring River, this does not seem far-fetched. Our guide says, "This is where he wrote 'Cold ground was my bed last night, and rock was my pillow, too.'" Frank knows the song, of course: "Talkin' Blues."

This is the main source of drinking water for miles around; divers once went 175 feet down the deep blue pool in front of us and never found the bottom. Our guide brings us fresh leaves to smell and taste. "Puts lead in your pencil," he says.

We end our morning sitting on a hillside under a tin roof, where a Rasta named Richard is cooking a fresh vegetable dish over an open fire. The fellow hands Frank his drum to play, and my son pounds out a good beat before accepting a plate. Richard cuts us a big stalk of sugar cane in a field below and we chew it as we drive away.

Later Jackie tells Frank that they used to keep slaves in the caves at Roaring River. "That's what I thought," Frank says. To escape, according to Jackie, the slaves would crawl seven miles on their bellies through a tunnel to safety on the other side.

Franklin loves it here, and doesn't want to leave. "After I get back to Boston, I'll be coming back—as soon as I have the money," he says at our last dinner at Jackie's. Be careful about telling Frank what to do, she counsels me privately; he's a grown man and will resent it. "You do pretty well, though," she adds.

When Winston shows up the following morning, Frank grabs his bags and quickly hops into the backseat. "Don't I get a hug?" Jackie asks from outside the window. He reemerges to give hugs to her as well as the Reiki treatment lady, who's shown up suddenly and whispers to me, "I had such a good session with him."

For much of the ride back to the airport, Frank does his "automatic writing" of hieroglyph-like characters. Our lunch waiting to board the plane is a quiet one. "Are you sad to be leaving?" I ask. "No," he says quickly. He's already distancing himself on the inside, including from me it seems. As we prepare to board the first leg to Orlando—Malidoma's hometown, I realize—Frank drops his passport. "You don't want to lose that," I say. "I know that!" he retorts. This angers him, rightfully so. I'm treating him like a kid.

He continues to draw for the entire plane ride. "You look like you're writing a whole book," I seek to engage him as we're about to land. Frank says nothing. "Are you not speaking to me?" I ask. "No," he says, "I'm concentrating."

We must go through immigration and customs in Orlando. As we disembark, authorities hold dogs on leashes to sniff everyone's carry-ons, apparently for drugs. In the long passport line, a woman is directing people with U.S. passports one way and those with visas in another direction. Suddenly Frank pipes up: "I have a visa. There must be some misunderstanding." The woman motions him to the wrong line. "Frank, will you follow me please," I say exasperatedly, and manage to quickly convince her that he's an American citizen. Then, at customs, after I say that Frank is my son, a woman begins to question us and asks what he does for a living. "He's a teacher," I lie, which is what Frank had said on the way out of the states. She turns to him. Frank stammers around, unable to answer when asked what he teaches. Finally he says, "I don't know. Art. Asian art." Somehow we're waved on through.

Waiting for our Boston flight to be called, I ask if he'd like a sandwich. "I don't know, Dick, I just want to get home and continue my writing." Finally aboard the plane, we're all the way to the rear in the middle and window seats. And almost from the moment we sit down, he starts going into a rant. "It was an alright trip, but it could have been better," he begins. How so? I ask. "Because I don't understand your language."

Then, in quite a loud voice, Frank starts rattling off geographical locations where he came from and Indian tribes that he was part of, and how he'd been Nelson Mandela for twenty-seven years (the exact amount of time, I later realize, that Mandela was imprisoned) and negativity about white people, whose presence dominates the plane. He's said "fucking" several times. The man seated next to me, whose wife and kids are across the aisle, asks Frank not to "use the 'F' word," and Frank says he's sorry.

I tell Frank I'm going to read, and the man next to me says he's going to do the same. Frank keeps talking for a little while, but soon in a much lowered voice. I tell him that, just as he'd told me earlier *he* didn't want to talk, now I don't. He talks to himself looking out the window as the plane takes off, sometimes in his private language. "I'm not comfortable here," he says. "Well, you're going to have to put up with that for another couple hours, as there's nothing to do about it," I say.

Things could have gone from bad to worse, but about halfway through the three-hour flight, Frank cools out. It's getting late. I bring out his medication, and he takes it. A friend meets us at the airport. It's fifteen degrees in Boston, as opposed to the balmy weather in Jamaica.

Another world to accept. Another homecoming to wonder, *where do we go from here?*

And yet, something is different. I can feel it in my bones.

• • •

As a man, I felt I had no purpose. I've been lost and I have been found. As a man you create your purpose and your sense of it. It is growth that I am talking about. It isn't the growth of a nation that creates a man. It isn't material expansion or monetary development. It comes from inside. When there is nothing there is infinite potential for something. Where there is darkness, light is there to fill it.

—Franklin's Journal, 2002

Notes

1. Malidoma on collecting: *The Healing Wisdom of Africa*, Jeremy P. Tarcher/ Putnam, 1999 paperback, pp. 254–5.
2. "We need to communicate intimately….": Harner, *The Way of the Shaman*, p. xvi.
3. The Dogon are a tribe from Mali in West Africa, believed to be of Egyptian descent and with astronomical lore that dates back thousands of years.
4. "When the ceremony was over….": *Black Elk Speaks*, University of Nebraska Press, 1979 paperback edition, p. 193.

• • •

CHAPTER 22

Spanning the Gateway

Do we ever understand what we think? We only understand that kind of think-
ing which is a mere equation, from which nothing comes out but what we have
put in. That is the working of the intellect. But besides that there is a thinking
in primordial images, in symbols which are older than the historical man, which
are inborn in him from the earliest times, and, eternally living, outlasting all
generations, still make up the groundwork of the human psyche.

—C. G. Jung, *Psychological Reflections*[1]

AFTER JAMAICA, A SHIFT SEEMS to have occurred in Franklin's way of
being. He's more direct and rambles less. I apologize for having
sometimes treated him on our trip "like a kid, being too protective,"
and he acknowledges this unhesitatingly. Awhile later, it is he who calls
to apologize for not being nicer when we were there. "I'm not much
of a vocalist," he says. I tell him it was a great trip. "Really? We'll do it
again sometime. Love you. Bye." Another time when I bring up our
experience in Jamaica, he says he will "treasure it."

I mention my desire to travel somewhere else with him, maybe
to meet the "friendly" gray whales that approach small boats in Baja's
Laguna San Ignacio (and the subject of my book, *Eye of the Whale*).
But after some consideration, Frank says he knows that I might "get
emotional" about his response, but he really can't see making another
trip so soon, maybe next year. Besides, he could already see the whales
and could draw them for me. Later, he'll tell me that it's important to

travel during the right time of the Zodiac, such as Aries, Capricorn, or Cancer.

Malidoma emails me: "I'm glad to hear that Franklin is changing. There was more work done subspace than in this dimension when we met at Jackie's." He wants to follow up with regular phone calls to Frank over a period of time, and soon writes again that they've spoken briefly and he'll reach out once more before leaving for a month in Europe.

Word comes from Frank's house that he's doing great and has suggested I be sure to wear sunblock while back out in California. Once there, I do my water ritual again in Malibu. Upon learning that I've secured a contract to write this book, Malidoma writes me: "This is an unusual opportunity to explore a galactic spirit wrapped up in a small human body."

When I see Frank next in Boston and tell him about my plan to write a book about him and our relationship, he informs me that he's also writing a book, and that it's about *me*. He then leaps mercurially between subjects—recalling locusts that once descended on the farm in Kansas, and his having been a helmsman (presumably when he learned how to sail on Boston's Charles River while attending Commonwealth School). At a bookstore, he picks up a magazine on sailing and a volume on "brain teasers."

He says he spoke with Malidoma a few days ago. "What did you talk about?" I ask. "The Memba Tribe in Nigeria," he says, and spells out Memba for me. All I can find online about the "African Memba Tribe" are a series of carved figures being auctioned by a U.S. gallery. "The Membas follow Nyingmapa Tibetan Buddhism and have their own script, Hikor, which is derived from the Tibetan," the reference says.

That's interesting to me, because of Frank's long-expressed fascination with Tibetan Buddhism. Being among the Memba, Frank had also said, is "a good place for Russells, as long as you don't spread any Ibogaine product." He was nervous about my writing down anything about that. I knew that Ibogaine is a hallucinogenic substance found in plants in Africa. Looking it up later, I learn that it was first discovered by a group of Pygmies, who taught Ibogaine-containing preparations to the Bwiti peoples of Gabon. The word *Bwiti* translates as "dead" or "ancestor." During Ibogaine rituals, initiates are said to undertake long journeys to the land of the dead.

Next time I see him, Frank asks for my notebook and draws out a pattern. What is it? I ask. "The pure milk in the glass," he says. Might he be referring to the water ritual with the organic milk that I've been conducting on his behalf?

On a Saturday drive, things become "curiouser and curiouser," as Lewis Carroll once described going through the looking glass. I'm taking Frank to New Hampshire to visit one of the young men in our family with whom he'd shared a common interest in science and mechanics, and to meet his fiancée. Pulling up to a sprawling nineteenth-century house right off a village green, a friendly cat named Olive greets us at the door. "That was my mother's name," I tell our hosts. "I thought its name was Lemon," Frank says. This turns out to be what they already planned to name their next pet. We hike through deep snow around their thirty-three-acre pond, inhabited by beaver and deer and stocked with several kinds of fish. Frank treks rapidly along as if he's wearing snowshoes, not simply rubber boots.

On the hour-long drive back to Boston, Frank says he'd like to live in China and attend either an astrology or culinary school. "You could look Chinese if you got a facial," he informs me. Then he starts weaving a strange historical tapestry. I've recently been reading a book titled *A Secret History of the World*, but I haven't discussed this with Frank. Now, as he speaks, it's as though he is picking up images from the book. I can't help but jot some notes as I drive—about Arabic tribes being "timekeepers of the world"; "Cain wasn't as bad as people thought"; Jesus and Muhammad bearing many similarities, but only one carried with him a genie; David, "prince of peace," was a later Adam. Another important figure was Harran, to whom Buddha gave "the sacred dust."

Did I know that the Maasai were descended from Canaanites? Franklin asks. Now, as I write this chapter, an Internet search reveals that Enkai, the Maasai creator god, bears very close etymology to Enki, creator god of the Sumerians; also to Enoch, the Canaanite hero (and son of Cain) who stormed heaven; and to Inca, divine leader of an ancient Andean civilization. But could my son possibly have read (and memorized) all of that?

As he speaks, I'm shaken by what seems to be coming through him. "So which planet are you from?" I find myself asking him.

"Sirius, the Dog Star. That's a beautiful constellation," he says. Then he continues: "There never was a beginning. It was atrophy." In the beginning, there lived a hermaphrodite type of . . . Bear. He himself was a reincarnation of the early fish-man. "The ocean was beautiful—bright, shiny," he says.

"When I was a fish, you were a fisherman," he says.

Another later Google search:

> In the Bible, the god of the Philistines was represented as half fish and half man. The Babylonians believed that such a being once emerged from the sea, appearing to them in the early days and teaching the people various arts. The likeness of this fish-man has been found among the sculptures of Nineveh.

The day after the trip to New Hampshire, I have a phone conversation with Malidoma. When I tell him about Frank's "secret history" lesson in the car, I can visualize the shaman shaking his head. "The way he's tuned into you and what you do, particularly when it comes close to the kind of thing that is alive in him—it's amazing. You know how to get his attention one way or another. You dwell on these types of subjects, and sooner or later you're gonna cross paths in the imaginal world."

At the same time, I've been struggling with a chapter about Frank's years in therapy with Dr. L. Not since 1999, fourteen years, have the therapist and I spoken. But an online search reveals that he's still in the Boston area, and I decide to try to touch base. I leave a phone message, and he returns my call. Dr. L. is pleased, but not surprised, to hear how well Frank is doing after all this time. And I'm curious what he might say about my son's seeming psychic abilities. The therapist replies: "I do find a capacity for acute perception in folks with this particular way of being in the world. They are less defended and consequently more sensitive to some essential things happening that the rest of us have a capacity for, but obscure by our ability to defend." It's surely a response of Western medicine—a world apart from Malidoma—but it's one I find worth contemplating.

In late March 2013, Etta comes to Boston for a visit. Frank wants to go to the Museum of Science, and I join them. As we walk down the hall toward the Omni Theater, he puts an arm around both of our shoulders. We watch together a forty-five-minute show about the Serengeti, wildebeest fording a crocodile-infested river, numerous larger-than-life visuals of Maasai. Frank tells Etta, privately, that he'd like to go back to Africa—but next time with her. And when I next pick him up from his music therapy, he tells me he had a dream about Tanzania.

Then a very strange "crossing of paths" occurs. I'm going through a box in the basement of my house trying to locate some of a friend's old diaries that she's requested. There's a date when something happened that she's looking to pin down. I pick up a diary with "1986" on the cover, and flip right to a page that begins: "Franklin got his finger smashed today from Riley jumping on a board—got a few stitches, lost some of the end of his finger." I hadn't been present, but this is one of the two painful childhood incidents that Frank brought up the night of his monologue in Tanzania. It's as if, somehow, I need to see it for myself in black and white.

• • •

Late that April, I arrive at the airport in LA, rent a car, and drive to Ojai. Malidoma is there again doing a workshop and divinations. We greet each other like old friends. He says he was just about to call Franklin today, but then his phone rang—and it was me instead. While a woman who's hosting him at the retreat center opens some red wine and grills up some lamb, Malidoma and I converse. He describes a boy in his village in Burkina Faso who was in similar straits as Franklin. The tribal elders followed the boy everywhere, writing down things that he said. Several times, Malidoma says, he's brought out the drawings that Franklin gave him in Jamaica. He just likes to meditate upon them, sometimes for as long as twenty minutes. I've brought along a folder of more drawings, all executed on the same day in Jamaica. Malidoma now spends some time leafing through them. "I like to call them glyphs," he says. "They are not random; they contain more than they appear. He puts a whole book on one page." Of one, he adds: "That's not even his hand, that's some spirit hand." And says of a few that depict faces: "These are beings that he sees."

Back with Franklin again a few weeks later, I mention Malidoma saying he sometimes simply sits and studies his drawings. Frank is delighted, and laughs. "He's a good guy," my son says, with a familiarity as if talking about a relative. "Do you want me to write some things in your notebook like I always do?" he asks. He proceeds to fill a couple of pages with words and glyphs. I can pick out "Navajo" and

"Jung" among these. One page bears a musical score labeled "Singer Machines." He speaks briefly, too, about ancestors.

My cell phone rings, and it's Dr. Reiner. I've begun helping Larry put together a memoir about growing up in Africa and all of his safaris, and he's wondering when we might meet to talk more about this. Frank asks to speak with him. "How's Marshall?" he asks, inquiring about Dr. Reiner's psychiatrist son, whom Frank saw one of the last times he was hospitalized. He says he'll send the doctor "some stuff."

The first volume of my biography, *The Life and Ideas of James Hillman*, is published in late spring. In New York, I attend a memorial tribute for him. Several hundred people are in the audience, while a host of friends and colleagues from as far away as Japan read poems, play music, and reflect upon Hillman's legacy. His tap-dance instructor is on hand—he'd taken lessons for twenty-five years—and the footage of Hillman's impromptu performances at various functions is heart-rending. I cry as I watch, missing the man and his remarkable vitality into old age.

When I see Franklin not long thereafter, pulling into his driveway he turns to me and says, "You should get into dancing." What kind of dancing? I ask. "Tap dancing," he says.

"Frank, you're always right in tune," I say. He grins.

In the car, Frank asks how I'm doing. "A little tired," I admit. He then makes reference to my astrological chart. While a Leo always has to be creative, he says, having my natal Sun square to planets in Taurus and Scorpio can make it tough to get work done. I shake my head. "Yeah," I say, "you're probably right."

Considering where things stood a year ago when Frank went back into the hospital after quitting Lincoln Tech and seemed for a while in worse shape than ever, Etta describes what's happening now as "a semi-miracle." Frank has a terrific music therapy session—"the Franklin we know and love," his instructor tells me.

Taking an art class would be good for him, Malidoma had recently told me "because what comes out of him on paper is out of some strange world that is potentially deeply exciting. That gateway or doorway has to be made bigger." I ask Frank what he thinks about taking some instruction in art, and he's interested. So I enroll him for the first of several weeklong classes at the Boston Museum School of Fine Arts. His drawing teacher emails me afterward: "Franklin did very well in the class. He created a ton of work and really enjoyed figure drawing and collage. He usually took what we were doing and branched off in his own direction, which was perfect. He was very self-motivated." Franklin's next teacher at the Museum School tells me that he is "having a ball," and finds his glyphs (which Frank tells him are Japanese) to be fascinating. The downstairs walls of Frank's house are soon decorated with his artwork: an elaborate glyph; drawings of a castle in Florence; racks containing cheese, honey and other foods; a cell phone, and a Jedi Knight. From a small black "doctor's bag," as he terms it, Frank brings forth to show me a series of metal sculptures that he's melded together.

Another time, he's waiting for me holding a large three-ring binder with a black-and-white geometric pattern for a cover. The opening page has *Crow History* as a headline, then a depiction of Crow Dog and a group of Sioux dancers. The Native American theme, it seems, is often at the forefront of Frank's imagination.

We had continued to kick around other places that we might travel together. At Malidoma's impetus, one was certainly Egypt. I came close to booking a "sacred journey" cruise down the Nile, exploring various ruins. But in July 2013, the country exploded after the military ousted the elected Muslim Brotherhood president and the tour had to be canceled. Frank was still keenly interested in China, and we also considered Machu Picchu. And there remained the possibility of visiting Malidoma's village in Burkina Faso, where the shaman spoke of bringing my son "face to face with what will look like peer energy to him."

In Jamaica, Malidoma had envisioned a desert-like area that Frank ought to visit. Once, when I mentioned the Mayan ruins as another potential destination, Frank replied: "Yeah, but I'd prefer maybe somewhere in this country—like an Indian reservation or something." He'd other times expressed a desire to see the Southwest. Perhaps this conjures up our trip to the Lakota Sioux reservation when he was twelve, to which he'd been imaginatively drawn back many times since. Or maybe it's something else.

Notes

1.   "Do we ever understand what we think?": C. G. Jung, *Psychological Reflections*, Princeton University Press, 1970 paperback edition, p. 47.

CHAPTER 23

. . .

Coming to Ground in New Mexico

It was the Indian manner to vanish into the landscape, not to stand out against it. . . . They seemed to have none of the European's desire to "master" nature, to arrange and re-create. They spent their ingenuity in the other direction; in accommodating themselves to the scene in which they found themselves. This was not so much from indolence . . . as from an inherited caution and respect. It was as if the great country were asleep, and they wished to carry on their lives without awakening it; or as if the spirits of earth and air and water were things not to antagonize and arouse.

—Willa Cather, *Death Comes for the Archbishop*

IT SO HAPPENS THAT I'VE received an invitation from Patrick Toomay to take us on a tour of the area in proximity of his home in Albuquerque, New Mexico. As with Malidoma, Toomay is another connection made in the course of my research toward writing the biography of James Hillman. The two men had met in Dallas in the early 1980s, shortly after Toomay's retirement from ten years of playing professional football in the NFL. Toomay was also a writer, having published an irreverent memoir, *The Crunch*, about life with the Tom Landry–era Dallas Cowboys, and later a novel (*On Any Given Sunday*) about the shadow side of the pro game and later made into a major motion picture directed by Oliver Stone. Since his college days, Toomay had been a seeker drawn to esoteric works of philosophy and poetry, which was how he'd encountered Hillman. I'd interviewed Pat over the phone for my book, and we'd hit it off over a breakfast meeting when he later visited Boston. He intuited that Franklin would find something of value roaming for four days "through rez lands, anasazi lands, lava fields, and tubes."

I knew little of the "sacred lands," as Toomay referred to them. "Out here," he told me, "the landscape is the shaman." Initially we'd scheduled a rendezvous for the spring, but something came up on his end and it had to be postponed. Now we are planning on late September 2013. As the date approaches, Frank becomes increasingly excited about going.

On the eve of our departure, I dream about being on a hike when coming upon a difficult downward passage through a body of water; my shoes get stuck in the mud and I need to retrieve them, but I manage to do so. In a second dream, Franklin is behind the wheel of a car and pulls up alongside me.

"We'll be doing some hiking on the trip, eh?" Frank asks on our way to the airport.

He brings along books on needlecraft and welding (the day before, he'd taken his first class in the latter). But for most of the way, my son remains silent, sullenly so. As we change planes in Dallas, he's moving his lips as if talking to someone. When I try asking before we board again why he is so uncommunicative, Frank replies: "You're so demanding. I try to talk to you, and you say, 'what?!'" I tell him I'm getting old, and maybe going a bit deaf.

No matter the situation, it's become obvious that Frank doesn't like flying, and is always defensive when I ask how he's doing during flights. On our last leg, I'm wondering why I've bothered to bring my son on yet another such sojourn, and I fear his rudeness might carry over to our hosts. After we land in Albuquerque around seven that night, Pat Toomay awaits us near the baggage claim. At sixty-five, he's a year younger than me, a tall bespectacled man who retains a football player's physique. Frank at first greets him brusquely, accelerating my worry, but soon becomes quite animated. We're driving toward town when Pat points out three volcanoes on the horizon, along with speaking of how New Mexico is the poorest state in the union. "Do you read a lot?" Frank asks him, adding, "Because you seem to know a lot of things."

For the first night of our stay, we check into the Nativo Lodge. From the entryway, Frank gazes long at the various shields of Indian chiefs that decorate one wall and begins listing off the names of their tribes. The next day, Toomay would tell me that, while my son didn't have the identifications correct, he may have been tuning in to the fact that they'd all once taken the same migration route from Asia. Frank has also said to Pat of his white BMW wagon: "This is a $16,000 car." That was the exact price Toomay had paid for it, significantly the first car he'd owned after having driven his father's for many years.

After depositing our bags, we ride over to Pat's nearby adobe house in Albuquerque's North Valley. Walking through the front gate, Frank points to a stacked pile of stones and asks, "Is that your totem?" It's a cairn, Pat replies; if you stack the stones properly, they'll remain in place. We are greeted in the kitchen by his partner, Lynn Haynes, a psychotherapist in private practice. Following a brief cordial visit, and examining the two guest rooms available to us, my son and I gratefully agree to move over here the next morning from the lodge.

Pat picks us up after breakfast. While Franklin settles in downstairs, I take a walk with Pat and Toby, their friendly Rhodesian ridgeback. We pass by ditches once dug by the Spanish for aqueducts. Pat describes a mystical experience he'd had in New Mexico in 1989, being drawn one moonlit night to the "charged" ruins of a thousand-year-old sacred Indian site. He knew then that he'd be back. He and Lynn had met on a mountain walk and been together for the decade since.

Our destination this first day is a trek up the nearby Sandia Mountains to a waterfall canyon. Mircea Eliade, the great scholar of shamanism and comparative religion, had spoken of four elements needed for sacred sites; these, Pat recounts, are rock, spring, tree, and ultimately shrine. Here we would see a piñon pine that seemed to grow out of the rock with a spring below—"a contained sacred space"—but first we'd traverse the Piedra Lisa "fairy trail."

"I haven't been up there since all the rain," Pat says, "so we'll see what it did to the arroyo. Should be pretty green. It's protected from the wind, so that won't bother us."

We set off mid-morning as the sun breaks through the clouds. A small herd of bison graze near the side of the road as we enter the

Sandia Reservation. According to Pat, "it would have been built out long ago but was preserved for national forest on this side. It's ponderosa forest all the way up the mountain." Frank says, "It's beautiful out here, shiny clouds, buffalo clouds. There's a good water system, right?"

"Yeah, a lot of water comes off of here and goes underground down to the city." We turn left onto a dirt road. "Thirteen minutes out the door and you're entering another world," Pat says. "See that formation up there? It's called 'The Shield.' We'll be going in its orbit." Pink granite embedded with quartz greets our eyes as the range grows ever more complex. Frank lists off all the colors he sees: blue, green, brown, yellow. "We'll look for bear scat," Pat continues as we approach a ravine full of large boulders. "If a bear shows up, stay calm and make yourself big. Don't run." They're likely to be brown bears, my son adds. The road turns bumpy and rutted. "Up here people live off the grid," Pat says.

There's only one other car in the gravel parking lot. It's a beautiful day, barely requiring a jacket. When we stop, Pat assembles walking poles for each of us. He hands me two canteens of water to strap around my waist, one of them filled with electrolyte, because there's little humidity to cause a sweat at the 7,500-foot altitude we'll be reaching, making it easy to get dehydrated without realizing. We walk up the dirt road toward the trailhead. Pat pulls off a needle of sweet-smelling piñon pine and holds it up to each of our noses, telling us that sometimes the smoke from burning these will hang like incense over a village. Cholo cactus, whose toxin is medicinal, blazes yellow. The Apache Rose, with its pink and lavender leaves, only blooms here in the fall.

Then Frank spots something in the dirt and calls our attention to it. "Snake skin," he says. It's so small, Pat thought it was a shoelace and I saw a piece of rope. "Want to pick it up, Dick?" Frank asks me. "No," I say. So he does. My son is right. Pat says it's the shed skin of a baby rattlesnake. That Franklin had not only seen it, but identified it as a snake, seems a marvel. He now mentions something obscure about China, and Pat notes that this is the Chinese year of the black water snake.

Looking behind us, Pat points out the Rio Grande Valley to the south. There is also a black band of lava and the three volcanoes again, seeming deceptively close but actually about twenty miles away. Past a sign for the Cibola National Forest, we turn right up the arroyo. "I'm having fun," Frank announces. "Good," Pat says with a laugh. Not another soul is in sight.

Beside a Gambel oak, Frank shows Pat the book he's carrying, *Natural Healing with Herbs*, along with his sketchpad. "That's a great thing to have with us," Pat says and adds: "The other thing about physical exertion in order to get to a sacred place, it drops your defenses—and the grandfathers can see what you're open for."

The trees loom above us as we climb, traversing a riverbed using our sticks. Coming to a rough spot that includes pushing ourselves up over a collection of boulders, Frank doesn't think he can make it any higher. But Pat coaxes him quietly that it's not that much farther—"see that little pine tree up there with its root in the rocks?"—and my son nods and starts forward again. We all then sit down beside a waterfall that flows through even larger boulders, the lonesome pine above us.

This is the "landscape of stones, water, and trees" that Eliade had described in the religions of many ancient cultures. "Stone stood supremely for reality: indestructibility and lastingness; the tree, with its periodic regeneration, manifested the power of the sacred in the order of life. And when water came to complete this landscape, it signified latencies, seeds, and purification."

I hear my son say, "Good hike. Nothing like the mountains. The smells are unbelievable. If you ever want to take a break and get away from things, this is the perfect place."

"Absolutely!" Pat enthuses. "If you're ever wound up too tight, come here."

When we set out again for higher elevation, the effort becomes more difficult. Not only boulders to climb, but a hanging tree limb above a clearing that requires propelling ourselves ahead with our hands against an adjacent rock face. "Look at the vertical on that," Pat says, pointing to the sheer cliff beyond. Frank points ground-ward to what he thinks might be some mint, calling it "a lucky omen." But soon he says he just can't keep ascending, so we stop and rest again.

I'm remembering a little over a year ago, the last time Frank was hospitalized, and a conversation where out of the blue he'd brought up the outdoor education organization, Outward Bound. "I couldn't climb the rock face—out of respect," he'd said, with no frame of reference. But which, at the time, had reminded me of something Robert

Whitaker, author of *Anatomy of an Epidemic*, told me over lunch: that rock climbing was something which, to everyone's surprise, groups of schizophrenics did successfully. "If I try to climb and put a dent in that rock, the whole mountain would fall apart," Frank had continued that day in the hospital.

As we now somehow get on the subject of different varieties of burials, Frank mentions bogs—and Pat notes that bogs are where Irish kings were once buried, the oldest bog in the world having been discovered only a few days ago.

"How do we get down from here?" Frank asks.

"Use your pole to lean on and take a step," Pat says.

"They should have double ones, with a stretchy spring in the middle. I'll invent one."

"Okay," Pat says, with a smile.

While initially tough, the descent soon becomes easier. Still, it requires vigilant attention to retain one's footing and, while recounting a story to Pat from my days as a *Sports Illustrated* reporter, I let my mind slip. Bringing up the rear, I break a backward fall with my left hand and, upon landing, a branch draws blood just below a knuckle. My son turns and moves toward me, alarmed. "I'm all right," I assure him. My flesh wound dries quickly. Later, Pat calls it a "blood sacrifice." Later, too, Franklin will say, "The mountain was too Gaelic for you." Both Pat and I have Irish Gaelic heritage, and we laugh heartily.

My son also wonders whether the mountain doesn't like my taking a certain picture. And, as we continues our descent, he mentions something about nuclear physics, which curiously was what Pat's late father—an Air Force major general—had once worked on for the Pentagon. A mountain blue jay, the only bird we see, sings to us from high in a nearby tree.

"I liked the climb," Frank says as we reach the gravel path again. "There were snakes all through there." Pat says that the rattlers, as well as the bears, should be heading toward hibernation about now. "I want to write about the golden cliffs," Frank goes on. "And about how would you ride a bike with rubber tires up this cliff?" That would make a good animation, says Pat. Frank turns back with a look of wonder crossing his face as the fog rolls in above the mountaintop. "Fog, it gets lonely," he says, "but people like it . . . I've got fuel for my writing now—the grass, the trees, the dirt, the rocks. I got to see Dick travel his path alone—but it was nice as a group, a nice thing to do."

What does he mean by alone? My fall? A revealing of my vulnerability? No matter, I've never seen Franklin enjoy being out in nature so much.

Back in the car, Pat suggests we add some green chilies to our lunch to clear the head after a trek like this one. "Ceremonial," Frank says, "you can also eat Szechuan."

"Exactly," Pat says, "Korean food uses the same thing but red chilies."

How does Frank *know* all this? Where does he pull it down from?

That night, Frank turns in early. When I go to see him, he's lying on his bed with the light on. "Thank you for taking me on this trip," he says, "it's wonderful." He admits being quite tired from all the hiking and adds, "You did pretty good hiking, too." But if I need something for my cut, he could do that. Or my back, which he worries could be out of whack, and offers to give me a massage.

In the living room, Pat, Lynn, and I reflect on the vast difference between our plane ride yesterday and the mountain trip today. But, as Lynn points out, it made perfect sense that Franklin would retreat inward first—the anxiety of leaving the group home, all the people in the airport, the long flights. "If he goes *in*, he is still engaged," she says, and this strikes me as a lesson I need to heed.

Later that night, Pat recalls a story about his eldest son. Some years back, Pat had been given a drumming tape by Michael Harner, author of *The Way of the Shaman*, a book I'd read while in Jamaica. It was powerful music and, in the course of listening, he'd seen himself transported down to a flowing river. He decided to give the tape to his eight-year-old boy, in a little experiment to see what he might experience. An hour later, Pat returned to hear that not only had his son journeyed down to the river, but had worked his way back past scorpions and then bears. He'd had a shamanic type of experience. And it had changed the boy, and the way he saw things. He grew up to become a radiologist, with an uncanny ability to detect things in patients' X-rays.

• • •

The next morning, Frank walks into the kitchen bringing one fist down on top of the other and proclaiming, "Team spirit!" We head out shortly after mid-morning, west on Interstate 40 and across the Rio Grande and into reservation territory. Navajo live on the north side of the freeway, Acoma and the related Laguna tribe to the south. The storied Route 66, with its original two-lane pavement, meanders just to our right, and we soon pass the Laguna's Route 66 Casino.

"It's not usually this lush," Pat says, "but it's what they pray for. Now we're in the red zone," meaning the red-clay soil. He turns to Franklin beside him in the front seat and points ahead: "That's a volcano right there, with the meadow below, above the tree line. It's sacred to every tribe." The Anglos call it Mount Taylor, but the Acoma name is Snow-Capped, the Navajo's is Blue Bead, and the Laguna's is Women in the Mist.

About forty-five minutes beyond Albuquerque, we leave the highway and pause at a truck stop by a sign: "Acoma Sky City 15 Miles." The tribe has about 3,600 members, the majority of whom live in town. We stop to visit two friends of Pat's, spiritual elders and master potters. Frank finds them "really good people" and thanks him for the stopover.

The scrub appears endless as we drive on toward the ancestral Acoma Pueblo. It dates back almost a thousand years, to around 1150. "Theirs is a matriarchal society, passed down through families," Pat says. "Every year they elect five field chiefs who live on the mesa. They perform liturgical duties for the entire year. It's a huge honor, but also difficult."

Suddenly, coming around a bend, a sheer sandstone cliff shimmers purple on the horizon. This is the uninhabited Katzimo, the "Enchanted Mesa." Legend has it that, centuries ago when a storm caused a landslide that blocked a lone path to its apex, the Acoma had moved about a mile to the southwest. Here, 367 feet above the valley, stands the village where about fifteen Acoma families continue to live year-round. "It was strategically positioned to ward off invading tribes," Pat tells us. The panoramic vistas take the breath away, as do the animated rock faces greeting us as we approach. The first white man in recorded history to see this, Spanish Captain Hernando de Alvarado in 1540, had written in his journal of having "found a rock with a village on top, the strongest position in all the land, well fortified, the best there is in Christendom."

"There's still no electricity or running water up there. Everything is hauled up." This is reputedly the oldest continuously occupied village in the United States. At the visitor's center, we purchase our tickets and board a bus with a group of about twenty tourists bound for the peak, elevation 6,885 feet. It might have been the set for a Western and, indeed, John Wayne made several movies here. A guide about my son's age, identifying himself as Robert, meets the bus. We emerge, surrounded by a series of old adobe clay homes, some three hundred spread out atop the mesa.

We pause first at the cemetery just outside the mission church built by the Spaniards a generation after the Battle of Acoma that resulted in their conquest of the Indians in 1598. According to Spanish accounts, as many as five thousand tribal people resided here at the time. The cemetery measures 400 feet by 400 feet, and is 40 feet deep. Humps of clay adorn the walls, each with carved eyes, noses, and ears; seen from below, the Acoma's hope was that these would be imagined as soldiers guarding the rim. A hole hewn into the south wall is a return portal for children who had been sold into slavery. No one is allowed to take pictures here.

The San Esteban del Rey (St. Stephen's) Church, still used twice a year, is 50 feet high, built without nails but with 40-foot-long beams of Ponderosa pine carried here by the Indians from Mount Taylor, thirty miles away. From the altar, red candles representing the native religion and white ones to represent Franciscan Catholicism spiral toward the ceiling. This is the oldest confessional in America.

Franklin is reverentially silent until we all emerge from the shrine and church. Then he begins to engage our guide. "Do you live here?" he asks, and Robert says he was raised in this area but now resides ten miles to the north. "Cool," says Frank.

"I'm here a lot, though," says Robert.

"I used to live on the Lakota reservation," says Frank.

"Where are you at now? Albuquerque?" asks Robert.

"Yeah," says Frank, pointing to Pat, "I live with them."

After Frank asks Robert whether he's been to New York and do they have a McDonald's in the vicinity, the two of them walk ahead and I overhear Robert inquire whether my son is part Apache. "Three-quarters," Franklin replies.

We pause at a ceremonial kiva, an underground chamber used in pueblos for religious rites, reachable by a ladder and disguised on the surface. After some minutes looking out on the enchanted mesa, where Robert tells us that his Acoma name means Meadowlark, Pat approaches him and places a generous tip in his palm, whispering that he much appreciated the gracious way he handled all of my son's comments and questions.

We decide to continue west. Looking out upon the cliffs, I muse that "I always see faces in rocks." My son doesn't miss a beat. "That one right up there looks kinda like you." The Anasazi site we're moving toward is an outlier of the Chaco Canyon, located on the same meridian. "The orientation of Chaco Canyon is North to South," Pat says. "The Great North Road runs for fifteen or twenty miles. The people called it 'Womb of the World'; souls ingress and egress along it. This was the same migration route used by the Mayans who built the Mexican pyramids at Teotihuacán."

We leave the highway and turn left down a dirt road. This was the spot to which Pat had been drawn in 1989, the night he couldn't remember how he wound up driving through certain towns and couldn't find Chaco Canyon and a Navajo woman in a store instead penciled directions to what was once a ceremonial gathering place for this region. A fault line ran down it—"volcanoes are quintessential openings to the lower world," as Pat put it—and three elliptical hollows carved by erosion dominated a sandstone escarpment beyond the circular remains of a huge kiva.

The site is aligned with certain full moons, which pass directly overhead. Pat didn't know then it was a sacred site for the Anasazi, who lived here between 900 and 1100 AD. "I knew nothing. I parked here and climbed over two barbed wire fences to the top of a knoll where I came upon the ruins." Instinctively, he'd removed his shoes, tiptoed down what seemed to be a corridor, and found himself lying flat on his back in the circle of a kiva.

Pat had later written:

It was a gentle ascent to the foot of the hollows. As I started up, I was fixed on the formation, but then I turned around, looked back at the moon. Huge, brilliant, it was ever ascending. Shaking my head, I looked back at the hollows, into whose face the moon was beaming. And suddenly I felt I understood why the site had been located here: The hollows were moonbeam catchers, a natural dish focused on the heavens, to capture and hold them—to create a confluence—so that their essence could be imbibed by whoever the long ago people who lived here.

Pat stops the car when he sees a sign that reads "Casamero Pueblo." Not another vehicle, or another soul, in sight. We pass easily through an opening in some barbed wire and begin to walk through thousands of grasshoppers humming and leaping before us in the tall sage. Beyond the scant remnants of the big kiva, the three of us stand amid the sandstone slabs where the Anasazi once resided. It is banded masonry, small limestone fragments and broken pottery once used to craft the dwelling place. There had been a smaller kiva here, the spot where Pat paused in meditation on his initial visit. A marker denotes an area used for food storage—a small bin built into the east wall—and two other rooms that had supported a second story. Another marker describes the bones of a child being discovered in one room. "It's a charged place, don't you think?" asks Pat. It certainly is. We sit down in silence for a few minutes that feels like half an hour, amid dirt, rocks, earth, and kiva. Pat's words prior to the trip hung in the soft wind: "Out here, the landscape is the shaman."

As we reach the car again, Pat says, shaking his head: "This is a soothing, soothing place." We each feel quietly renewed. Franklin says he'd felt a "pretty extensive Chinese or Japanese influence up there," and Pat agrees.

On our way back to Albuquerque, he turns off the highway again at a sign for the El Malpais National Conservation Area. "We're going into the badlands," Pat informs us. Lava fields here extend out some thirty miles. Pat had once tried to traverse some of it, "but walking through lava is really hard. The surface is so uneven, it doubles or triples your time over a flat surface." Today, "because of the angle of the sun, this could be beautiful. We'll be driving along the cliff face."

For no reason I could fathom, maybe ten minutes into the badlands, Pat pulls off the road. He says nothing, but beckons us to follow him. We wander together into the cedars. We haven't gone far when Pat leans over and picks up a tan clay fragment. Several inches long, it has visible lines of blue paint. "Pottery shard," Pat says. "Possibly a thousand years old."

As a boy, Franklin had a knack for finding fossils. Now, continuing our walk, he soon pulls one shard, then another, up from the dirt. Some bear carved ridges, distinguishing them from ordinary stone. Starting back toward the car, my son hands them to me. We've gone about twelve miles altogether when Pat turns off-road again and stops at a remarkable overlook above a vast green valley covering the lava, with sheer sandstone cliffs all around blazing golden in the setting sun. "Nobody here either! Unbelievable!" Pat exults as I walk to the edge to photograph what I could of the cinder cones and shield volcanoes that you could see scattered in the distance. These, according to a plaque, were created by multiple volcanic eruptions over a hundred thousand years. Visible, too, was Mount Taylor, a composite volcano from 3.5 million years ago. And the sandstone was formed by sea deposits that periodically covered the area between 63 and 138 million years ago, the bluffs carved by millions of years of erosion.

Back in the car, Frank says, "You could trek up here, but you'd need the right kind of shoes. This is theatrical, I really enjoyed it."

Yes, very dramatic, Pat agrees.

• • •

The next morning, when I knock on Franklin's door, he's down on the floor "doing exercises." Later I find him outside standing quietly by a post, with Pat's dog Toby watching him quizzically. "I'm studying," Frank says.

It's early afternoon when we set out for the Sandia Mountains again. There, "The World's Largest Tramway" fills up quickly with Sunday passengers. Our female guide announces that we'll start at 6,559 feet and climb almost 4,000 vertical feet straight up to the peak at an altitude reaching 10,378 feet. This will take thirteen minutes, traveling twenty feet per second. A quarter-million visitors a year come here to do this, the first voyage having occurred in 1966. It's still the longest tram ride in the Western Hemisphere, but there's now a longer one in Armenia. "What's the name of that one?" my son asks, but our guide doesn't know.

We soar above the juniper and cottonwood trees, past the hovering red-tailed hawks and the still visible wreckage of a TWA plane that crashed on the mountain back in the 1950s. We pass over the solid rock, seven-story-high Totem Pole Pinnacle; over Big Canyon dotted with ponderosa pine; over Echo Canyon with its sculpted-looking rocks. From the top we'll be able to see 11,000 square miles, which is 9 percent of all New Mexico.

But as we ascend, I observe Frank holding tight to one of the poles toward the back, the expression on his face growing more agitated the higher we go. I realize that I had no clue he had a fear of heights. Could this also account for at least part of his reaction when he takes a plane? When we finally stop, he rushes off ahead of everyone with a kind of shuffling gait that he adopts sometimes when in a nervous hurry. Pat and I find him sitting down inside the waiting area. He throws a big smile at us and says, "Survival Techniques 101."

My son declines accompanying us on a hike along the mountaintop. "I don't like the air," he explains. As Pat and I traverse the railing-less edge to take some pictures, he says, "Yeah, Frank wouldn't like this." We return to find him looking at maps on the wall, saying he's doing okay, so Pat and I hike a bit longer on the other side, getting back just in time to catch the next tram down.

Frank is shaky. Pat takes his hand as we approach the tram, and then Frank grabs my arm as well to steady himself. Once inside, he grasps tight to a pole with both hands. I can feel him wincing as we pause briefly at the first of two transformer towers as the guide says, "Another swing and sway, folks." This is the clearest the weather has been in two months, he continues. But it's an interminable ten-minute ride for my son, who can't wait to be back in the car.

Once we're all safely inside, he says, "There were a few dips. Everyone felt so secure. But it was a pure helium atmosphere." Pat nods: "It *is* like pure helium. Did you ever see people when they swallow helium gas?" The two of them do a simultaneous imitation of the resulting high-pitched voices, and we all laugh.

At 4 p.m., we have an appointment to see Ashéninka Mino. He is a healer from the central Amazon jungle of Peru, who has recently moved to Albuquerque. Initially he'd lived just down the block from Pat, which is how they met and this came to be arranged. According to Pat, Mino's arrival is part of a transition of such things from East-West to North-South. Mino uses various indigenous techniques to work on someone's vital body. A brief Internet description says that he treats anxiety, stress, tension, depression, rage/anger, as well as helping those who lack energy and confidence or suffer from physical ailments like headaches or back pain. I am hoping that Franklin will agree to experience Mino's treatment.

Bernadette, his short, dark-haired, attractive partner, greets us at the door of a modest house in a residential neighborhood. Mino is a youthful-looking fifty-three, with a kindly face and dark hair that flows straight down his back almost to his belt loops. They invite us to come out to the backyard, where tobacco and "holy basil" are growing under plastic row covers. Nearby is a plywood shack with a roof and one wall open to the outside, where Mino has set up a makeshift treatment room. We're invited to sit down across from him in folding chairs. Next to Mino's is a long table containing stones and eggs and pipes—his "altar," Bernadette will later call it.

She will do the translating. Mino is starting to learn English, she says, and Franklin suggests he could take classes on the Internet. Frank also speaks of having lived with the Iroquois—and the Lakota—and of various foods he can prepare, tamales and chicken of example, and something he calls "Sapura." I mention that we've considered making a trip to Peru and the Incan ruins of Machu Picchu, and Frank speaks of Apache guides that he hopes could take him there "on my own sometime, not with my stepfather." (Twice in reference to me, he will correct "father" and call me "stepfather," which he's not done in some time.) "Que bueno!" Mino exclaims.

I ask what part of Peru he comes from. A community near the Perine River, he says, in the central Amazon. Snake territory. "My language is Snake," Mino says. Frank says he speaks the language of Koala, the bear. But Mino stays with the subject of the snake. Some come out of the mountains, he says, others go in the water. "Coral? Black snake?" my son queries. Various colors including black, Mino says. "Black ones will chase you till they bite you," he continues.

"There were a few pythons I saw," my son tells him. Mino responds that the pythons in his land grow to be three or four feet long, including a very colorful one shaped rather like a boat. "In my culture, a certain snake comes when somebody is to pass away. It's a warning. Others *no son malos*. A boa when hungry gets long and skinny. This is why the natives carry machetes. Once you are living there, you become aware."

Pat has been trying to move the conversation away from the snake and back to the treatment. "Mino works on you energetically," he says, glancing over at Frank. But my son's response is quick: "I don't want to do it today. If you want to do it, Dick, go ahead."

For a moment, I hesitate. *I didn't come here for me*, I think to myself. I take a deep breath. "Okay," I say. Pat suggests that he and Frank go for a walk or wait inside the house. They depart.

Through Bernadette, I ask if it's possible for Mino to work through me on my son's behalf. He shakes his head. No, it must be individual; but relationally, the treatment helps someone to be more grounded and to heal inner turmoil. Then let's go ahead, I say. I pass him a pack of American Spirit cigarettes, as Pat had suggested for an offering.

Mino explains that he works with tobacco, using a delicate mixture from the previous year that has been prayed over. "It is used to open [someone], people ask what does that mean?" He draws comparison to a key opening a lock. "I use tobacco to open you up for access. There are things your body does not need that I take out. From the top of your head to the bottom of your feet. There are five steps. These are not techniques, but you might also call them pathways." He uses stone—obsidian works well and sometimes volcanic rock—as well as the point of an egg, "kind of like a flashlight that enables you to see at night," to find things inside someone to be removed. Once the space is open, he uses his hands above the physical body. As confirmation he might also utilize a few oils or a candle to help concentrate the energies of the session.

He doesn't pay attention to the clock, although treatments normally last about an hour and fifteen minutes. "Be very relaxed and breathe," Bernadette translates. "If you feel him lift your hands or your feet, let him do the work. If the reaction of your body is crying or laughing, let it come out. Don't hold onto anything. You might feel like you are falling asleep, but you aren't.

"You have asked to help your son, but there could be other things deeper to work on. Memories of childhood, or more recent ones, may come up. You want to place these things together in a box, basket, or bag, and mentally take this to the water and see yourself putting it into the water. The water can be a river, a lake, wherever you feel comfortable. Our spiritual brothers will be there working in the water."

If I need to empty my bladder during the session, just say so. I'll do that right now, thank you. As I walk into the house, my son looks up from a couch and offers some advice: "Be careful when he puts that snake medicine on you." Despite his smile, there is a hint of real concern in his voice. Franklin glances at Pat and adds, "We'll give him a chant, I guess. A nurture dance. Lakota for 'Good People Dance.'"

Pat says, "We'll bring a stretcher for you and carry you home."

Frank says, "Clean him out—all those tacos, man!" That's a reference to our lunch, just prior to arrival here. Pat cracks up as I head for the bathroom.

It takes Mino about ten minutes to set up the space outside. When I return, he has changed into a white cloth tunic with a checkered pattern, reminiscent of Malidoma during our divination. I take off my shoes, my watch, and empty my pockets. At a fold-out massage table, Mino asks that I lie down on my back. He places a cloth over my eyes, then another one as I fold my arms across my chest. The sweet pungency of tobacco fills my nostrils as he moves slowly around my outstretched torso, dispensing the smoke into the air and then blowing on it.

Sometimes flies buzz around my head or land on my hands. I also occasionally hear barking dogs and, at what feels like propitious times, the singing of birds. Mino moves, too, with a hard egg, and then a stone, gently lifting my arms and placing the object in each of my hands before setting the arm back down again.

An image arises from long ago, with the African medicine man in the small village of Anansu, who shed his robe, stripped to a decorated loincloth, and knelt to pray as the apprentice grabbed an egg from a bucket and put it on the ground. "He can look at this and see what is coming," the apprentice said.

At times I feel Mino's hands leap suddenly off of whatever part of my body he is working on, as though releasing something. And, indeed, twice I place memories in a basket and deliver them to imagined ocean waves. Both, I realize later, relate to the transitional age of thirteen. The first is the painful recollection of the physical confrontation I had with Franklin, after I'd barred him from listening to rap music and he lashed out at me. The fight that he'd brought up again, that night of "the snake god" in East Africa.

The second recalls something that happened to me at that same age, when a worker in my father's office—a Native American in his twenties—tried to molest me. We'd just moved to Kansas City, and I had few friends as yet, and after meeting me one day he'd asked my dad if he could take me to a matinee movie. It was *Swiss Family Robinson.* After his first unsuccessful attempt while taking a walk, we sat in the front row of the theater and I clung to a popcorn box on my lap. A few days later, he sent a gift of a head-dress home with my dad. I stashed it away, high on a closet shelf. I never could bring myself to tell my father, even after he later asked me whether anything strange had happened that Saturday afternoon. On my walk with Pat here this morning, the memory suddenly returned and I'd felt compelled to tell *him.*

As Mino works on my chest, I experience powerful exhalations and a feeling of rising and falling. My body twitches in various places at different times, which seems like releases of energy. I become more and more relaxed. I notice that one shoulder feels different, very good in fact, not that I'd noticed anything wrong before. Finally I hear Mino whispering something about "very slowly" in my ear, and realize he is telling me that the session is over. Shortly thereafter, he removes the blindfolds and I am shocked back into the late afternoon sunset. I feel an intensity, an aliveness, in my surroundings. I've no sense of time, but my watch says I've been lying on the table for more than an hour.

Mino brings Bernadette back outside and, through her, asks me a series of questions about how I'd felt during the treatment and anything I might have experienced in the back of my neck and head, or my shoulders, chest, and stomach. "Que bien," he says, nodding after a number of my answers. Then he says: "We worked things up, broke open several things—in your head, your throat, strong in your chest and abdomen. A lot of things got released. *Your male energy has come to you and you will be able to move forward.*"

Bernadette tells me that, during the session, inside the house Franklin had said he wanted to talk to her, which they did for some time. "He really wanted to communicate. I did not always understand him; there were different subjects all packed into one." Had Mino conducted the session with Frank, she adds, it would have been about giving him calmness and tranquility. But he would need something deeper, and probably Mino would have referred him to someone in Peru, where his sister is a naturopathic doctor and his personal guide lives in the same area of the Amazon jungle. Bernadette says, "While he worked with you, he asked that the work be connected to your son." Mino closes by giving blessings to me, my family, and my community. I am asked to place my "gift" on his altar next to the ceremonial objects. As Pat had earlier instructed, I leave sixty dollars there.

As we say our good-byes and return to the car, Pat says: "We kept seeing puffs of smoke coming out of there periodically. In the meantime we had a great chat, also with Bernadette, about plants and stuff." Frank looks at me and says: "Did he play a magic kazoo?" and adds: "He put Dick in a sleeper hole." This cracks Pat up.

"Well, he didn't use the snake medicine on me," I reply.

"He probably pulled the snake *out*," says my son.

We stop at a grocery store so I can pick up some limes, carrot juice, and orange juice to mix and drink in the morning for the ensuing eight days prior to eating anything: "On the physical level, this will help remove what was manifested energetically," Mino had said. I also buy a bottle of Red Ghost Pines Wine, which feels appropriate to share this evening.

Back at the house, Frank disappears quickly to his room, exhausted. I hang out with Lynn and Pat. "Frank said he wished you would treat him more like a peer than his father," Pat says of their time at Mino's. "He talked nonstop. He talked a lot about race in the home where he lives. It was really unbelievable." Pat considers a moment, then continues: "Mino and Bernadette met him where he was, like our guide did yesterday at Acoma. They were all people of color. And it was an environment where he felt safe." Not that Franklin doesn't need to be held and watched, but he has a desire to move out of an infantilized space. Hence his referring to me as his stepfather from his need "to collapse the father-son dynamic, which, of course, is difficult for you." I am struck by the echo of James Hillman's similar advice to me almost a decade before.

Of my having done the healing session with Mino rather than my son, Pat adds: "Often you think you are doing something for someone else, and it's actually you."

"You've got to go through it first," says Lynn, "then it opens the space for him. And he's saying to you, 'if you are out *here*'"—she extends her arm—"'and are not flexible, open, and fluid, *I* can't move.' It's like family therapy, in that sense."

Of the two memories that I cast into the waves, Pat notes that Hexagram 24 of the Chinese oracle, the *I Ching*, is "'Return by way of the old place to the new.' But it's a spiral." When I return, Pat recalls Franklin mentioning the "Gaelic mountain" having caused my fall up there: "Brought you to earth—it's all archaic stuff—brought you to your knees. We imagine we are the alchemist, but really we are the retorts."

He goes on: "The return is major. We went to Acoma, starting with the Indian elders. Then up came your story today about what happened when you were thirteen, also with an Indian: the linear, profane experience. You have an experience here with the Indians, and a memory comes back that was verbalized. Our logic would be that the event at thirteen was a sentimental thing that you willed. Whereas the reversal was engineered for you here—the landscape as the shaman—self-organizing nature doing her work, something unwinding and opening up."

He offers up a quote from an Irish writer named John Moriarty: "Out of a healed past, a healed present will flow."

I take a break to check in on Frank. It was "a good day," he says, and he's going to sleep.

During the night, an image returns. I am seventeen, with my parents and younger brother on a fishing trip off of Puerto Vallarta, Mexico, when the boat's motor conks out. While our guides try to get it started again, we're rowed ashore to a deserted island that we set out to explore. Like the Swiss Family Robinson, I muse. Which, as I now recall, was among my favorite stories as a child. Before the Indian took me to the movies . . .

On my morning walk with Pat, he notes how Franklin is "associating all the time and picks up a lot of signs." Like yesterday, when he mentioned the wall markings in his room, after which Pat pointed out similar markings in the landscape as we journeyed up the mountain in the tram. Frank is up by the time we get home. Over breakfast, when I speak of Mino and Bernadette as being good people, he says, "Active lifestyle." He turns to Pat and comments on how people from Peru have cool hair. "And he had wide set eyes, too," Pat says. He puts on a CD that Frank had been intrigued by yesterday, a Kashmiri chant that Pat often played while visiting the site of the Anasazi ruins. My son returns to his room to listen. The chant moves from sadness and longing to the ecstatic.

It seems to be a laid-back final day in New Mexico. Frank decides to stay home and work on some drawings. As I sit outside on the porch with Pat, suddenly a sharp-shinned hawk swoops into our conversation between two Russian Olives, right in front of our faces, and soars on. We decide to drive a few miles to an organic farming field, Los Poblanos Open Space, where locals plant corn to feed the migrating sandhill cranes. We hike to a four-cornered crossroads, where at sunset the view of the mountains is apparently to die for. We get talking about Gaelic legends and of our both having visited the site where poet W. B. Yeats is buried in western Ireland. Pat recalls the epitaph marker on Yeats's grave:

> Cast a cold Eye
> On Life, on Death.
> Horseman, pass by!

As we reach the end of a path, a horse sculpted out of welded metal stands at the base of a cottonwood tree. I recall that the first thing Franklin said to me this morning was: "There are horses here." There is a particular cottonwood around the bend that Pat wants me to see. To the Indians, these trees are sacred because they signify that water is nearby. They're called "the rustling tree," for the sound they make in the wind. This one is said to be hundreds of years old. Yet as we approach, the tree is down—part of it anyway. A worker with a chainsaw is cutting a massive dead limb that's fallen across the path. "A wounded cottonwood," Pat says, almost in a whisper.

We pause to marvel at the stately gnarled presence where the healthy part of the cottonwood arches skyward. "Look at the size, like a big anaconda," Pat says. "It probably got too heavy and toppled. So it goes." We walk on. Later, he'll speak of the sadness that initially overcame him. Thinking of the "part of the structure that had to go in a different direction": A sadness for one of his grandchildren, who suffers from a congenital disease. And for Franklin as well. "But the tree man was there, doing his work," Pat will say.

• • •

That night, I go to visit some other friends in Albuquerque, who live high on a mountaintop. Pat and Franklin stay home and are watching one of the *Star Trek* movies in the living room when I return. Frank's had a difficult night, Pat informs me. He'd had severe chills and taken a hot shower for a long time. But now he seems to be fine. On our walk the next morning, Pat elaborates: my son's hands were shaking so badly he could barely hold a cup of tea. He'd vomited in the shower. "He's speaking, like nature, in signs," Pat says. "You pulled away, and Frank cratered a bit."

It's leaving day. On the way to the airport, Pat asks Frank about his welding class and he responds animatedly about the various things he's learning—"circular tube . . . wire mesh . . . acetylene." Everything he says is crystal clear, concrete. Obviously, my son feels very connected to Pat. I can see how deep it went by the way Frank warmly smiles and shakes hands good-bye outside the airport. "Thanks a million," I say to Pat. I don't think I've ever used that phrase before. I would not soon forget the former football player's quiet empathy with both my son and me.

After going through security easily, I get smoothies at Frank's request for the two of us. "What was your favorite part of the trip?" I ask him as we wait to board.

"That hike up the mountain," he says unhesitatingly. "That was wonderful."

On the plane, while Frank sits quietly drawing or reading his welding book, I ponder: *Should I not have gone to my friends' home on the last night? Or was it perhaps important for Frank to know that someone like Pat would indeed take care of him when I wasn't around? Was it perhaps important for Pat, too?* All unanswerable questions, and perhaps excuses on my part. I can't say.

Now, alone together again, are my remarks and offerings to Frank still too overbearing and parental? It starts after the change of planes in Houston, when I tell him that he needs to sit in the middle seat where he's been assigned. "Not the window, eh?" he responds angrily, and adds, "I don't want to talk bullshit." When the stewardess comes down the aisle later with the cart, I ask if he wants something to drink. "I just want to read my books," Frank says. But when I order a margarita, he gets one too.

The next day is his welding class, and I go to pick him up. Frank is in a back room of the Fine Arts Center on a computer. He looks up and greets me with a huge smile and a resounding "Hi!" He's had a great class, shows me four or five pieces that he's done, including one very interesting long creation with curved wires welded cleanly to each other.

Despite the warm Indian summer weather, Frank is still wearing a heavy jacket and wool cap, as though about to climb another mountain. We set out on a few errands, and I tell Frank that I'm trying to treat him more like a peer than a son, but I don't always do that well. "You're doing pretty good," he reassures me. We stop at a bookstore where he picks out a book on astrology and another titled *The Genome*—which I'd been perusing myself only moments before, unseen by him.

Then, as I walk into a gas station to retrieve the keys to a car that I've just had inspected, I notice upon reaching for my wallet that my left hand is covered with blood. The wound from the mountain has reopened. I wrap my hand in a Kleenex to stanch the flow. Back home that afternoon, I call Pat Toomay again to thank him, and happen to mention my still-bleeding hand. "It *was* a kind of bloodletting," he says, "revealing vulnerability—and how important that is. What happened here was huge, and a lot of it was meant for you. Which is very delicate with Frank's condition. But it's like at Mino's: that kept some pressure off of him with more taken on by you. You are thereby granting him something."

I call Etta. She's had a talk with Kaye Lawrence, who is having her obtain a "grounding stone" called hematite. I look it up online. The name hematite derives from the Greek word for blood. Shiny black on the outside, if you break open the stone, the inside bears a deep blood-red color. Hematite is almost 70 percent iron, making it a popular healing stone for blood-related disorders.

Etta continues that one of the spirits whom Kaye had encountered while "journeying" with her was a woman singing beautiful Gaelic music. Perhaps, Kaye thought, this was either someone closely associated with Etta or even Etta herself in a past life. Etta has always wondered where her love for Irish and fiddle music originated and why she felt so comfortable while traveling some years ago in that part of the world. I tell her what Franklin said after I fell down that day in New Mexico: "The mountain was too Gaelic for you."

She says Franklin had earlier texted her asking, "Where are you?" When they then spoke on the phone, he told her that he was drumming and would call back. "Love you," he said, instead of good-bye.

In the weeks ahead with Frank, our coming to ground in New Mexico will linger. "How did you like the weather there?" he asks me. Pretty good, I say. "But you fell," he says. I show him the scab on my hand, which has pretty much healed.

Then, at his welding class, Frank cuts his hand. It, too, is a minor wound, but he points it out to me and, while we're getting him some winter clothes in a department store, it starts to bleed again. I then display to my son a new cut on my middle finger, obtained while closing a door the other night.

"Pat Toomay might say these are more blood sacrifices," I tell Frank, and he nods his head.

I have a dream about Pat and Frank being out there somewhere, kneeling down together in the dirt.

CHAPTER 24

• • •

Invoking the Ancestors

The cry is not yours. It is not you talking, but innumerable ancestors talking with your mouth. It is not you who desire, but innumerable generations of descendants longing with your heart.
—Nikos Kazantzakis, *The Saviors of God: Spiritual Exercises*[1]

ANCESTORS ARE APPEARING MORE CONSISTENTLY at the forefront of Franklin's thoughts. The Russell ancestors, he says to me, are "really good at inkblots." Also known as the Rorschach test, psychologists have used inkblots for many years with patients in an effort to determine personality characteristics and emotional functioning. The test has proven particularly useful in diagnosing underlying thought disorders and in differentiating psychotic thinking where a patient is reluctant to openly admit to it.

A few months earlier, Frank had asked if I wanted to come up to his room for a minute. Sure, I said. "You don't have to," he said. No, I want to, I said. His room was still cluttered, but in better shape than before. "I'll play you a few riffs on the guitar," Frank said. "This one is Clarence." After a minute or so, he paused and then resumed, saying: "And this one is Olive." The melody for my mother was more melodic than the one for my father. I flashed back to my mother giving him some piano lessons as a boy. Frank moved over to his piano keyboard and produced a few innovative riffs.

During my first divination with Malidoma in Ojai, in addition to the water ritual I was given to do, the shaman had instructed me about something else. It was toward the end of our ninety minutes together, and referred to what I'd shown him of Franklin's writing as a young teenager:

> "Two faces—one black and one white represent the two parts of me learning to live with each other."

Malidoma had his eyes closed when he spoke. "The task that I am seeing here is, there is a need for reconciling ancestors. It's not like introducing him to your ancestors, it's more like you are the child presenting a great-great-great-grandchild to them—because this person, who is intimately part of your life, is wanting a seat in the family tree. And only you can do that."

I'd felt my heart start to pound in my chest as Malidoma continued: "You have to bring Franklin to this spiritually. It's not like grabbing him by the hand. It is all in utterances, words that you say to your ancestors, about his protection . . . his sense of belonging: that they *have to find a way to include him in the tree.* Because he comes from another dimension and he cannot be considered as a guest, with you being the host—no, there has to be a full entitlement to the genealogical tree."

As to what Franklin wrote about the "two faces," I was responsible for reconciling the white one. "The black face is one that Africa has what it takes to reconcile. That's when a sense of wholeness becomes possible." I interjected that Frank's mother's ancestors came from West Africa. "Okay. So eventually this is going to have to be the other task." Meaning, I presumed, that Malidoma would need to meet Etta.

Looking again at the shell pattern I'd created on the divination cloth, Malidoma went on: "It's part of a very complex maneuvering." First, however, my son had to be inserted properly into his Caucasian lineage. "There is a tremendous amount of love that is going to come out of this initiative. Do you see this little heart?" Malidoma uncovered a stone at the far end of the pattern. "You have to solicit the love that your own ancestors have for you, to be extended unto *him.*" Franklin needed to stand at the forefront of a long line of ancestors. The sense of belonging would, in turn, give him the strength to reach for the other half of his heritage.

Malidoma continued: "This is something that requires some test drives. The first most obvious one is discursive, to take the form of words—something that you utilize as the receptacle for the encoding of discourse. You will need something that comes from your own grandparents and great-grandparents, an object that still carries a trace energy, that is put in a sacred context—with a red burning candle symbolizing the vitality of the place and the moment. This would come as a good start."

The initiative that I took would be felt as a healing, as symbolized by a black object on the table in front of me. Malidoma said: "He may feel like he belongs to nothing but *way* out there. So however this is done could amplify the self, and match the sense of belonging that he feels in the *other* world. The job will be for him to see this part of his chemistry as authorized, with the option of backing out if he chooses to. But he needs to know that he is part of this, so that he can make the choice of embracing it, or not."

• • •

Before this, I'd been aware of the importance of ancestors primarily from the psychology I had read. C. G. Jung viewed fears, behaviors, and thoughts in both young and old as remarkably similar across time and cultures. More than coincidence, Jung called this the "collective unconscious." It was comprised of archetypes, primordial images inherited from our forebears. Under certain circumstances, Jung believed that certain hereditary units could become activated, allowing the spirit of an ancestor to "take over" one's actions.

"I know no answer to the question of whether the karma which I live is the outcome of my past lives, or whether it is not rather the achievement of my ancestors, whose heritage comes together in me," Jung wrote in *Memories, Dreams, Reflections*. "Am I the combination of the lives of these ancestors and do I embody these lives again? Have I lived before in the past as a specific personality, and did I progress so far in that life that I am now able to seek a solution? I do not know."[2]

Malidoma put it like this, in his book *The Healing Wisdom of Africa*: "Ever since Christianity unearthed the gods and goddesses and sent them far away above the clouds, many people in the West have been left standing on the ground feeling abandoned, staring longingly at the sky wondering when God will come. In contrast, indigenous people see the divine as arising from below. Indeed, the ancestors, who dwell under the earth and form a vast pool of energy, allow us to walk upon them. Thus the divine is right under our feet and directly connected to us through the earth."[3]

I knew that I was a mixture of European bloodlines, with great-grandparents originally from England, Ireland, Germany, Norway, and, earlier, France. My mother, Olive, wished I had known my grand-mother, who died before I was born. We shared, my mother said, a common interest in "the mystical." Apparently my maternal grand-mother possessed an uncanny knack for seeing into the future, and did both numerological and astrological charts. The latter was, of course, an ability that Franklin also possessed.

There seems to have been a "traveling gene," too. My mom's father, and later her brother, had worked as station agents for the Min-neapolis and St. Louis Railroad. And on my dad's side, the possibility of Spanish gypsy blood dated back centuries. As a boy, I remember being fascinated by my father's olive-skinned cousin with the strange last name, Galajikian.

> Beauty is in her eyes, the eyes of a gypsy. Oh placid face let me reach out and embrace you.
>
> —Franklin's Journal, late '90s

I didn't know much more about my ancestors and certainly never considered invoking their spirits on my son's behalf. And I had no idea where to begin, for nothing of theirs had been passed down to me, not even their pictures. My younger brother, who'd taken care of our father toward the end of his life, had all that.

There was something else Malidoma wrote in his book, which stuck in my brain; perhaps because it was such an unusual thing to consider: "Ancestor rituals *help to heal the ancestors themselves* [author's italics] and our connections with them."[4] Rummaging through some papers that I'd saved, I came across a handwritten short piece that my dad, Clarence, had written about his father. It turned out that my grandfather's name had been Frank, though I'd never known him and wasn't consciously aware of his name when my son was born, our hav-ing instead named Franklin after FDR.

My dad began: "Father was a dreamer of big dreams—who couldn't quite make his dreams come off. His father had been a barber, who insisted his son become a barber." My father went on to describe how Frank Russell hated being a barber, which brought to mind Franklin's altering his hairstyle especially when he was going through a change in his life. My dad's father, who "had a fine creative mind and did a lot of reading, much of it along the lines of 'mind power,' etc." envisioned establishing a breakfast cereal business and received some financial backing. He created both a hot and a cold cereal and "put freshly minted pennies in each package as an incentive to youngsters. . . . He drove house to house and out to farms selling his product from a horse-drawn buggy. Also in grocery stores in relatively nearby towns. But World War I brought grain shortages. Wheat all went to government needs." The company went into bankruptcy.

"Dad was never quite the same," my father continued. He dreamed up a soft drink with a cherry-like flavor that he called Pep, but had no financing to bring it to the marketplace. So Frank Russell unhappily returned to barbering and then took another job as a traveling salesman. "We didn't spend a great deal of time together as I was growing up because he was away so much of the time," my father wrote. The last time they saw one another was in the mid-1930s. Frank "headed for California soon after" and "just seemed to drop from sight."

I vaguely remembered my father talking about some of this, but reading it now, several things surfaced in my mind. I thought of my son's penchant for invention and all the big dreams he'd had, ever since he was small, and how he could never quite bring these to fruition. I recalled my mother telling me that her parents had also separated. I thought of my own parental absence much of the time during Frank's early years.

My father went on to write about his parents having encouraged him to sing. He had an operatic tenor voice and my mother was an aspiring concert pianist when they received a scholarship to study in France. While there, my dad was offered a film contract by MGM but chose to postpone it. When World War II broke out, my parents were forced to catch the last boat back to the United States.

> Listen, listen, do you hear it pounding, ounces of music. Beats, relevant beats, beats nationally known, right now, flow the beats.
>
> —Franklin's Journal

In 1996, I took a trip to visit my father in a nursing home in Denver. It had been seven years since my mother died. When I called to tell him I was coming, suddenly my dad said: "Dick doesn't need to be ashamed of marrying a black girl." My father seemed to be speaking not to me, but to someone else—perhaps, I wondered afterwards, to my mother on the other side? My brother was in the room and, embarrassed for me, had taken the phone back from him. Later, Bob would forewarn me that long-suppressed racial anxieties were surfacing regularly in the father I thought I knew.

He's turned ninety and is in a wheelchair now, the walls of his room lined with photographs of what used to be, what almost was. One picture shows him and my mother all decked out, standing beneath a theater marquee in Minneapolis with SYMPHONIC CHORUS: THE RUSSELLS emblazoned above their heads. That was before I was born, when my parents organized and directed the Twin Cities Symphonic Chorus during the Second World War. It was a biracial chorus, rare for those days. I remember them speaking of a black friend named Worthy.

Out of the blue, my dad begins telling me the story of his and my mother's shipboard voyage back from France in 1939. Paul Robeson happens to be on the same boat. He invites my parents for cocktails. They knew who he was, of course—a world-renowned black singer, actor, and activist. My father doesn't know that I just took my son to see a Broadway show about Robeson's life, or that I intend to write about him in my book on *Black Genius*. In fact, in the course of my research, I have become friends with Robeson's son, Paul Robeson Jr.

On the boat, my mother doesn't want to accept Robeson's invitation. She'd grown up in Houston, Texas, where the only black people she knew were servants—third-class citizens who stepped off the sidewalk to let whites pass, sitting in the back of the bus, and using separate toilets in railroad stations. She was, she'd admitted to me once, terrified of blacks and couldn't face the idea of a social occasion even with an African American of Robeson's stature. A shipmate says they will be missing a tremendous opportunity. So, with trepidation, they go, and end up spending a wonderful evening talking about the history of folk music and spirituals.

My father tells me that meeting Robeson "turned everything around for us." But did it really? This becomes painfully evident as my father keeps bringing up a "conspiracy" to remove him from his room in the nursing home. Gradually, I gather that the imagined perpetrator is a black man who comes periodically to assist the patients in taking their showers. He also speaks of a woman across the hall who had fallen one day, and been helped up by "two nigger boys." Never in my life have I heard my father use the "N" word.

I flash back to my boyhood in the 1950s, hearing my parents tell me never to say that, coaching me: "Eeny meeny miny mo, catch a *rabbit* by the toe, always say rabbit, even if the other kids don't." I recall looking into the wishing well that graced our front yard in suburban Chicago, repeating the phrase to myself, saying "rabbit" and wondering about the other word. I also recall the "colored cleaning lady," as my mother called her, who came once a week to dust and vacuum our house. Racial attitudes, try as one might to bury them, ran deep.

In an unpublished memoir that my father wrote, there is a passage about the meeting with Paul Robeson on the ship back across the Atlantic from France. Twice that night Robeson had offered to help my dad continue to pursue his promising musical career after they docked in New York. But my father contracted severe pneumonia upon landing and, told by a doctor not to sing for a year, went back into advertising. Although Robeson followed up by writing him two letters, they never saw one another again. And my dad never fulfilled his dream.

In the nursing home, often things jumble together in my father's mind. I am his brother, my brother is his father, and sometimes he admits to getting my brother and I confused. Although clearly this is part of his advancing dementia, I realize now that it is not unlike Franklin's thought process. Over the years with Frank, the subject of ancestors periodically came up in this way. Once my son discussed having been *my* father through various centuries, and even had a whole family tree built up. Another time, Frank mentioned Clarence as one of his children and thought I should marry Olive.

In the nursing home, Dad tells me that it was my mother who initially had difficulty with my having gotten together with "a black girl," and then having a racially mixed child. But he adds that she had come to accept it. They had visited Franklin several times when he was a boy. I remember my mother giving Frank some piano lessons and dedicating one of her compositions to him. When I depart, my father asks that I give his love to Etta and "your little boy."

He tells me, too, that Franklin had written him a letter saying, "I don't know who I am."

Three years later, simultaneous with Franklin having just been hospitalized for a second time, I would see my father once more. We would listen to a cassette from 1955 of him singing while my mother accompanied him on the piano. We would cry together. Two weeks later, he died at the age of ninety-one.

Even then, long before Malidoma entered my life, I thought of what is passed on invisibly between generations. I'd wondered whether the offer from Paul Robeson that my father seemingly turned away had become part of my own subconscious, compelling me somehow to try to redeem what my dad could not.

· · ·

A long-ago memory of a relationship. Her name is Vanessa, we are in third grade circa 1955 in suburban Chicago. She is the only "colored girl" in the entire grade school and seems to have no friends. I don't really know why I befriended her on the playground. Perhaps I felt her loneliness, perhaps how different she was merely fascinated me, perhaps unconsciously I was motivated to know her by the hidden prejudice in my parents, or some combination of all of these. I became her confidante.

One day her mother came to school, a black patch over one eye. And I asked Vanessa why. Her father beat her mother up, she said, he gets drunk a lot and it's happened more than once. I was shocked, didn't even know such situations existed in life; my own parents had one glass of sherry with dinner and, as far as I knew, almost never fought. I questioned Vanessa, didn't believe her at first. She insisted it was true. In that moment, she had opened my eyes to a world beyond my understanding, a world of violence and pain. And it both attracted and repelled me.

There was a game we played. At one corner of the playground, in a small square corner against the concrete wall of the building, Vanessa would take me prisoner. Holding the jump rope taut as far as her arms could stretch it, blocking any attempt at escape, my pleas half-hearted, part of me rather enjoying what I now view archetypally, the bondage of centuries played out in a role reversal, her delight implanted in my memory alongside my growing discomfort as the game continued day after day until the bell rang ending recess.

After her mother came to school that day with the patch over her eye, I didn't want to play the game anymore. I began to run. Vanessa pursued me, incessantly, indefatigably, both of us weaving in and out of the other kids who never even seemed to notice this private ritual. My recollection is, the chase went on for days. I was a boy, I was faster, she couldn't catch me but stayed close enough behind to keep me moving, farther and farther away from the little cell at the corner of the school yard.

I hear her laughing behind me. I turn my head to look, am I about to be captured? Suddenly I am falling backward onto the concrete. I have smashed into the back of another boy's head. I am seeing stars. I stand up quickly and turn away, placing my hand to my mouth. It is bleeding badly and I've nearly knocked my two front teeth out. I run crying into the principal's office. My mother is called to the school.

That day marked the end of my relationship with Vanessa. I don't remember if we ever spoke again. I remember only an image on a school bus. I'm watching her from off to the side, an empty seat next to her as she stares out the window. Most of the time I walked to school. Once, with some other boys, I remember hiding in some bushes outside the fenced house where Vanessa and her parents lived. But we saw no one behind the windows.

I look back across the years and wonder, does the fact that I grew up in a still-segregated society shade my memories, make them assume a mythic quality they would not otherwise have? Weren't we, couldn't we have been, simply two children playing the games that children play? Maybe I ran away from Vanessa forever simply because I'd been hurt and embarrassed. Maybe I recall this incident so vividly because, through my entire youth, she was the only person of color I ever really knew.

Years later, a close acquaintance hearing this story would suggest that perhaps my guilt over rejecting Vanessa's friendship might have later played a role in my attraction to Africa and then to Etta.

• • •

When Franklin was thirteen, and in the eighth grade, one afternoon after school we had a long talk that I wrote down:

> He was talking about a black guy who'd spoken to his group of boys that day, in a kind of "men's session" congruent with Frank's taking part as an escort in a beauty pageant. The fellow had talked of how he sees

little hope, with most black teens turning to selling drugs because they can't get jobs. How the guy held up a picture of black slaves picking cotton, then of a black man picking up bottles and cans off the street—what's the difference? We still have indentured servants, Frank says. But he personally does have hope, that some kind of job is out there if you want it. And that it's a matter of educating the kids.

Frank does not like the word "minority." He used to see it as a means of referring to African Americans and Hispanics as inferior because of the word "minor," whereas majority did not have the same connotation. Then somebody told him that minority was not a bad word. But when Frank used it around a black guy, the fellow didn't like it and asked him why he was using it.

He says he does not care for Afrocentrism, though he understands where its adherents are coming from, because Frank feels unity is what is important and not emphasizing separation and differences. He says blacks in this country are not Africans any longer.

It has been hard for him, he says, to relate to other kids in the Roxbury area because his upbringing has been so different from theirs. He does not have the same problems. He is not out on the streets as much as his friend J----. He sees J---- being offered drugs on the street, something which has never happened to him. He didn't even used to want to be out on the hilltop, but has become curious and concerned about what is going on around him. Sometimes he wishes he'd grown up in a "normal" little family, but realizes he hasn't. We talk about the perspective living in this kind of extended family has offered him.

The realities of racism in the world came as a great surprise to him because he was simply not raised in such an environment, had been immune to it. He said he felt one reason that racism has existed for so long (in white people) was because many black people are so beautiful. "They are afraid of beauty. . . . And of darkness (maybe he said "blackness") and grace . . . coordination." He finds himself more attracted to black girls and Hispanic girls, but finds only a few white girls really beautiful. He thinks about the child he will have someday, wanting he/she to be beautiful.

He says one of these days he is going to speak out about what's on his mind—because he feels he has something to say—but he hasn't yet because he doesn't want to face embarrassing questions about the way he lives, his parentage, etc. But he has strong views, concerns about society and its direction.

This conversation we had was a real eye-opener to me. He is not my "little boy" anymore.

Even then, my son was in a sense my teacher. A few years later, we were talking about my book, *Black Genius*. I was concerned that the subject was over my head. So what would you want to know? I asked Franklin.

About spirit, he replied. About what drives a person to go beyond themselves.

What does it take to make a genius? There have been so many. So many too become geniuses because of a disability. For example Thomas Edison couldn't hear that well because of an accident where he had his ears yanked when pulled back onto a moving train. He was responsible for inventing the lightbulb, phonograph and moving picture. Helen Keller invented Braille. She was deaf, and blind. George Washington Carver was somewhat deaf and this helped him concentrate on his plant world that he came to know so well. Genius comes in all different levels.
—Franklin's Journal, written shortly
before his breakdown at age seventeen

• • •

When you were a young child, you dreamed of climbing. Experiences of euphoria you couldn't explain. Events unfolded in your life. Things hurt you and things held you back. Moments brought you to the epitome of emotions. What was it that made you evacuate from your soul, anyway there is a direction home. Do not be shocked when I say it isn't necessarily death. It is work. I once heard that if you can't find something to live for, find something to die for. And some days you'll feel like a pin cushion filled with sorrow. Or a voodoo victim. Pick it up. Maybe try a dinner invitation.
—Franklin's Journal, at age twenty-three

How can I find a way for my ancestors to include him in the tree, as more than a strange guest at the table? I fly to Idaho to see my brother Bob and gather what I could find about those who preceded me into this world. My brother's wife and my nephew, Paul, a musician with whom I've always been simpático, meet me at the airport. I recall that, when Paul paid a surprise visit to Boston on my fiftieth birthday (he was then twenty-three), I'd taken him upstairs to show him a studio where we sometimes played and listened to music. He'd walked all around clapping his hands to test the acoustics, and then asked if he could play the piano. My nephew had sat down and started wailing on precisely the favorite song Franklin loved to play, Scott Joplin's *Ragtime*.

Before dinner, we listen to a tape that our parents sent Bob for his thirtieth birthday, a compilation of various musical moments as we were growing up. This opens things up between us. I tell the story of my trip to Africa with Franklin and then about my shamanic quest and taking him to meet Malidoma in Jamaica. For purposes of my ancestral ritual, my brother and his wife agree to loan me a beautiful metronome from the 1840s that had graced my mother's piano, as well as a handwritten original of a poem written in German by my great-great-grandmother on my father's side. I spend all the next day immersed in a family archive, scanning photos of ancestors onto my computer.

Back home in LA before going to sleep, I feel "visited" by images of certain ancestors on my mother's side, in particular her older brother and my Irish great-grandfather (who fought with the North in the Civil War). I then dream about taking Franklin to visit an Indian reservation. I show Alice the photos of my forebears and I write to Malidoma.

It's time to do the ceremony. Late that afternoon, I bring the metronome, the poem, and printouts of many of the pictures down to a quiet room where I can be undisturbed. I carry, too, a carved wooden fertility doll that I'd picked up years ago traveling in West Africa, once used by the Ashanti medicine man whom I met there. I light two red candles as I call my ancestor's names and turn their photographs face-up, one by one. I read a translation of my great-grandmother's poem aloud and ask that they provide my son a place at the ancestral table, accept him not as a guest but a family member, and provide him protection as well as a sense of belonging. At the end, I thank them all. I can feel their presences and find myself deeply moved. Closing my eyes, I sit in silence for a time. There are tears in my eyes when I open them again.

I've never gone through anything like this before. Yet I don't feel foolish in the slightest. The ritual seems like a perfectly normal thing to do. But after this, my dreams indicate a shift in psyche. In one, I am with a black man who seems to be a clinician for Franklin, and we open a box of material that includes a bundle of letters my son has written. The man says he doesn't know if he can trust me to read them. Yes, I respond, I have to be able to trust you as well, and it isn't easy.

Then I tell him how I am hoping to redefine schizophrenia through writing this book.

I conduct the ritual again over the coming days and, in a follow-up phone conversation with Malidoma, ask whether I should continue. He says it's a good idea: "You have to find a rhythm for it, though, no steady mathematical frequency or regularity associated with it, but if you follow your intuition." He goes on to say that, when he's back home in Africa, "I talk to my ancestors pretty much every morning because that is *their* home, and on the road every day too before I go to work because I feel the appropriateness of it. Always, in the end, it is quite settling."

Malidoma continues that, in reading aloud the translation of my great-grandmother's poem, "see the poem as like a baton that is passed on to you . . . like an edifice that would benefit from your own architectural contribution. Usually in African tradition we call every individual addressing ancestors an artist, a contributor to continuity, a subtle underpinning of artistic contribution to what has already been done by predecessors."

He believes it's important that Franklin see their pictures, "because in this context he is more connected to them than even you. You are only the moderator, like a DJ in concert of the relationship, so you become this ongoing weaving spider connecting the dots and the knots. Usually a person of your type is one with high intuitive frequencies, which means anything that comes to you looking at the outset like an idea is actually an order from your ancestors. They won't come in this kind of patriarchal way, but maybe you feel like you're getting some ideas, some imagery. This is in keeping with your authenticity. They want you to own what comes to you, as an artist."

The next time, the ideas and imagery center around the racial attitudes that my mother grew up inculcated with in Texas. Late one afternoon, I seclude myself with a photograph of my mother reading to me when I was a little boy, some of her jewelry and the metronome that had pulsed the beats atop her grand piano. I close my eyes and address all of my ancestors aloud, allowing a long moment of silence before then speaking directly to my mother. I tell her that I believe she had ultimately come to terms with her racism, by teaching Franklin piano and even dedicating a composition to him. But perhaps her own ancestors had not, and could she ask them to do so, on his behalf.

We should come together. Families should talk. Tribalism should be entertained.
We were once one with our creator and we should be again. . . . Why can't we
obliterate the notion of race. . . . We could use the mistakes of the past to learn
from them. We could create a new renaissance in art, music, religion.
　　　　　　　　　—Franklin's Journal, among the last entries from 2002

Notes:

1. "The cry is not yours....": Nikos Kazantzakis, *The Saviors of God: Spiritual Exercises*, online at http://beachprophet.blogspot.com/2013/08/the-cry-is-not-yours-nikos-kazantzakis.html
2. "I know no answer to the question....": C. G. Jung, *Memories, Dreams, Reflections*, Vintage Books, 1965 paperback, p. 317.
3. *The Healing Wisdom of Africa*, p. 190.
4. "Ancestors help to heal....": *The Healing Wisdom of Africa*, p. 195.

CHAPTER 25

• • •

Descent of the Panther, Flight of the Pigeon

Enlighten that dark blood of your ancestors, shape their cries into speech, purify their will, widen their narrow, unmerciful brows.
— Nikos Kazantzakis, *The Saviors of God: Spiritual Exercises*[1]

SHORTLY AFTER FRANKLIN AND I returned from Jamaica, Malidoma had said to me: "I think the African ancestral component will have to kick in soon in order to bring Franklin permanently to this side of consciousness and to his purpose. I'm still struggling with the logistics of that in my mind."

At that time, Etta admitted to me that the idea of seeing Malidoma frightened her. Then, in April, she emailed that after seeing some pictures I'd sent her, he felt surprisingly familiar—and she would indeed like to seek a divination with him at some point soon. Etta had already been communicating with Kaye Lawrence, to whom she mentioned two concerns. The first was how to be a better mother to Franklin and more sensitive to his needs as a grown man. The second was a large chunk of memory loss surrounding her early years, of which she could recall only isolated instances.

Their second phone conversation had lasted for more than an hour. "Your heart is very hurt," Kaye told Etta, then spoke for a long while about what she called "soul loss"—how the soul divides and splinters off when hurt occurs that can't be understood or tolerated, and how those pieces must be found and slowly reintegrated into the person. Kaye asked about her family, and Etta described some of the dysfunctional parts as well as her parents' desire to raise a good family.

Etta wrote me: "One of the very significant things that Kaye said to me was that there is a huge wound that has been carried through generations in my family on my mother's side. A lot of the work that she did had to do with that, and consulting with her guides to find a way to make a healing."

After that, following a visit with Franklin, I wrote to Kaye about him. He'd had what staff at his house called an "awesome week," energetic and engaged. But something abruptly changed and I was very concerned. He was uncommunicative, wouldn't look me in the eye, and had a difficult time organizing his thoughts to the point of starting to take a bite of food and stopping in mid-air. His music therapist, too, found Frank much more distracted than usual. Frank would only say that he was fine. "Is it possible something was stirred up energetically with Etta that could be involved with this?" I asked Kaye.

She responded: "I only had time for a very quick check-in last night, but this is what I got: Franklin IS feeling the shifts and re-visitations of his mother to the time of his childhood. He is going there, too. The word that kept coming up was 'lost' to describe how he felt then. . . . Without doing a formal retrieval, my guides and I asked [his "spirit animal"] Bear to be with him. This seemed to comfort Franklin, particularly for the protection Bear offered him. The work that Etta is opening to seems very important."

Almost simultaneously, an email arrived from the staff person in charge of Frank's house, which I was very relieved to read: "Franklin came down this morning for his medication, which staff administered, and he is in a good mood. He greeted staff with a big smile. He told staff he showered and he is ready to start his new program."

And, after another phone session with Kaye, Etta wrote again: "Seems like so much is possible now that Franklin is more engaged in forging the direction of his life. The image of his animal spirit, the bear, has been coming to me a lot, especially since I worked with Kaye last Saturday. I am glad that it is the weekend again now and I have a little more space to meditate on the journey we took."

Memories from Etta's childhood are beginning to return. She's also been learning more about her ancestors. Etta was descended from a very large American family whose heritage included African,

European, Native American, and Asian populations. Many of them were quite successful professionals, of the middle and upper middle classes. Many had also lived in Maryland, not far from where Etta now resides. Yet her mother, while she worked hard to instill decent values in her four children, for many reasons moved away from both her own and her husband's family, leaving the kids relatively isolated from their larger heritage.

Kaye Lawrence had not planned to do an ancestral "distance journey" with Etta, but that's what transpired during an ensuing lengthy session over the phone. Etta has granted permission for Kaye to speak freely with me about this, and I've driven up to Maine to meet her in a coffee shop that she frequents.

Kaye had hesitated to use the word *possession* with Etta, but she tells me that "this could be said to have been possession by the ancestors, though not with the intention of harming her. They had been following the generations and attaching to the lineage. Not only of Etta, but other of her family members."

A storm with gale-force winds had blown across the Northeast the day of the distance journey. "I learned that we would be going to the Lower World for part of the healing," Kaye continues. "This is a world filled with compassionate beings and does not correspond with the Christian concept of hell. I was holding Etta's feet and singing." A spirit whom Kaye refers to as Mother was present. "We combed out the relatives from Etta's energetic field. Mother had gathered all of the ancestors who wanted to come. As we descended to the first level of the Lower World, the ancestors kept singing about going home."

Accompanying Kaye and Etta were Mother and Crow. I flash back to the black binder of Franklin's drawings and writings that he had shown me recently, with the words "Crow History" on the opening page. Kaye brings out a black notebook and begins to quietly read aloud from her notes of the session.

"The four of us were poling a raft down a swollen thick narrow river. It seemed very tropical, I could smell the ocean. We came upon a village with a big hill in the middle. We saw a light on land ahead—a whole tribe—a big reunion and celebration. It was absolutely beautiful.

"And in another level of the Lower World, there was a tall tree with a black panther at the top, and a three-year-old stretched out on its back. That was Etta."

The image seems to sear the back of my eyelids, I can envision it so clearly. I experience a chill as Kaye continues to read. "The panther had the girl under her right arm, and then this *enormous* panther climbed down and sniffed all of us. Crow was startled, and flew onto my head. The panther turned and licked the three-year-old's face, with its rough tongue, but very loving. This meant further healing was happening. . . . I drummed and sang."

In Kaye's experience, anytime a black panther appears, it is a spirit animal very dedicated to its own mothering, a remarkably protective and nurturing being. Black panthers are an ancient and powerful totem, symbolic of the feminine and the dark of the moon. In rites of ancient Egypt, a panther tail was worn around the neck or waist to help strengthen someone. The panther also signifies death—and rebirth.

After their journey, Kaye had sent Etta a voice recording of drumming accompanying a journey to the Lower World, to help her connect again with the black panther that had protected her as a small child. But Etta found that, while she could sense the presence of Franklin's Bear, she could not readily contact her own "spirit animal."

I feel myself drawn not only into the story, but taken outside time, into an archetypal realm that James Hillman wrote about, and where Franklin often resides. A realm where parallel lines between our 3-D reality and the imagination merge into the "breadthless length" described in Euclid's geometry.

· · ·

In September 2013, after a frenetic schedule of almost two full months abroad—half of it spent in his African village—Malidoma arrives in Baltimore. He will be giving divinations in Randallstown, less than half an hour outside the city. It's a perfect opportunity for Etta to see him, and I've asked Malidoma's secretary to put her on the schedule. When I manage to reach him on the phone, he hasn't realized that Franklin's mother would be coming on Saturday. He says he will look forward to it.

A few months earlier, Kaye Lawrence had told Etta: "The spirits know that we are getting close to a divination and will be paying attention."

The nondescript house where Malidoma is staying is in a quiet and secluded suburban neighborhood. As Etta drives up at mid-morning, she can't quite get it through her head that an African shaman is actually inside performing divinations. She parks, walks up the driveway, and rings the bell. A tall, medium brown-skinned woman opens the door. "Hi, I'm Bobbie. Are you here to see Malidoma?" Etta answers affirmatively and introduces herself. "Yetunde will be back soon to greet you. She had to do an errand. Just come in and have a seat."

Removing her shoes, Etta walks up a short flight of stairs and into a living room area to the left. Bobbie disappears into another part of the house. Etta finds a seat on a sofa near a window facing the street. It feels quite strange. Two gentlemen are sitting with their eyes closed on another sofa and a woman with long blondish hair and large blue eyes sits in an armchair gazing into space. They all appear to be in a deep state of meditation.

After a few minutes, during which Etta is afraid to breathe too loudly, Bobbie comes in. Etta tells her she's afraid of disturbing the others, and Bobbie laughs. "Oh, it's just fine," she says. (Etta will later learn they had each already seen Malidoma and were probably simply napping while waiting for Yetunde to return with some supplies he had ordered for them.) Bobbie says Malidoma is almost ready to see her and Yetunde should be back any minute to take her in.

Coming from somewhere in the house, Etta hears a man's voice—so warm and immediate that she knows it must be Malidoma—and a woman's response with the same lighthearted tone. What a relief. Etta no longer feels so anxious. Finally it's time. Yetunde has not returned, so Bonnie leads her back through the house to the room where Malidoma awaits her. When she opens the door, he is looking out a window, his back to the door.

Malidoma turns as Etta enters. "Ah!" he exclaims. "I see. Now I know!"

They exchange warm greetings and sit down facing one another. "When I saw Franklin, I didn't know," Malidoma continues. "But I see now that you are the key." Etta proceeds to move the beads and stones on the divination cloth. As Malidoma studies the pattern, she turns on her tape recorder. Another journey commences.

"You have a wonderful connection with the other world," Malidoma says. "The world of spirit is pretty much wrapped around you. The problem that shows is this part. Do you see how this green area of the cloth is almost empty? That shows the obstacles, woundedness, that is part of an inheritance. At an early age is when this happened to you."

"That's what Kaye Lawrence said," Etta whispers her response.

"Oh, so this is not the first time you are hearing that. So as a result, yours has been a hard uphill battle, to try to preserve the essence of your being and your integrity, your gifts and so forth. Now you find refuge in what they call here the mineral, which you have been able to translate as music. Sound is a healing place for you, like an outfit that you put on. A place that we call, in general, art—the same thing that Franklin is doing, in order to be able to transcend his situation.

"It's taking him awhile for the dust to settle around his life, so that his genii can have a social function. Just like you. You had to wait thirty-five years in order to have a kind of life that you could call reasonably stable. He's heading closer and closer to that edge. The one important thing is for you to stop blaming yourself, feeling like there was something you could have done that you didn't. It's not like that. When you are weighed down by your own process, insufficiencies, incompleteness, wounds to the soul—there are things that require a completely whole person to be able to accomplish. You were not whole, at that point, to do the kind of things you are blaming yourself for. So something is now demanding you to see your healing as *his* healing. And the transformation is very close."

Malidoma pauses and looks again at the pattern. "You tried at least to make beauty where there was none, to create peace where there was turmoil, and to restore stability where everything was topsy-turvy. You did *do* something with your life, thereby setting a precedent that he's going to ride on. That's why it's a time for expressing gratitude. You say that you teach music. Music speaks heart language, universal language, and young people pick it up just like this!" He snaps his fingers. "You are planting seeds in them. You are doing the work of the ancestors, as messenger and storyteller. It's like every time you stand there to teach, you are doing a ritual. Every time you grab an instrument and start to play, you are contributing to a cleansing. And cleansing the good beyond you onto Franklin. Every moment that you play with his picture in your mind—yes, that's what I saw—you are contributing to that."

Etta indicates that is precisely what happens to her. "Because you are showering this wall of his psyche with beauty," Malidoma continues. "And beauty and love are the best healing that can be bestowed, besides any pill or concoction. It's the love of your heart that never wavers for him. That's what is keeping him strong and growing."

Etta says she is always telling her young students stories about Franklin. "He's there with you. He's always been there with you, and that is something really profound, really deep," Malidoma says. When she left the family on Fort Hill, Etta tells him, she thought she would return. But then she met Kamal, who taught her how to sing and eventually became her husband. "I had a sense of ancestral family meeting him," she says, "which gave me a sense that I didn't have in my own family."

Malidoma says, "You see, that is why your leaving the community was ordered by your spirits, by your ancestors. What are the chances that you would then encounter a teacher who would show you all these things that you have never let go of since? It's the kind of thing that comes as a blessing."

He points to a circular pattern on the divination cloth, where the rings contain a number of different shells. "Now let's talk about this. I think what is still in need of attention is the retrieval of your total authenticity. *When you experience early in your life some form of trauma, your soul separates from the body.*"

At the time I transcribed the tape of Etta's divination session, I hadn't yet heard from Kaye Lawrence about the black panther that held the three-year-old Etta in the Lower World. Etta had told me about the memory loss surrounding her early years, and of Kaye having also spoken to her about the soul splintering off when great hurt occurs at a young age. "It seems that your greatest need is your own healing," Kaye had told her.

Now Malidoma says: "It's like, once upon a time something happened; you're wheezing and you haven't exhaled yet. As long as that is the case, the pattern stays like it is. So a mechanism needs to be put in place, where you can be reunited with your core being. It is close to you but can't get in the door, simply because the space has not been ripped open."

"That's why I feel like this," Etta says.

"That's right, sometimes you feel like there is a shell. Because the other you has not come home yet. And that other you was chased out because of something that rocked your world, damaging in essence."

Another pause, before Malidoma continues: "When something like this happens, it takes a special ritual retrieval, or ritual sweep, in order to get this piece back in. The method, in your case, will require either a pigeon or a dove and a black chicken. And because I am here, I would like you to find me this so that I can work on you before I leave. I don't want to assign this to somebody else."

Etta's sucking in of breath is audible. "Okay," she says.

"It's in the night that I do this. Therefore, put all effort necessary to bring this together. Yetunde will help you. Then at least you may hope that your integrity being complete will accelerate Franklin's process of self-recovery. I've contemplated taking him to Africa, but no, I needed to see you. I had to see both parents in order to make an assessment. I realize, for you, it is this. If this is resolved, then the loop is complete."

"You know," Etta says, "I thought that I would have to die in order for everything to be okay."

"Etta—" Malidoma interrupts.

"I mean, I really did."

"Yet it shows here, you are gonna be in this world for a very long time. Because you're going to be holding grandchildren, a sign that fundamentally speaking you did something right. That's something you will live long enough to be able to verify. This ritual has to do with homecoming, coming home to yourself."

"That's what I always say. I tell Kamal, I want to go home. But it isn't home *here*."

"No, it's not home as a structure, as a place somewhere. It's home as a kind of feeling that settles you, inside of yourself. This emptiness is causing all the longing, the feeling that something is incomplete. Of course it is. It's not healthy to be walking side by side with your soul, because you are the *temple* of your soul, your spirit. That's why I need this chicken, and this bird. The chicken is for you, the pigeon or the dove is for Franklin. This ritual is for both of you, and it is so delicate that I prefer to be the one doing it."

If she can locate these by that night, they should meet again around nine o'clock. Otherwise, the following evening would be all right. "You should go out there and talk to Yetunde while I finish up."

"Okay," Etta says. "This is great."

"It was meant to happen at all costs," Malidoma says.

• • •

In many ways the belief in many gods is much more interesting than the belief in one god.

—Franklin's Journal, late '90s

After seeing Etta, Yetunde goes to find Malidoma and returns with his orders to purchase an assortment of birds for various post-divination rituals, including two for Etta's. Etta is getting ready to go home for a bit when she realizes that she's being included on the bird-seeking trip. She leaves the house with Yetunde and Bobbie, who is concerned about putting live birds in her new car, but they finally settle on the fact that Bobbie's is nonetheless the best to use.

They drive for miles out into rural Maryland, bound for an alpaca farm where the owner raises many animals, among them chickens, guinea hens, doves, and pigeons. Finally they reach an idyllic farm setting that reminds Etta of the years she lived in Kansas. Apparently various people, including religious sects, routinely make this trek, sometimes for large numbers of fowl. The owner knows Bobbie well and takes them on a tour of the premises. All of his animals look to Etta like characters out of a wonderful children's book. They roam freely among one another within a large fenced area—huge fluffy cats, an overfriendly billy goat who constantly seeks to be petted, and many types of birds.

When it comes time to select theirs, an intense discussion ensues about whether it should be hen or rooster, big or small. Etta ultimately finds a young rooster—a beautiful, mostly black rooster with brilliant green and blue overtones in his tail feathers. He kicks up quite a fit upon being selected. No doves are available, so they settle on a white pigeon for Franklin's ritual. Etta's rooster and pigeon become roommates in a cardboard box. The pigeon makes no fuss whatsoever, but the rooster hollers all the way back to Bobbie's house.

Once they get there, Etta goes home to Kamal, who's been feeling under the weather. It's dusk when she returns again to where Malidoma is staying. A different group of people has assembled. The women talk shop—very respectfully, Etta feels. What is about to transpire seems like old hat to them, but she will learn later that none has personally experienced a "ritual sweep" before, although a few had observed the ceremony. At one point, Etta sees a very quiet, darkly clothed man pass through the room. It takes her a moment to realize that this is Malidoma, minus the beautiful tribal dress and flashing smile.

As time for Etta's ritual approaches, Yetunde asks if she's going to take off her clothes. "What?! Do I have to be naked out there in the cold with folks watching!" Yetunde looks at Etta calmly and shrugs: "That's the way I've always seen it done. But I've never had a problem getting naked."

At this point, Etta is in so deep that she'd have done just about anything. But Yetunde checks with Malidoma, who says the participants can wear their clothes so long as no one ever used them again. Etta sheds everything down to her undergarments and wraps a blue blanket from her car around herself. Yetunde thinks Etta looks so great that she does likewise in preparation for her own ritual, using a sheet that Bobbie graciously donates to her. (Both blanket and sheet will be discarded afterward.)

The only illumination is dim light from inside the house and streetlights in the front. Two people precede Etta with their rituals: Yetunde and a woman who came from Washington, DC, with her husband. Several others bear witness, standing on the porch in the dark and watching the ceremonies unfold in the backyard.

When it is Etta's turn, Malidoma motions her to stand in the center of a ring of ashes. He brings forth her black chicken from a box on the porch. He holds it firmly and asks Etta to lay her hands on its back. It's somewhat chilly outside, but the chicken is warm and she can feel the life in it. Malidoma prays and makes incantations as they hold onto the bird together.

Finally he has her let go. He dunks the rooster's head first into a bucket of water next to him. He then takes the bird and passes it along Etta's outstretched arms . . . over her head . . . down her front and back several times—all the while uttering incantations in a soft voice that occasionally rises while he passes the bird seemingly faster and more urgently over her, resting it for a long time on the top of her head. The rooster, dunked more than once, is good and wet.

A week later, it is still difficult for Etta to describe how she felt. Definitely frightened, but not in the sense of fearing imminent harm. Everything seems to rush to her head, as if trying to push out the top. Standing still within the circle, she finds herself wanting to fly away.

"Step away!" Malidoma exclaims, and she moves outside the circle of ashes.

By this time, the tears start coming, a shaking and crying that Etta cannot seem to stop. She walks for a few minutes around the yard. Malidoma asks Yetunde to be with her. She stays to make sure Etta is okay. The tears won't cease. But after a time, she can sit still. And after what seems an eternity, she goes back into the house and finds her way into the bathroom, where she removes her wet garments and cleans up.

Malidoma spends some time in the kitchen washing up. Gradually, everyone makes it to the upstairs. There he opens a bottle of wine, takes a glass for himself, then brings the bottle to the dining room table where everyone has gathered, and offers it to any who wish to partake.

> *For as soon as he is in ecstasy the manang goes down to the underworld in search of the patient's soul. Finally he captures it, and suddenly rises, holding it in his hand, then replaces it through the skull. . . . The cure ends with the sacrifice of a chicken.*
>
> —Mircea Eliade, *Shamanism*[2]

• • •

The night passes. First thing the next morning, Malidoma has told Etta that he himself must move the divining shells, without looking, in relationship to the ritual performed. "If it worked, then it will show me," he has said. At that point, they could move on to a healing ceremony especially for Franklin.

And so they do. First Malidoma instructs Etta concerning what to say to the white pigeon. She must ask it to take the healing that she has experienced to her son. The bird must carry back to Franklin his medicines and his gifts and all the people who have helped him through the years, along with all the love she holds for him. "You will *feel* that the bird is listening to you, and when you let it go, that it is carrying something else out there. This is to facilitate his recovery, his getting into clarity about his life so that then he can become as active as possible. This is a piece that I can only tell *you*. Mother knows things about their children that no one else can."

Malidoma picks up the white pigeon and shows her how to hold its legs tight together with one hand, while keeping the other hand up under its breast and wings so that it cannot fly. Then he places the bird in her hands. At one point, the pigeon begins to make little popping noises and Malidoma has Etta hold it a little looser. He begins stroking the pigeon's head repeatedly, incanting prayers to Franklin. Except for the utterance of hers and Franklin's names, Etta cannot understand the language. After a while, Malidoma indicates it is her time to pray to the bird. She looks directly into the pigeon's pink eyes, which grow huge before her gaze, and talks about Franklin's needs, asking the bird to find him.

Etta would later recount: "I fell in love with the bird as I talked, and finally I sat him down so that he could fly away. I heard Malidoma say, in a very quiet and gently reproaching voice, 'Etta, you were supposed to release it into the air, so that it will *know* to fly away.' I looked at the bird, which was now walking away, and asked Malidoma if I should try to catch it again. He said that the bird would never allow itself to be caught again.

"The bird didn't fly. Just calmly walked about. I followed, praying and beseeching it to fly to Franklin. It looked at me from time to time as I walked alongside it. Malidoma said that it was fine to follow it, that the bird was just getting its bearings since it hadn't been guided into flight. Finally the bird flew up to the fence that surrounded the backyard, sat there for a while, then walked along the fence, all as I kept talking to it and gesturing for it to fly away. I heard Malidoma behind me saying, 'So graceful.'

"Finally the pigeon flew up into a huge pine tree in the adjoining yard. I was so relieved. Malidoma laughed and said again, when I fretted that my pigeon hadn't flown very far: 'It's just getting its bearings.' He walked back into the house, still chuckling and saying, 'You made me laugh today.'

"I kept watch on my beautiful messenger for a long while. It stayed fluffing its wings and then shifting to rest upon a different and higher branch of the tree. I finally had to leave and trust that it would find its bearings and take mine and Malidoma's prayers and blessings to Franklin.

"When I picture the bird, I feel happiness. I can feel him in my hands and now still, in quiet moments, hear the powerful rustling of his wings in flight."

Her scheduled forty-five-minute divination had lasted for twenty-four hours.

• • •

The following weekend, Etta writes me an email: "This past week I have felt very strange; like something is gone and there is space wherever that was. It's almost like a waiting time, and hard to get my bearings. I have a busy work schedule which keeps me focused in the hours I spend with the kids. But in spare moments, I keep spacing out, and have to be careful with doing even simple things, especially driving. Like I'm high, but I'm not. . . . I can say for sure that this visit with Malidoma was a life changer. Thank you for making this first divination possible. I could never have imagined that taking this step could open so many doors."

I dream that I see Franklin and then Malidoma going by in a vehicle, when Etta appears to my surprise and we walk together down the street.

Etta has written to Kaye Lawrence about her time with Malidoma and tells me that I should feel free to tell Kaye more. When I do, Kaye speaks of how she and Malidoma see similar things but use different methods. "Etta is a beautiful soul," she says. "The ancestors were trapped and were taking away from her, without meaning to. Now she is experiencing herself." She pauses and then adds: "They are supporting her now."

> *Beauty. How do we measure beauty. . . . Beauty is sought after, fought about, taught through culture, and inherent. I am black and white. Where does that leave me? I look at myself and see a black man as I suppose others do, too. Does that make me beautiful, superior, or even ugly. Well I tricked you, I am grey— white and black, French, German, and African man. . . . I hope I can live up to my status as citizen of the world.*
>
> —Franklin's Journal, late '90s

Notes:

1. "Enlighten that dark blood. . . .": Nikos Kazantzakis, *The Saviors of God: Spiritual Exercises*, online at http://en.wikiquote.org/wiki/Nikos_Kazantzakis
2. "For as soon as he is in ecstasy. . . .": Mircea Eliade, *Shamanism*, p. 351.

CHAPTER 26

• • •

Light within the Tunnel

Now patience; and remember patience is the great thing, and above all things else we must avoid anything like being or becoming out of patience.

—James Joyce, *Finnegan's Wake*[1]

IN THE MONTHS AFTER ETTA'S divination and my trip to New Mexico with Franklin, the themes he and I have been learning to play together continue to resound. "This is for the book," Frank says as we drive along. "When Jesus was younger, he practiced magic on the ancients." I dutifully bring out my notebook. Having an Asian beer at lunch, he adds: "One additive to beer is molten dolphin sweat." What an idea! The notebook comes out again. "Dolphins come in all shapes and sizes," my son adds.

He travels quite a bit to other countries in his dreams—back to Tanzania, another time to Greece. In one of my dreams, I am going somewhere with Franklin and happen upon a single-spaced sheet of paper, which I believe to be the key to "curing" his mental illness. I'm trying to locate this again in what seems to be the back of a car.

But what, I wonder later, constitutes a cure? Would I even want to "fix" a son who can speak of Jesus practicing magic on the ancients and adding molten dolphin sweat to my beer? A friend poses the question this way: "Should we have given Prozac to Van Gogh and called it a day? Are we snuffing out the variation in the human condition that causes genius?"

Yet, of course, there are still the "bad days," the cutting-edged accusations and innuendoes that put my appreciation as well as my tolerance through a shredder. Accompanying him to his bimonthly appointment with Dr. K., I make the suggestion that Frank try taking his medication on his own again rather than have the house staff administer it. This, to my way of thinking, would accelerate the process of independence that's been so in evidence on our New Mexico trip. Almost immediately, Frank shifts into an accusatory gear. The KGB are experts at hypnotizing people—"you'd know all about that," he says, pointing across the room at me—and they're also good at poison: "Do you know how to do that?" As often, there are just enough elements of truth to get to me. I'd once researched the KGB's and CIA's "mind control" techniques.

Given my son's reactions, obviously the doctor changes nothing in terms of how Frank takes his medication. As we pull into his driveway, Frank is talking about slaveholders and how he wouldn't be a slave to anyone. I'm once more being too controlling. Why did I feel compelled to bring up taking his meds on his own, when *he* hadn't? *What did I expect?*

Two more dreams: I'm with Franklin when one of Malidoma's magical "little people"—the Kontomblé—seems to have shown up, although when daylight comes in the dream, I can't remember seeing it. . . . I'm at a big outdoor party with my son. He has wild Afro hair and is doing a solo dance, and I figure that he's probably been drinking. Then I can't find him.

After talking for years about his interest in welding, Frank loves the weekly class, using a blowtorch to unite the molten metal into a unique coalescing of designs. He even goes to the Fine Arts Center on Saturday mornings to practice what he's learned. I pick him up there. "Are you a man of prayer?" he asks at lunch. I think for a moment, then say, "Sometimes I am, yeah."

"Do you like totem poles?" he asks.

Trying to remember where I first saw a totem pole . . . I recall that they were a childhood object of fascination to me. I didn't know then, of course, that totem poles symbolically represented shamanic powers among certain Native American tribes. Or that some of the carvings symbolized the exploits of animal spirits like Raven, or a woman (Kats) who married a Brown Bear.

I dream about being on a train and disembarking in Baltimore, but I'm not sure if this is the right station to get to Etta and Kamal's house for something I have planned with Franklin. I try calling them, but the connection is terrible.

• • •

In early November 2013, Alice and I take a train to New York, where I'm lecturing at the Jung Institute and her brother is running in the city's annual marathon. From there we fly back to LA. How long I'll stay west depends on how Frank is doing. Good news on the health front: his latest blood tests show normal blood sugar and no signs of lingering diabetes.

When Etta comes to visit him, he brings along for their outing a few books, including a large tome on minerals and an esoteric work about yoga. Frank asks his mother a number of questions: "Were you interested in astrology when you were young? You and Kamal have been together for about twelve years, right? You wanted to be a geneticist?" He recalls all his times in the hospital and when they began. The next morning, he brings another big book—this time, on pharmacology. She asks whether he's looking up the medications that he's taking, and he nods affirmatively. "So he's really thinking about a lot of things—trying to put the pieces together," Etta writes me. Going shopping, "he was really chipper—literally jogging from aisle to aisle looking for stuff." She concludes: "God knows, the main thing is that he is interested and searching. . . . It was like we were meeting for the first time—in a different space. He's grown—and so have I."

After Etta described to Frank some about her divination session with Malidoma, Frank replied that he likes him too—but doesn't feel ready for another visit yet. There has been discussion among all of us about Frank's possibly returning to Jamaica when Malidoma goes again in January, and going this time with Etta. But Frank, who's equivocated for a while, now says he doesn't want to do it. The shamanic realm, though, remains very much in evidence. On the first day of 2014, I've just been writing about Malidoma in the book when a text message comes over my phone. It's him, wishing me a happy New Year.

Every time I speak with Franklin over the phone, I'm struck by how different he sounds: more alert, more engaged, asking me to hold on for a moment so he can grab a piece of paper to write down the phone number for an adult gymnastics class that I've found for him. He's consistently courteous—something his mother has also observed—and thanking me for my help. He wants to pursue finding a job, or maybe returning to school, rather than making another trip this winter. Even when the heat on his floor goes out, amid bone-chilling temperatures in Boston, Frank is sanguine about temporarily relocating to another group home until it gets restored.

In the middle of the night, I experience what the psychologists call a "big dream." I lie in bed for a bit reflecting on it, holding Alice's hand while she sleeps, our cat Oliver dozing between us. Then I get up to write down the details while it's still fresh. I'm with Franklin in a hospital setting, and report to a female nurse that he's been saying some profound things and seems much better. Then a boy in the next room escapes and starts running down the street and I run after him. I realize that this is the rap singer, Tupac Shakur (who was shot and killed in a drive-by shooting in September 1996, the month before Franklin had his breakdown at seventeen). We feel very connected, and he to Frank, and I'm not afraid of him. I then see Etta and Kamal sitting outside on a porch. I pause to tell them Frank is in the hospital and I've seen him and also that to my surprise I'd run into Tupac, but I can't stay. Somehow, though, I am drawn back to them. In a different setting, I thank Kamal for everything; he has metamorphosed into an older drummer. Now I need to catch a train, but I've forgotten a briefcase of papers and must return a second time to retrieve them. Two black boys appear in my path, and I think they will stop me—but they don't.

> I exist in the depths of solitude
> pondering my true goal
> trying 2 find peace of mind
> and still preserve my soul.

—Tupac Shakur, "In the Depths of Solitude"

While he nods his head a bit, to his Tupac CD, he thinks of what it is like to be a gangster. He writes his own song and sings it aloud. "Never grown up in the ghetto, but I have heard all the songs of torture though. Some songs speak of the four devils. They go lust, greed, envy, and such and such, it'll make you want to bust, it doesn't take a genius to know that much. Although I know of the life of grief and sometimes brief, I wonder, where would I be, would it take me under?"

He sits, satisfied with his freestyle rap, still wondering. Stepping out into the cloudy morning he walks over to the coffee shop across the street. He orders a coffee and stares out of the window. There he sees people of all different colors walking by. He thinks to himself, what a rich heritage America does have. He wonders, have we truly reached the land of the free?

—Franklin's Journal, late '90s

• • •

I take a day-trip with Alice to Catalina Island, twenty-six miles into the Pacific from Long Beach. For the first time in quite a while, on one of the island beaches I decide to do my water ritual for Franklin. It's a windy day and the waves are strong. On my first toss of the organic milk, I lose my footing somewhat. The bowl slips out of my hand and breaks in half on a rock. I finish the ritual without it, holding onto the two pieces. Alice is waiting nearby on some steps leading down to the beach. When I've finished offering to the ocean the apple cider vinegar, the vodka, and the kernels of corn, I show her the broken bowl.

"Do you think it's a bad omen?" I ask.

"No," she says, without hesitation, "you just need a new container."

Early in February 2014, soon after Franklin's thirty-fifth birthday, I return for several weeks to wintry Boston. Etta has seen him again and expressed concern about some shakiness that he's complained about as well as some short-term memory drop-outs. But by the time I arrive, Frank seems to be fine and is very glad to see me. "In the book," he says, "you can talk about my being in the hospital because at that time it was very dangerous on the streets."

At a Thai place for lunch, Frank selects what we'll *both* have to eat, including (only for me) a listed shot of "Cobra's blood" Vodka that's been distilled in Chinese herbs. How could I say no? Had any interesting dreams lately? I ask him. Yes, one about martial arts and another about a garden growing beets and cabbage. He gets a big kick out of my telling him that I'd dreamt the night before about onions. "Vidalia are good ones," he says.

Home again—maybe I'm going completely off the deep end—I Google "onions and mythology." It turns out that the word is derived from the Latin *unio*, which means "unity or oneness." The layers of onions have often been mentioned in literature as a metaphor for discovering multiple facets of something or uncovering a truth. Ancient Egyptians viewed the onion's circles as a symbol for eternity, and placed onions over the eyes of the dead. So sacred was the vegetable to the Egyptians that oaths were sworn by placing the right hand on an onion. Carrying well beyond the days of the pyramids, the link between onions and eternity is reflected in the onion domes of Russian Orthodox churches. And, as a young generation of Americans will tell you, from the movie *Shrek*: "Ogres are like onions. Onions have layers. Ogres have layers. We both have layers."

A Cambridge lawyer who sees Franklin for a yearly evaluation toward his treatment plan tells me: "He's the best I've ever seen him." What is most encouraging, as far as I'm concerned, is his openness to having a real conversation concerning his desire to return to school at Franklin Institute, where he completed more than thirty credit hours in mechanical engineering back in 2002. He listens carefully as I explain that he'd need to take out another student loan, even though I'm still paying back the loan for Lincoln Tech where he didn't complete the program. Frank then volunteers that he doesn't want to fail this time. Finally he suggests that he start by taking only one class and seeing how that goes. He then adds that he's grateful to be talking about all this. I call the school, and the admissions director says one class would be fine and Frank could do it in the summer.

I'd earlier written asking Kaye Lawrence if she might "check in" on Frank sometime soon, given Etta's concerns about his health. As I'm describing in the book the moment that Alice and I first pulled up to Kaye's door in Maine, I decide to look at my email and she's just responded. Kaye had observed that, while she could "feel some anger connected with Franklin's struggle to live his human experience," Kaye also "learned that the shamanic work is grounding him more in his human life and is progressing well. There didn't seem to be anything more to do energetically at this time."

I drop Frank at his weekly music therapy session with his teacher, Patrick. When I return toward the end, I'm expecting to hear my son pounding away on a new drum machine that we've picked up. Some-one who sounds like they've had a lot of training is playing the piano, and I figure this must be Patrick. I'm wrong. When I peek in the door, he's the one sitting on the floor with the drum machine and a xylophone, trying to keep up with Frank on the keyboard. Franklin's jazz riffs are remarkably inventive, fingers flying from lower to higher octaves as if he's channeling his grandmother.

"Wow!" I say when they stop, poking my head in all the way. "Frank, that was incredible! I had no idea you could play like that!" My son smiles broadly.

"This is his instrument," Patrick says. "Frank reminds me of Thelonius Monk. He's starting to play in patterns and shapes."

In the car again, the question pops out of me: "Hey Frank, what would you think if you became famous someday?"

He doesn't answer right away. "I'd have to work at it," he says, then adds: "Is that what you want for me?"

I feel foolish having asked. "I'm not sure," I say, truthfully.

"I'm actually quite happy being kind of a jack-of-all-trades," Frank says.

We return to his house to try to get a new desktop computer working. His adopted user name is Rembrant, without the *d*. He's either written down the password wrong or forgotten it, as I can't get the machine to turn on properly either. "I screwed up," Frank says. An admission that, not long ago, he wouldn't have been able to make. Then he says: "But, well, neither of us really knows what we're doing." Which is so true, and cracks me up. I contact the computer store, which says simply bring it in to tech support.

After I pick him up following his art therapy, Frank says a curious thing. Besides the sweatpants and a shirt that he'd like to get at Target, "they now carry angel pants."

Angel pants? I ask.

"They're related to honoring the dead," Frank says.

• • •

My friend Melinda, so in tune to Frank all his life, writes me: "Franklin has memories older than most of the human race, so you have to draw them out into the Light of your life. . . . He needs to start the memories coming. They will not seem like memories to him, most likely they will seem like future possibilities, and it's up to you to make it possible for them to happen—Give him a Future! The dimensions you are moving through here are unknown and unfamiliar to you. . . . But for him, it's like getting a bicycle, then much later a car . . . getting a small apartment and much later, maybe a house. The future is blocks of incomparable Time, arranged however you need to arrange it in order to 'Live and Love.' Time is made to be shaped into blocks by each soul, so they have somewhere to live."

It's dusk when I arrive in Ojai in April 2014. Malidoma is making his biannual trip to conduct divinations for individuals as well as a West African group ritual. I hadn't anticipated seeing him for another divination, but it feels like something is unfinished that I need to learn about. This relates to ancestral questions. With, as Franklin said, "honoring the dead." Into, as Melinda wrote, "unknown and unfamiliar" dimensions.

Candles light the small room. "I think there is indeed some more to dig out," Malidoma says, as I spread the shells and stones clockwise on the table between us. Studying the pattern, he continues, "You have barely scratched the surface of ancestral issues." This is no longer about mending the relationship with my biological ancestors, but an enormous "can of worms" that ties into "the larger family, the race relations, connecting you through Franklin and his mother to the ancestors of the Middle Passage and all the way to Africa. . . . Ancestors of this land and ancestors that were made subservient to other ancestors. Through this it is possible to trace all the way down to what Franklin is an embodiment of."

On the male Russell side, I recall later, there was a gap predating Franklin's great-grandfather Frank, who "just seemed to vanish from sight," as my father wrote. He'd set down that earlier generations of Russells had settled in Virginia, before migrating to Illinois. Etta will tell me that some of her ancestors lived in Virginia, too.

As Malidoma puts it, I need to be an architect; moderating the handshake between the two lines of ancestry, excavating "to find those hidden truths that are useful in contributing to any lasting change. . . . You will see that the rabbit hole is deep." The intervention is designed to bring a sense of belonging out of what currently remains an "incomplete homecoming."

For Franklin, the dual nature of his heritage "is causing him to perhaps become the embodiment of the relational crisis that has historically become prevalent between these ancestors. This is something a sensitive being like him cannot avoid. Simply because it is a radical gesture of honesty and integrity for him, as an advanced spirit, to be

able to carry it—however painful, however difficult, however tormenting that will be. . . . It is amazing that somebody can be such a cradle,
as if he has the metabolic power to reconcile all this."

He continues: "The conflict has to do with the European grandi-
osity that calls itself the 'High Culture,' the one that knows everything,
that knows better. And then the rest of the world, namely Africa, that
knows nothing. It is suggested that you have a role to play, to help dis-
sipate that, to be able to intervene in such a way that this point of con-
tention is removed from the equation—thereby allowing a direct flow
between two ancestries that are warring themselves within a person."
He doesn't need to add that that person is Franklin.

I point to a stone at the edge of the circle and ask what it signifies. "This is radical change, the snake zone that symbolizes radical change." Again, the snake. Malidoma points to a small key facing
toward the deep-orange ancestor stone near the middle of the circle,
calling this "a kind of access to the ancestral vault . . . part of the journey into the unknown."

I gaze deep into the pattern spread out before me, mesmerized by
the cluster of objects. The assorted stones and shells seem possessed by
an internal vibrancy in the subdued light. My insides are churning. A
part of me hasn't really wanted to hear this. A part of me has hoped that
the ritual work both I and Etta have done is enough. Yet Malidoma
is saying that this is all far from over, that indeed the effort has only
begun. And another part of me feels ready for whatever that next step
requires.

A visit to Malidoma's village remains to be fulfilled. "Had you
been already to Dano," he is saying, "you would have been subjected to
certain kinds of rituals that would have ripped open this whole thing.
And Franklin would have had a chance to be really—I don't know—
amused by it. But first, there is this incompleteness, this unresolvedness.
I'm not ignoring the fact that you have already been to Africa, but that
part you still need to go, the western part, is as close to the origin of
Franklin's ancestors as you can get. How to make it happen, at what
time, is a practical organization that is totally different from the rel-
evance of the whole concept we've been discussing."

In the meantime, I have a new water ritual to undertake. This
time, at the Atlantic Ocean, where the ancestors landed, where the
handshake across the divide needs to happen . . . where, as Malidoma

says, something "could be revealed to you about the circumstances that Franklin has been the expression of. There is something about that which is still a mystery."

> *And so we beat on, boats against the current, borne back ceaselessly into the past.*
> —F. Scott Fitzgerald, *The Great Gatsby*

• • •

As I look back across the years—the promise of Franklin's youth, the painful onset of his illness, the hopelessness accompanying its persistence—I find myself amazed at the endurance of his spirit and that we were ultimately able to find a torch-lit passageway through a long dark tunnel by way of travel and shamanic experience.

I don't pretend that it's light at the *end* of the tunnel. There is no way to know exactly where we are or what may come next. As I write this, Franklin is considering a move out of the group home and into his own place, maybe in Boston and maybe even somewhere else. On the one hand, that represents a big step. On the other hand, it raises new worries and fears. Always a what-if?

I still struggle with my parental "control issues." Perhaps any parent would, whose grown child has problems that preclude "normal" developmental stages in education, vocation, and relationships. But I'm working at this, and Franklin seems to think I'm generally allowing him more room to be a man. He also knows that I'll be there to support him, as will his mother.

I have a certain faith in the process that the three of us embarked on together; a faith based on what I see manifested in Franklin and between us. He has changed and, best of all, seems hungry for more. The isolation that long accompanied his difficulties is no longer chronic. It could be said that he "knows his own mind," and better accepts his limitations while still being able to dream. If some of those dreams exist only in the imaginative realm, so be it. I've learned the importance of this for him.

Through it all, I've come to appreciate who Franklin is, his unique essence: his integrity, his empathy, his humor, his psychic capability. I've been led away from conventional thinking and down a more metaphysical path, one that he already traverses. Along the way, a psychologist friend put it like this:

To the extent that psychosis involves the creation of an alternate reality, the goal is to enter that world, empathically and imaginally, in order to establish a bond that allows the psychotic person to gradually blend their world with the world most of us think of as real. There's also a recognition, of course, that the world we think of as real is actually infused with aspects of the Other—or Under-world—that there is a mysterious interpenetration or even an underlying unity.

In what became a shared adventure, Franklin and I joined hands across those two realities.

More than thirty-five years ago, when our son was born, a friend said to his mother after seeing a picture taken when he was a day old: "I think Franklin is really your teacher." How true, in many ways, that has proven to be. I would otherwise never have thought much about my ancestral heritage. I would not have paid as much attention to my dream life. I doubt very much that I would have traveled again to Africa, and I doubt if I would have sustained a friendship—assuredly, not as deep a one—with Etta.

Just as I sent this book off to the publisher, an email popped in from Franklin – the first email he had ever sent me. It contained two lines:

justice is for all
see you around

So what's next? Who can say. But, as Malidoma suddenly exclaimed at our recent get-together: "The story goes on, for God's sake!" This phase of the odyssey with my mysterious son draws to a close, very much "to be continued."

> *I decided to do a little experiment of my own with "reality" versus "imagination" when I was home visiting my village . . . I brought with me . . . a Star Trek tape titled "The Voyage Home." I wanted to know if the Dagara elders could tell the difference between fiction and reality. The events unfolding in a science fiction film, considered futuristic or fantastic in the West, were perceived by my elders as the current affairs in the day-to-day lives of some other group of people living in the world. The elders did not understand what a starship is. They did not understand what the fussy uniforms of its crew members had to do with making magic. They recognized in Spock a Kontomblé of the seventh planet . . . and their only objection to him was that he was too tall. They had never seen a Komtomblé that big.*
>
> —Malidoma Patrice Somé, *Of Water and the Spirit*[2]

Notes:

1. "Now patience, and remember patience....": James Joyce, *Finnegan's Wake*, p. 108.
2. "I decided to do a little experiment....": Malidoma Patrice Somé, *Of Water and the Spirit*, p. 8.

There was a boy
A very strange, enchanted boy
They say he wandered very far
Very far, over land and sea
A little shy and sad of eye
But very wise was he.
And then one day,
One magic day he passed my way
While we spoke of many things
Fools and Kings
This he said to me
The greatest thing you'll ever learn
Is just to love and be loved in return.

—eden ahbez, *Nature Boy*

• • •

Beyond Diagnosis:
Schizophrenia and Shamanism

Where schizophrenia is common, magico-religious healers are not—and where shamans practice, insanity becomes spiritual.
        —Joseph Polimeni, *Shamans Among Us: Schizophrenia,*
        Shamanism and the Evolutionary Origins of Religion[1]

IN A PHONE CONVERSATION NOT long after my first meeting with Malidoma, I asked Kaye Lawrence how she would define the difference between shamanism and schizophrenia. "The difference is grounding and the choosing," she said. "Always tethered in some way, the shaman chooses to go out and come back." But it wasn't always easy. "I was locked outside my body once in a journey, and it was very frightening," she went on. "Hovering in my healing room and not being able to get back into my body, going through the house above the ceiling and the kitchen, looking at the colors of the rug and seeing things so clearly, I wondered if it was a schizophrenic experience. Thankfully, I was finally able to reenter my body, but I was shaken up for a couple of days."

After this conversation, I embarked on a course of research. In older textbooks, according to Dr. E. Fuller Torrey, there existed many accounts of surgeons being able to do appendectomies and similar procedures on some schizophrenics with little or no anesthesia—as if they were *already* having an out-of-body experience.[2]

It turned out that, for a long time among Western anthropologists and psychiatrists, there was a "schizophrenia metaphor" for the shamanic state. An early paper on Siberian shamanism drew the comparison with "nervous disorders, especially the various forms of arctic hysteria." In 1924 and 1937, scientific studies equated shamans with epileptics and hysterics. In 1940, the practice was compared with psychosis. Then in 1949, the world-renowned French anthropologist Claude Lévi-Strauss said in a key essay that a shaman was actually a kind of psychotherapist—the difference being that "the psychoanalyst listens, whereas the shaman speaks." The shaman cured people by transforming their "incoherent and arbitrary pains" into "an ordered and intelligible form."[3]

Then in 1961, George Devereux, a pioneer in ethno-psychiatry, took the matter back to square one, saying: "Briefly stated, we hold that the shaman is mentally deranged."[4] And in 1967, Dr. Julian Silverman of the National Institute of Mental Health published a study in the *American Anthropologist* journal that postulated shamanism as a form of acute schizophrenia. The two conditions, Silverman contended, have in common "grossly non-reality-oriented ideation, abnormal perceptual experiences, profound emotional upheavals, and bizarre mannerisms." Silverman attributed the decision to become a shaman to an inability "to solve the culturally defined basic problems of existence."[5] A few years later, in 1970, American ethnologist Weston La Barre contended that "the shaman is one who has suffered an authentic nervous ailment or mental illness."[6]

However, the pathological view of shamanism began to shift with a paper by Dr. Richard Noll published in 1983 in the *American Ethnologist* journal. Noll's aim was to demonstrate that the schizophrenia metaphor "is unfounded and that it falsely evokes a medical model, which, in turn, clouds our understanding of shamanic experience." It was true that the "initial call" of some shamans occurred after having gone through "profound emotional experiences" or "miraculous self-recoveries from a serious condition." But the biggest distinction between the shaman and the schizophrenic had to do with volition: "The shaman voluntarily enters and leaves his altered states of consciousness"—this was found to be true in a study of forty-two different cultures—"while the schizophrenic is the helpless victim of his."[7]

The shaman, as Michael Harner, founder of the Foundation for Shamanic Studies, was quoted, "operates in non-ordinary reality only a small portion of his time, and then only as needed to perform shamanic tasks."[8] While a schizophrenic has trouble distinguishing between outer and inner, or ordinary and non-ordinary, states of consciousness, this is not true of most shamans. In 2001, Australian psychiatrist Roger Walsh concluded that the shamanic state clearly differed from schizophrenia, especially in terms of awareness of the environment, concentration, control, sense of identity, arousal, affect, and mental imagery.[9]

All this was a validation of Mircea Eliade's classic 1964 book on shamanism in various countries around the world, where the Romanian scholar noted: "Today the bona fides and psychological genuineness of a considerable portion of shamanistic states is generally recognized.[10] Also a validation of a much earlier statement by England's Edward Burnett Tylor, considered the founder of cultural anthropology, writing in 1871: "Everyone who has seen visions while light-headed in fever, everyone who has ever dreamt a dream, has seen the phantoms of objects as well as persons. How then can we charge the savage with far-fetched absurdity for taking into his philosophy and religion an opinion which rests on the very evidence of his senses?"[11]

• • •

Suddenly my whole being was filled with light and loveliness and with an upsurge of deeply moving feeling from within myself to meet and reciprocate the influence that flowed into me. I was in a state of the most vivid awareness and illumination. What can I say of it? A cloudless, cerulean blue sky of the mind, shot through with shafts of exquisite, warm, dazzling sunlight. [12]
—An individual describing the ecstatic bliss of "peak experiences" in *Surviving Schizophrenia*, by Dr. E. Fuller Torrey

At the same time, there was considerable research in recent years going beyond the medical model of schizophrenia. "Walking Between the Worlds," a paper by Serena Roney-Dougal of the Psi Research Centre in England, drew parallels to the shamanic and even psychedelic realms, in all of which "one experiences reality in mythic archetypal patterns, often called primary process thinking." This is also experienced by all humans nightly when we dream, yet "a large majority of schizophrenics complain of poor sleep" (including my son). Thus, I thought, perhaps that "natural" avenue is denied those afflicted with schizophrenia more than with "normal" individuals. The paper went on: "Both psychotics and those taking a psychedelic trip have difficulty expressing thoughts: rambling, incoherent, word salads become charged with symbolic meaning so that one may affect a union between the word and its object." As with dreams and on a mind-altering drug, psychosis is likewise a "chaotic condition in which various ego states succeed one another without a common reference point. . . . All three show an altered experience of time: timelessness, time standing still or time slowed down."[13]

As anthropologist Jeremy Narby writes in his book, *The Cosmic Serpent*:

> During the 1950s, researchers discovered that the chemical composition of most hallucinogens closely resembles that of serotonin, a hormone produced by the human brain and used as a chemical messenger between brain cells. They hypothesized that hallucinogens act on consciousness by fitting into the same cerebral receptors as serotonin, "like similar keys fitting the same lock."[14]

It is known that a shamanic state can be precipitated by psychotropic plants such as ayahuasca or peyote, which activate the brain's serotonergic (also called 5-HT) receptors. Initial hypotheses in the 1960s concerning the possible relationship of 5-HT to schizophrenia were based on the effects of LSD, which is structurally related to 5-HT. But there were problems with this idea: LSD produced primary visual hallucinations, not the auditory ones involved in schizophrenia. Also, paranoid delusions, conceptual disorganization, and disturbances in memory were common with schizophrenia, but not under the influence of LSD. Still, as Joseph Campbell put it, the LSD phenomenon "is an intentionally achieved schizophrenia, with the expectation of a spontaneous remission—which, however, does not always follow."[15]

The primary theories about a biological cause for schizophrenia do point toward aberrant neurotransmission systems (dopamine or serotonin) that affect cognitive functioning. Interestingly, the highest concentrations of 5-HT have been found in the pineal glands of schizophrenics. "A serotonin hypothesis of schizophrenia," a paper published in June 2013 out of the SUNY-Downstate Medical Center, concluded that "chronic widespread stress-induced serotenergic overdrive in the cerebral cortex . . . is the basic cause of the disease."[16] Similarly, MDMA, more generally known as Ecstasy, is known to activate the serotonin pathway.

Back in 1965, at the height of the psychedelic era, a German research team announced that they had isolated a compound called dimethyltryptamine, or DMT, from human blood. DMT was known to be a very powerful psychedelic chemical, an active ingredient of ayahuasca, a hallucinogen used by Peruvian shamans. Previously, researchers had found DMT crystals in plants and then in the brains of mice and rats, tracing pathways by which those animals manufactured DMT. This turned out to be the first endogenous human psychedelic, a compound formed within the body and found in human brain tissue, urine, and cerebrospinal fluid.[17]

Perhaps not surprisingly, given the proliferation (and fear) of mind-altering drugs at the time, the first studies of DMT focused around whether humans with higher levels of the naturally occurring chemical might be more prone to severe mental illness. In 1976, a study of 122 recently admitted psychiatric patients and 20 normal subjects detected DMT in the urine of 47 percent of those diagnosed as schizophrenic—and only 5 percent of the normal subjects. Yet, as described in Dr. Rick Strassman's 2001 book, *DMT: The Spirit Molecule*, the National Institute of Mental Health discounted the theory of a DMT-psychosis relationship, leading to the demise of human DMT research. Strassman believed "the data begged for further clarification. Instead, these federal scientists distanced themselves from an extraordinarily promising field and encouraged others to do the same."

In the mid-1990s, Strassman received permission to conduct the first federally approved psychedelic research in almost a generation, specifically on the DMT compound. According to one summary of what happened to Strassman's subjects while under the influence: "Though expecting mystical raptures and deep psychological insights, in his study he was astonished to find many of his volunteers reporting unexpected encounters with strange and sometimes disturbing alien beings with advanced technology in what amounted to classical UFO 'abduction' experiences. Unable to explain away the volunteers' experiences, he began considering whether these were genuine encounters with independent sentient beings in otherwise normally invisible dimensions."[18]

The subjects seemed to be propelled temporarily into another world.

Although these are exceptions rather than the rule for brilliant and creative individuals, it's noteworthy here that Albert Einstein's son, James Joyce's daughter, and Pablo Picasso's mother were all diagnosed schizophrenic. So was the son of James Watson, Nobel Prize–winning co-discoverer of the DNA molecule. But what in the gene pool differentiates the genius of an Einstein from the mental illness found in one of his children?

In a 2009 paper by Andrea Kuszewski, "The Genius of Creativity: A Serendipitous Assemblage of Madness," she examines this question at some length. The distinction has to do with cognitive control. As the author puts it:

> The highest potential for cognitive success seems to have the highest risk for cognitive debilitation, when looking at schizotypal traits. . . . In Schizotypy, the brain takes metaphorical leaps from domain to domain, making remote associations, using a broad attentional set. These are some of the hallmark characteristics of creativity.
>
> Such traits or genes taken to an extreme, paired with high cognitive control, lead to an Einstein, Joyce, or Picasso. However, those same traits paired with low cognitive control manifests as Schizophrenia, the wide range of thoughts without the executive function to assess appropriateness.[19]

Autism falls at the opposite end of the spectrum from schizophrenia. Extreme traits characteristic of autistics, writes Kuszewski, are "narrow interests, literal thinking, and perseverative attention to stimuli . . . without the control of cognition to maintain appropriateness." Yet this often comes paired with high cognitive control that manifests as mathematical genius (the savant-like nature of many autistics; think Dustin Hoffman in *Rain Man*). As Kuszewski says, such mathematical genius "is creativity without the divergence of thought, but still with the superior critical thinking skills. Intensely convergent thinking with high cognitive control leads to perseveration on an idea or subject, which can be beneficial in mathematics."

So the "serendipitous assemblage of madness" theory is one where the gift of cognitive control is at the heart of things. There is "optimal expression of . . . debilitating genes" also found in depressives ("extreme sensitivity and empathy...interpersonally gifted") and narcissists ("extreme confidence and belief in one's abilities . . . motivational speaker or natural leaders")—other variants of creativity.

Earlier studies in Iceland had revealed that "both patients with schizophrenia and their relatives had about double the chance of being a high school honor graduate than the general population," and also held more doctorate degrees per capita.[20] A recent article in *Scientific American* on the link between creativity and mental illness reported the findings of a new long-term study—that first-degree relatives of patients with schizophrenia "were significantly overrepresented in creative professions." "Positive" schizotypal traits such as "unusual perceptual experiences, thin mental boundaries between self and other, impulsive nonconformity, and magical beliefs": all these, to some degree, I could apply to myself. The idea, as earlier outlined in the Kuszewski paper, is "that overlapping mental processes are implicated in both creativity *and* psychosis proneness."

Schizotypal traits are also evident in studies of contemporary cult figures. As Oxford sociologist Bryan Wilson pointed out in a study of charisma: "If a man runs naked down the street proclaiming that he alone can save others from impending doom, and if he immediately wins a following, then he is a charismatic leader: a social relationship has come into being. If he does not win a following, then he is simply a lunatic."[21]

> *Have I not told you that what you mistake for madness is but over-acuteness of the senses?*
>
> —Edgar Allen Poe

A fascinating alternative theory about schizophrenia appeared in a long chapter in a 1976 book by an American psychologist, Julian Jaynes, called *The Origin of Consciousness in the Breakdown of the Bicameral Mind*. Jaynes's work followed the discovery, in the 1960s, that the human brain has at least two very different "thinking modes." The left side of the brain tends to deal with language and logic, and the right side with art, mathematics, and music, although each hemisphere controls the opposite side of the body. The selective, focused, methodical left brain filters information so that we are able to see the big picture.

However, the way Jaynes explains it, these characteristics of self-aware consciousness as experienced by most people today did not always exist. Before humans began learning rudimentary language as recently as three thousand years ago, the cognitive functions of the human brain were once divided into a part that seemed to be "speaking" and another part that listened and obeyed (a bicameral mind). People back then, especially under conditions of stress, responded to hallucinated voices in the head, arising in the right hemisphere but heard by the left side. Believing these mental commands came from external "gods," they dutifully obeyed. Until approximately the era of Homer's *Iliad*, music and poetry literally emanated from the heard voices of muses. Jaynes built his case through studies of ancient art forms and literature, including the Old Testament prophets. The sense of need for external authority in making decisions—as well as religion, hypnosis, possession, *and schizophrenia*—Jaynes called remnants of the bicameral mind.

He lay out this vivid description of what's experienced by the majority of schizophrenics, in the "florid unmedicated" condition: "We hear voices of impelling importance that criticize us and tell us what to do. At the same time, we seem to lose the boundaries of ourselves. Time crumbles. We behave without knowing it. Our mental space begins to vanish. We panic, and yet the panic is not happening to us. There is no us. It is not that we have nowhere to turn; we have nowhere. And in that nowhere, we are somehow automatons, unknowing what we do, being manipulated by others or by our voices in strange and frightening ways in a place we come to recognize as a hospital with a diagnosis we are told is schizophrenia. In reality, we have relapsed into the bicameral mind.[22] . . . According to our theory, we could say that before the second millennium B.C., *everyone* was schizophrenic."

Nowhere in the early bicameral civilizations, Jaynes noted, is there "any depiction or mention of a kind of behavior which marked an individual out as different from others in the way in which insanity does. Idiocy, yes, but madness, no."[23] Jaynes referenced Plato, who in the *Phaedrus* called insanity "a divine gift, and the source of the chiefest blessings granted to men."[24] In Plato's *Dialogues*, the Greek philosopher delineated Socrates' four kinds of insanity, all of which were linked to the gods: "prophetic madness due to Apollo, ritual madness due to Dionysus, the poetic madness 'of those who are possessed by the

Muses'….and, finally, erotic madness due to Eros and Aphrodite. Even the word for prophetic, *mantike*, and the word for psychotically mad, *manike*, were for the young Plato the same word, the letter *t* being for him 'only a modern and tasteless insertion.'" Jaynes mentioned another correspondence in the ancient Greek word for insanity, *paranoia*, which "literally meant having another mind alongside one's own."

He also harkened to something Malidoma had spoken to me about: the "little people." Daniel Paul Schreber was a distinguished German jurist who suffered a series of psychotic mental collapses and wrote a book, *Memories of My Nervous Illness* (1903) first utilized by Freud and then by Jung in his pioneering early study of *dementia praecox* (later called schizophrenia). As Jaynes recounted, Schreber's voice-visions of "little men" were "suggestive of the figurines found in so many early civilizations. And the fact that, as he slowly recuperated, the tempo of speech of his gods slowed down and then degenerated into an indistinct hissing is reminiscent of how idols sounded to the Incas after the conquest."[25]

But something had changed in ancient Greece. By the time of his later dialogues, writes Jaynes, "the elderly Plato is more skeptical, referring to what we call schizophrenia as a perpetual dreaming in which some men believe 'that they are gods, and others that they can fly,' in which case the families of those so afflicted should keep them at home under penalty of a fine. The insane are now to be shunned. Even in the exotic farces of Aristophanes, stones are thrown at them to keep them away."[26]

Jaynes continued: "What we now call schizophrenia, then, begins in human history as a relationship to the divine, and only around 400 B.C. comes to be regarded as the incapacitating illness we know today. This development is difficult to understand apart from the theory of a change in mentality"[27]—in sum, the breakdown of the bicameral mind. Jaynes added something later that I had observed over the years with Franklin: "Hallucinations often seem to have access to more memories and knowledge than the patient himself—even as did the gods of antiquity."[28]

Irwin G. Sarason, author of the textbook *Abnormal Psychology*, wrote in 2004: "Many schizophrenics have attested to an experience that is spiritual, professing that they are god, preaching that they have communicated with a god, or saying that they are a messenger from god, etc."[29] In this context, consider the admittedly schizophrenic "interpreter" who somehow got onstage in 2013 alongside world leaders paying tribute to Nelson Mandela, proceeded to use an invented sign language to reach any deaf ears, and later said he'd heard voices in his head during the event while hallucinating visions of angels flying into the stadium.

Jaynes also asked: "And why is 'hearing voices' universal throughout all cultures, unless there is some usually suppressed structure of the brain which is activated in the stress of this illness?" Jaynes wrote that "the genes that were in the background of the prophets" would today be labeled by "conscious men" as "an enzyme deficiency."[30] (Recalling to my mind the moment soon after arriving in Africa when Stephan said, "We always let nature to take place" and Franklin responded, seemingly out of nowhere, "The enzymes.")

In a section titled "The Advantages of Schizophrenia," Jaynes raised the "genetic inherited basis to the biochemistry underlying this radically different reaction to stress. And a question that must be asked of such a genetic disposition to something occurring so early in our reproductive years is, what biological advantage did it once have?"

Dr. Joseph Polimeni, an associate professor of psychiatry at the University of Manitoba and an internationally recognized evolutionary psychiatrist, posits a similar question in his 2012 academic work, *Shamans Among Us*. He views schizophrenia as "not a traditional medical disease," but rather as possibly representing "a vestigial behavioral phenomenon that was once advantageous to ancient hominids."[31] Unlike Jaynes, however, Polimeni's focus is genetic: the heritability of schizophrenia and its relationship in that sense to shamanism, dating back to hunter-gatherer subsistence societies. Present-day schizophrenics are viewed by Polimeni as "evolutionary selectees who [once] served the important societal function of communication with the supernatural."[32] As with someone struck by mental illness, Polimeni notes, becoming a shaman "is often perceived as something that overcomes an individual"—and is often marked by a temporary insanity around the same age as schizophrenia's onset. And as with the shaman, schizophrenic psychosis often shows "fixations with religious ideas." In Polimeni's theory, religion is considered evolutionarily advantageous and shamans have served as generators of that religious content (Polimeni himself is an admitted atheist).

Polimeni cites several fascinating experiments, including one where "patients with schizophrenia outperformed control subjects by a wide margin during a very specialized visual-perceptual task." This had to do with estimating "the number of lines in various configurations," which favored the schizophrenic patients when "displayed in a disorganized fashion." In another study, patients with schizophrenia were also "less deceived by the distorting effects of adjacent images [and] much less vulnerable to....optical illusion."[33] This, again, would seem to indicate a brain function that long ago paid dividends, but no longer served such purpose.

In September 2007, a study was published in the British *Proceedings of the Royal Society B*, concerning the evolution of genes linked to schizophrenia. As *Scientific American* reported: "After analyzing human DNA from several populations around the world and examining primate genomes dating back to the shared ancestor of both humans and chimpanzees, researchers reached a striking conclusion that several gene variants linked to schizophrenia were actually *positively* selected and remained largely unchanged over time, suggesting that there was some advantage to having them." The study team "focused on 76 gene variations most strongly related to schizophrenia. By comparing these combinations with the evolution of other genes known to affect neuronal processes, the researchers determined that 28 of the schizophrenia-associated genes have been evolutionarily preferred in recent years by either Caucasian, Asian or African populations." A co-author of the study, evolutionary biologist Bernard Crespi, was quoted: "You can think of schizophrenics as paying the price of all the cognitive and language skills that humans have—they have too many of the alleles [variations of genes] that taken individually...might have positive effect, but together they are bad."[34]

Their announcement, which admittedly surprised the scientists, reinstated some of what Jaynes had written about the bicameral mind. In neurological studies, Jaynes pointed out, the electrical activity of the brain for most people over an extended time frame "shows slightly greater activity in the dominant left hemisphere than in the right hemisphere. But the reverse tends to occur in schizophrenia: slightly more activity in the right." While most of us switch between brain hemispheres about once every minute, in schizophrenics tests have shown that "the switching occurs only about every four minutes, an astonishing lag." Schizophrenics "tend to 'get stuck' on one hemisphere or the other and so cannot shift from one mode of information processing to another as fast as the rest of us. Hence their confusion and often illogical speech and behavior in interaction with us, who switch back and forth at a faster rate."

As the "primitive" bicameral mind experienced auditory hallucinations with an "often religious and always authoritative quality, the dissolution of the ego....and of the mind-space in which it once could narratize out what to do and where it was in time and action," so with the modern schizophrenic. "In effect," Jaynes concluded, "his is a mind bared to his environment, waiting on gods in a godless world."[35]

More recent neuropsychiatric research by Dr. Iain McGilchrist also addresses the question of our divided brains, hypothesizing that *as a culture* we have oriented toward the left hemisphere—"relatively rigid, rule-bound and abstract in its view"—to our detriment. "Instead of distinct mechanisms," McGilchrist has written, "the right hemisphere sees interconnected, living, embodied entities. In communication the right hemisphere recognizes all that is nonverbal, metaphorical, ironic or humorous, where the left is literalistic."[36] It might be suggested then that the "schizophrenic remnants" of the uncontrolled bicameral mind are worth paying attention to, since such brains favor the "unusual" verbal associations of the right hemisphere as opposed to little activity in the left.

Colin Campbell, a traditional *sangoma* (healer) in South Africa, more recently put it like this: "Those who are more on the horizontal axis (air-water; the existential, non-physical axis), embody those parts of the culture that have become marginalized and will start acting out what is missing in our culture. The culture needs to listen instead of 'shuff' these people into institutions. They have a function to wake the culture up." Campbell also said: "It is the schizophrenic who can self-heal and reintegrate who has the makings of a shaman."[37]

Mythological scholar Joseph Campbell, in a 1970 paper titled *Schizophrenia: The Inward Journey*, summarized: "The inward journeys of the mythological hero, the shaman, the mystic, and the schizophrenic are in principle the same; and when the return or remission occurs, it is experienced as a rebirth: the birth, that is to say, of a 'twice-born' ego, no longer bound in by its daylight-world horizon. It is now known to be but the reflex of a larger self, its proper function being to carry the energies of an archetypal instinct system into fruitful play in a contemporary space-time daylight situation....The whole problem, it would seem, is somehow to go through it, even time and again, without shipwreck."[38]

Or, perhaps, as psychologist Richard Noll wrote of schizophrenics, "it would be closer to the truth to see most of them as voyagers who have been shanghaied, for unknown reasons, on a ship which never reaches port."[39]

· · ·

Before his breakdown forced him to leave the Commonwealth School, Franklin's favorite pastime had been learning to sail with his class on the Charles River. In the years since, he'd often expressed a desire to build boats—something, I learned, not uncommon among those diagnosed schizophrenic. "We know that water generally is a symbol of the collective unconscious," as Jungian psychologist Marie-Louise von Franz wrote, "therefore the ship has always had the meaning of being something that keeps you afloat and makes it possible for you not to drown in the unconscious."[40]

During the early years after his diagnosis, Franklin had consistently drawn mandalas, which sometimes featured a fragmented center, but with the chaos often compensated by a symmetrically ordered circumference. His later drawings sometimes resembled pictographs, or prehistoric art. As Polimeni points out in *Shamans Among Us*, similar "elongated or grossly distorted body parts and collage-style scenes" are not only seen in contemporary shamanism but in the early and more elaborately fluidic artwork that suddenly appears in the archaeological record about 40,000 years ago, following modern humans' migration into Europe out of Africa.

After meeting Frank in Jamaica, Malidoma had brought up a phenomenon I'd not heard about before: "He is almost like one of those, what do you call them, *indigo children*—a new breed of spirit [that's] come into this world carrying a completely different paradigm."

My subsequent Internet search revealed that "indigo children" were first described by a San Diego parapsychologist, who noticed kids with an unusual vibrational color (an indigo aura) surrounding them. This was later observed nationally in particular children born after 1978 (Franklin was born at the end of January 1979)—children with high IQs, keenly sensitive and intuitive, and who did not like to be touched (Franklin possessed all such characteristics). Many were labeled ADHD in school systems that didn't know what to make of them (one mother changed Attention Deficit Hyperactivity Disorder to mean instead "Attention Dialed Into A Higher Dimension.") Sometimes diagnosed with autism or even childhood schizophrenia, they were often telepathic with their parents, as Franklin certainly could be with me and his mother. A documentary film described a boy of three talking about knowing Michelangelo in a previous life and a little girl telling her mother that she'd been watching her for some time "before I chose you" to be conceived by.

One "indigo child" offered this self-definition: "Indigos are strong, passionate and sometimes thought to be aggressive or 'naughty.' However, this is just who they're supposed to be. They have to be willing to go against authority because they're here to change things. They are good with people; they love to talk and communicate, but they can't stand chaos—it overloads them."

Of course, there are many skeptics. Dr. Russell Barkley, a clinical psychologist and internationally recognized authority on ADHD, was quoted in a *New York Times* article on indigo children: "All of us would prefer not to have our kids labeled with a psychiatric disorder, but in this case it's a sham diagnosis. There's no science behind it. There are no studies."[41]

So was I still grasping at straws in an attempt to better understand my son? Nonetheless, people had come into my life who used a different language than the medical model . . . a language much more akin to what Franklin subscribed. As Malidoma told me at my initial divination session: "Here it shows that special powers are derived from nature, the intention being to bring greater fluidity in the human evolution, to make it easier to evolve by kicking in a chunk of the brain that is dormant."

In Malidoma's eyes, Franklin potentially had "a role to play in the world that can become extremely useful to like-minded people—because he is on the path to survive the label of 'schizophrenic.'"

Notes:

1. "Where schizophrenia is common…." Joseph Polimeni, *Shamans Among Us*: *Schizophrenia, Shamanism and the Evolutionary Origins of Religion*, 2012, p. 232.

2. Schizophrenics and anesthesia: Torrey, p. 41.

3. Levi-Strauss: quoted in Jeremy Narby, *The Cosmic Serpent*, p. 15.

4. George Devereux quoted on shaman as mentally deranged: *The Cosmic Serpent*, p. 15.

5. Julian Silverman: Stanley Krippner, "Conflicting Perspectives on Shamanism: Points and Counterpoints," http://stanleykrippner.weebly.com/conflicting-perspectives.html.

6. La Barre on shamans: Krippner paper

7. Richard Noll, "Shamanism and Schizophrenia: A State-Specific Approach to the 'Schizophrenia Metaphor' of Shamanic States," in *American Ethnologist*, Vol. 10, No. 3 (August, 1983), 443–459:

8. Harner quoted in Noll paper.

9. Roger Walsh: See his book *The World of Shamanism: New Views of an Ancient Tradition*, Llewellyn, 2007.

10. Mircea Eliade: *Shamanism: Archaic Techniques of Ecstasy*, Princeton University Press, 1992 paperback. Also available online for free download.

11. Edward Burnett Tylor: Noll paper.

12. "Suddenly my whole being was filled….": Torrey, p. 39.

13. "Walking Between the Worlds" by Serena Roney-Dougal, www.psi-researchcentre.co/uk

14. Serotonin: *The Cosmic Serpent*, p. 49.

15. Joseph Campbell on LSD: "The Inward Journey," http://www.mindspring.com/~berks-healing/campbell-schiz.pdf

16. "A Serotonin Hypothesis of Schizophrenia": Arnold E. Eggers, *Medical Hypotheses 80* (2013), 791–794, available online.

17. DMT history: see www.spiritmolecule.com

18. "Though expecting mystical raptures….": "Voyaging to DMT Space with Dr. Rick Strassman, M.D.," interview by Martin W. Ball, http://realitysandwich.com

19. "The Genius of Creativity: A Serendipitous Assemblage of Madness," by Andrea Marie Kuszewski, March 1, 2009, METODO Working Papers, No. 58.

20. Studies in Iceland: Joseph Polimeni, *Shamans Among Us*, p. 84.

21. Charismatic leader: Bryan R. Wilson, *The Noble Savages*, p. 7.

22. "We hear voices of impelling importance….": Julian Jaynes, *The Origins of Consciousness in the Breakdown of the Bicameral Mind*, Mariner Books, 1990 edition, p. 404.

23. In 2003, a study was published examining material from Greek and Roman literature, from the fifth century BC to the start of the second century AD, seeking to identify schizophrenia and related disorders. The study found "no written material describing a condition that would meet modern diagnostic criteria for schizophrenia." This was "in contrast to many other psychiatric disorders that are represented in ancient Greek and Roman literature." Evans, K., McGrath, J. and Milns, R. (2003), Searching for schizophrenia in ancient Greek and Roman literature; a systematic review. *Acta Psychiatrica Scandinavica*, 107:323–330, doi: 10.1034/j.1600-0447.2003.0053.x

24. Plato on insanity: Jaynes, p. 405.

25. Schreber and "little men": Jaynes, pp. 415–6.

26. "the elderly Plato….": Jaynes, p. 406.

27. "What we now call schizophrenia….": Jaynes, p. 407.

28. "Hallucinations often seem….": Jaynes, p. 412.

29. Irwin G. Sarason: quoted in "Shamans Equal Schizophrenics," by Anthony Wilkins, Texas A&M, www.kon.org/urc/v8/wilkins.html.

30. "enzyme deficiency….", Jaynes, p. 426.

31. "vestigial behavioral phenomenon….": *Shamans Among Us*, p. 21.

32. "evolutionary selectees….": Dr. David Koulack, quoted on p. 2 of *Shamans Among Us*.

33. Experiments: *Shamans Among Us*, pp. 94–5.

34. "It's No Delusion: Evolution May Favor Schizophrenia Genes," by Nikhil Swaminathan, *Scientific American*, September 6, 2007.

35. "his is a mind bared to the environment….": Jaynes, p. 432

36. Divided brain: Iain McGilchrist, "The Battle of the Brain," *Wall Street Journal*, January 2, 2010.

37. Colin Campbell: "Shamanic Perspective on Mental Illness: The Icarus Project," September 17, 2008, online.

38. Joseph Campbell, "The Inward Journey," http://www.mindspring.com/~berks-healing/campbell-schiz.pdf

39. "it would be closer to the truth….": Richard Noll, "Shamanism and Schizophrenia," *American Ethnologist*.

40. Water and the collective unconscious: Marie-Louise von Franz, *The Cat*, p. 34.

41. Russell Barkley and indigo children: "Are They Here to Save the World?" by John Leland, *New York Times*, January 12, 2006.

Acknowledgments

Thıs was the most ıntımate book that I've ever tried to write, and I couldn't have done it without the strong help and support of my friends and family. The idea to do the book was the inspiration of Jessie Benton, while Franklin and I were traveling in Africa. I'd never have thought of going without the impetus of Dr. Marshall Lawrence (Larry) Reiner. My wife Alice, and my son's mother Etta Russell-Scott, read all of the chapters and assisted greatly in shaping the direction of the book. I am grateful to my publisher, Tony Lyons, and my editor, Jason Katzman, for believing in the project, and to my literary agent, Sarah Jane Freymann, for shepherding it along.

My initial readers of the first draft were both psychologists, Randall Severson and Ronald Schenk, and I am deeply grateful for their advice and enthusiastic response. George Peper and Ross Gelbspan offered, as with my earlier books, their astute editing eye on all the chapters. Chuck Burger smoothed out the edges on many a sentence. Patrick Toomay and Steve Ewert provided metaphysical and personal insights on every chapter. My thanks, too, to psychiatrists Scott Becker, Bradley Tepaske, and Joseph Polimeni. And for their very useful suggestions along the way: Devora Wise, Eben Given, David Gude, Ann Gelbspan, Jonathan Cobb, Andy Castro, Steve Boyda, Arnold Eggers, Orland Bishop, and Chris Henrikson (founder of the remarkable Street Poets organization).

Finally, my thanks to my brother Bob Russell and his wife Deborah for their support through the years, as well as Candy Guerin, Kay Rose, and Abby Rockefeller. At Franklin's current residence, my appreciation to Teresa and Ciatra for their appreciation and interest.